EUROPEAN PHARMACOPOEIA

Supplement 4.8 to the Fourth Edition

published 24th November 2003

The Fourth Edition of the European Pharmacopoeia consists of the main volume 4 dated 2002 and supplements 4.1, 4.2, 4.3, 4.4, 4.5, 4.6, 4.7 (*with a cumulative list of reagents*) and 4.8. The **supplements are non-cumulative** and are to be kept for the duration of the Fourth Edition.

To use the Fourth Edition, make sure that you have all the published supplements and consult the index of the most recent volume to ensure that you use the latest versions of the monographs and general chapters.

EUROPEAN PHARMACOPOEIA ELECTRONIC VERSION

The Fourth Edition is also available in an electronic format (CD-ROM and internet version) with all the monographs and general chapters contained in the book. With the publication of each supplement the electronic version is replaced by a new fully updated cumulative version.

PHARMEUROPA

Quarterly Forum Publication

Pharmeuropa contains preliminary drafts of all new and revised monographs proposed for inclusion in the European Pharmacopoeia and gives an opportunity for all interested parties to comment on the specifications before they are finalised. Pharmeuropa also contains information on the work programme and on certificates of suitability to monographs of the European Pharmacopoeia issued by the EDQM, scientific articles on pharmacopoeial matters and other articles of general interest. Pharmeuropa is available on subscription from the EDQM (see opposite).

INTERNATIONAL HARMONISATION

Refer to information given in chapter *5.8. Pharmacopoeial Harmonisation.*

EUROPEAN PHARMACOPOEIA

FOURTH EDITION

SUPPLEMENT 4.8

Published in accordance with the
Convention on the Elaboration of a European Pharmacopoeia
(European Treaty Series No. 50)

Council of Europe
Strasbourg

The European Pharmacopoeia is published by the Directorate for the Quality of Medicines of the Council of Europe (EDQM).

ISBN: 92-871-5106-7

Printed in France by Aubin, Ligugé

CONTENTS

Note : on the first page of each chapter/section there is a list of contents.

IMPORTANT NOTICE

NOTE FOR INFORMATION OF USERS OF SUPPLEMENT 4.8

A change in terminology has been introduced for the IMPURITIES section of monographs where the term "specified impurities", in conformity with ICH guidelines, is used for impurities that have a defined individual acceptance criterion. Monographs of the European Pharmacopoeia have been elaborated to take account of the specified impurities mentioned. It is recalled that monographs on specific substances are to be read in conjunction with the general monograph *Substances for pharmaceutical use (2034)*, a revised version of which is included in Supplement 4.6.

CONTENTS OF SUPPLEMENT 4.8

A vertical line in the margin indicates where part of a text has been revised or corrected. A horizontal line in the margin indicates where part of a text has been deleted. It is to be emphasized that these indications, which are not necessarily exhaustive, are given for information and do not form an official part of the texts. Editorial changes are not indicated.
Individual copies of texts will not be supplied.

NEW TEXTS

REVISED TEXTS

CORRECTED TEXTS

The texts below have been corrected and are republished in their entirety. These corrections are to be taken into account from the publication date of Supplement 4.8.

GENERAL CHAPTERS

2.7.2. Microbiological assay of antibiotics

2.9.1. Disintegration of tablets and capsules

2.9.27. Uniformity of mass of delivered doses from multidose containers

MONOGRAPHS

Monographs

Celiprolol hydrochloride (1632)

Ciclosporin (0994)

Cod-liver oil (type A) (1192)

Cod-liver oil (type B) (1193)

Flunitrazepam (0717)

Homatropine hydrobromide (0500)

Homatropine methylbromide (0720)

Pefloxacin mesilate dihydrate (1460)

Polymyxin B sulphate (0203)

Tributyl acetylcitrate (1770)

Verapamil hydrochloride (0573)

Homoeopathic preparations

Arsenious trioxide for homoeopathic preparations (1599)

TEXTS WHOSE TITLE HAS CHANGED

The title of the following text has been changed in Supplement 4.8.

Sodium iodide (^{123}I) solution, becomes :
Sodium iodide (^{123}I) injection (0563)

SUPRESSION OF TEXTS

*The following text was deleted on **1 July 2003**.*
Lypressin injection (0506)

*The following texts were deleted on **1 January 2003**.*
2.7.3. Assay of corticotropin
2.9.21. Particulate contamination: microscope method
Corticotropin (0759)
Human fibrinogen, iodinated (^{125}I) (0604)
Oxyphenbutazone (0418)
Sodium iodide (^{125}I) solution (0280)
Swine erysipelas immunoserum (0342)
Tinctures (0792) - *see Extracts (0765)*

*The following text was deleted on **1 April 2002**.*
Canine contagious hepatitis vaccine (live), freeze-dried (0446)

2.2. PHYSICAL AND PHYSICOCHEMICAL METHODS

2.2.32. LOSS ON DRYING

Loss on drying is the loss of mass expressed as per cent *m/m*.

Method. Place the prescribed quantity of the substance to be examined in a weighing bottle previously dried under the conditions prescribed for the substance to be examined. Dry the substance to constant mass or for the prescribed time by one of the following procedures. Where the drying temperature is indicated by a single value rather than a range, drying is carried out at the prescribed temperature ± 2 °C.

a) "in a desiccator": the drying is carried out over *diphosphorus pentoxide R* at atmospheric pressure and at room temperature;

b) "*in vacuo*": the drying is carried out over *diphosphorus pentoxide R,* at a pressure of 1.5 kPa to 2.5 kPa at room temperature;

c) "*in vacuo* within a specified temperature range": the drying is carried out over *diphosphorus pentoxide R,* at a pressure of 1.5 kPa to 2.5 kPa within the temperature range prescribed in the monograph;

d) "in an oven within a specified temperature range": the drying is carried out in an oven within the temperature range prescribed in the monograph;

e) "under high vacuum": the drying is carried out over *diphosphorus pentoxide R* at a pressure not exceeding 0.1 kPa, at the temperature prescribed in the monograph.

If other conditions are prescribed, the procedure to be used is described in full in the monograph.

2.3. IDENTIFICATION

2.3.2. IDENTIFICATION OF FATTY OILS BY THIN-LAYER CHROMATOGRAPHY

Examine by thin-layer chromatography (*2.2.27*), using as the coating substance a suitable octadecylsilyl silica gel for high performance thin-layer chromatography.

Test solution. Unless otherwise prescribed, dissolve about 20 mg (1 drop) of the fatty oil in 3 ml of *methylene chloride R.*

Reference solution. Dissolve about 20 mg (1 drop) of *maize oil R* in 3 ml of *methylene chloride R.*

Apply separately to the plate 1 µl of each solution. Develop twice over a path of 0.5 cm using *ether R.* Develop twice over a path of 8 cm using a mixture of 20 volumes of *methylene chloride R,* 40 volumes of *glacial acetic acid R* and 50 volumes of *acetone R.* Allow the plate to dry in air and spray with a 100 g/l solution of *phosphomolybdic acid R* in *alcohol R.* Heat the plate at 120 °C for about 3 min and examine in daylight.

The chromatogram obtained typically shows spots comparable to those in Figure 2.3.2.-1.

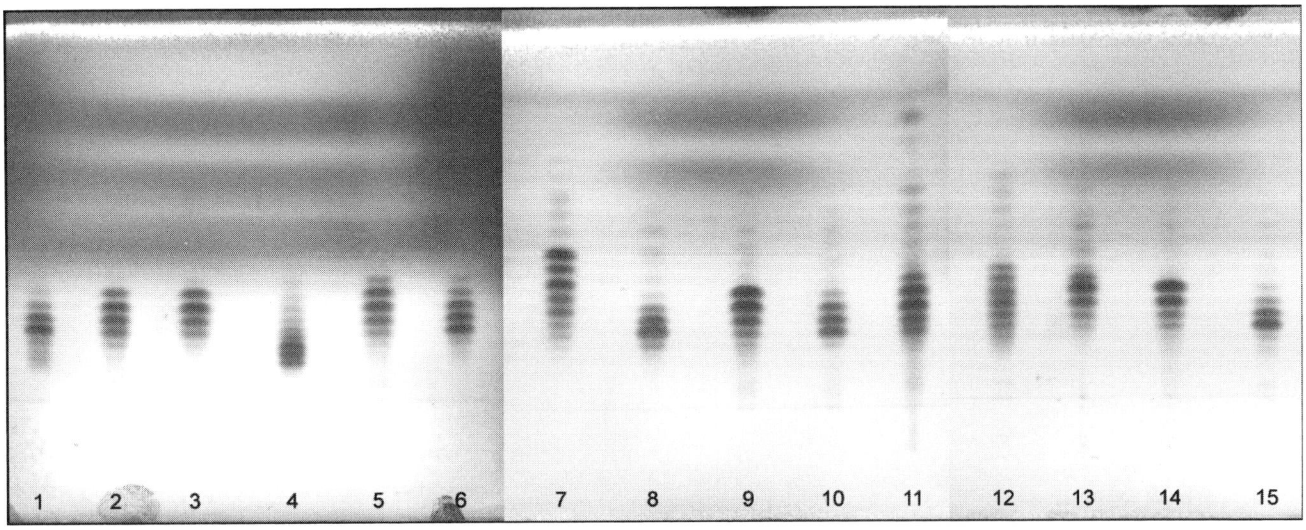

1. Arachis oil
2. Sesame oil
3. Maize oil
4. Rapeseed oil
5. Soya-bean oil
6. Rapeseed oil (erucic acid-free)
7. Linseed oil
8. Olive oil
9. Sunflower oil
10. Almond oil
11. Wheat-germ oil
12. Borage oil
13. Evening primrose oil
14. Safflower oil (type I)
15. Safflower oil (type II)

Figure 2.3.2.-1. – *Chromatograms for the identification of fatty oils*

2.7. BIOLOGICAL ASSAYS

2.7.2. MICROBIOLOGICAL ASSAY OF ANTIBIOTICS

The potency of an antibiotic is estimated by comparing the inhibition of growth of sensitive micro-organisms produced by known concentrations of the antibiotic to be examined and a reference substance.

The reference substances used in the assays are substances whose activity has been precisely determined with reference to the corresponding international standard or international reference preparation.

The assay must be designed in a way that will permit examination of the validity of the mathematical model on which the potency equation is based. If a parallel-line model is chosen, the 2 log dose-response (or transformed response) lines of the preparation to be examined and the reference preparation must be parallel; they must be linear over the range of doses used in the calculation. These conditions must be verified by validity tests for a given probability, usually $P = 0.05$. Other mathematical models, such as the slope ratio model, may be used provided that proof of validity is demonstrated.

Unless otherwise stated in the monograph, the fiducial limits of error ($P = 0.95$) of the assay for potency are not less than 95 per cent and not more than 105 per cent of the estimated potency.

Carry out the assay by method A or method B.

A. DIFFUSION METHOD

Liquefy a medium suitable for the conditions of the assay and inoculate it at a suitable temperature, for example 48 °C to 50 °C for vegetative forms, with a known quantity of a suspension of micro-organisms sensitive to the antibiotic to be examined, such that clearly defined zones of inhibition of suitable diameter are produced with the concentrations of the antibiotic used for the assay. Immediately pour into Petri dishes or large rectangular dishes a quantity of the inoculated medium to form a uniform layer 2 mm to 5 mm thick. Alternatively, the medium may consist of 2 layers, only the upper layer being inoculated.

Store the dishes so that no appreciable growth or death of the micro-organisms occurs before the dishes are used and so that the surface of the medium is dry at the time of use.

Using the solvent and the buffer solution indicated in Table 2.7.2.-1, prepare solutions of the reference substance and of the antibiotic to be examined having known concentrations and presumed to be of equal activity. Apply the solutions to the surface of the medium, for example, in sterile cylinders of porcelain, stainless steel or other suitable material, or in cavities prepared in the agar. The same volume of solution must be added to each cylinder or cavity. Alternatively, use sterile absorbent paper discs of suitable quality; impregnate the discs with the solutions of the reference substance or the solutions of the antibiotic to be examined and place on the surface of the agar.

In order to assess the validity of the assay, use not fewer than 3 doses of the reference substance and 3 doses of the antibiotic to be examined having the same presumed activity as the doses of the reference substance. It is preferable to use a series of doses in geometric progression. In routine assays when the linearity of the system has been demonstrated over an adequate number of experiments using a three-point assay, a two-point assay may be sufficient, subject to agreement by the competent authority. However, in all cases of dispute, a three-point assay as described above must be applied.

Table 2.7.2.-1. – *Diffusion assay*

Antibiotic	**Reference substance**	**Solvent to be used in preparing the stock solution**	**Buffer solution (pH)**	**Micro-organism**	**Medium and final pH (± 0.1 pH unit)**	**Incubation temperature**
Amphotericin B	*Amphotericin B CRS*	*Dimethyl sulphoxide R*	pH 10.5 (0.2 M)	*Saccharomyces cerevisiae* ATCC 9763 IP 1432-83	F - pH 6.1	35-37 °C
Bacitracin zinc	*Bacitracin zinc CRS*	*0.01 M hydrochloric acid*	pH 7.0 (0.05 M)	*Micrococcus luteus* NCTC 7743 CIP 53.160 ATCC 10240	A - pH 7.0	35-39 °C
Bleomycin sulphate	*Bleomycin sulphate CRS*	*Water R*	pH 6.8 (0.1 M)	*Mycobacterium smegmatis* ATCC 607	G - pH 7.0	35-37 °C
Colistimethate sodium	*Colistimethate sodium CRS*	*Water R*	pH 6.0 (0.05 M)	*Bordetella bronchiseptica* NCTC 8344 CIP 53.157 ATCC 4617 *Escherichia coli* NCIB 8879 CIP 54.127 ATCC 10536	B - pH 7.3	35-39 °C
Dihydrostreptomycin sulphate	*Dihydrostreptomycin sulphate CRS*	*Water R*	pH 8.0 (0.05 M)	*Bacillus subtilis* NCTC 8236 CIP 1.83 *Bacillus subtilis* NCTC 10400 CIP 52.62 ATCC 6633	A - pH 7.9 A - pH 7.9	30-37 °C 30-37 °C

Antibiotic	Reference substance	Solvent to be used in preparing the stock solution	Buffer solution (pH)	Micro-organism	Medium and final pH (± 0.1 pH unit)	Incubation temperature
Erythromycin estolate	*Erythromycin CRS*	*Methanol R* (see the monographs)	pH 8.0 (0.05 M)	*Bacillus pumilus* NCTC 8241 CIP 76.18 *Bacillus subtilis* NCTC 10400 CIP 52.62 ATCC 6633	A - pH 7.9	30-37 °C
Framycetin sulphate	*Framycetin sulphate CRS*	*Water R*	pH 8.0 (0.05 M)	*Bacillus subtilis* NCTC 10400 CIP 52.62 ATCC 6633	E - pH 7.9	30-37 °C
				Bacillus pumilus NCTC 8241 CIP 76.18	E - pH 7.9	30-37 °C
Gentamicin sulphate	*Gentamicin sulphate CRS*	*Water R*	pH 8.0 (0.05 M)	*Bacillus pumilus* NCTC 8241 CIP 76.18	A - pH 7.9	35-39 °C
				Staphylococcus epidermidis NCIB 8853 CIP 68.21 ATCC 12228	A - pH 7.9	35-39 °C
Josamycin	*Josamycin CRS*	*Methanol R* (see the monograph)	pH 5.6	*Bacillus subtilis* CIP 52.62 ATCC 6633 NCTC 10400	A - pH 6.6	35-37 °C
Josamycin propionate	*Josamycin propionate CRS*	*Methanol R* (see the monograph)	pH 5.6	*Bacillus subtilis* CIP 52.62 ATCC 6633 NCTC 10400	A - pH 6.6	35-37 °C
Kanamycin monosulphate Kanamycin acid sulphate	*Kanamycin monosulphate CRS*	*Water R*	pH 8.0 (0.05 M)	*Bacillus subtilis* NCTC 10400 CIP 52.62 ATCC 6633	A - pH 7.9	30-37 °C
				Staphylococcus aureus NCTC 7447 CIP 53.156 ATCC 6538 P	A - pH 7.9	35-39 °C
Neomycin sulphate	*Neomycin sulphate for microbiological assay CRS*	*Water R*	pH 8.0 (0.05 M)	*Bacillus pumilus* NCTC 8241 CIP 76.18	E - pH 7.9	30-37 °C
				Bacillus subtilis NCTC 10400 CIP 52.62 ATCC 6633	E - pH 7.9	30-37 °C
Netilmicin sulphate	*Netilmicin sulphate CRS*	*Water R*	pH 8.0 ± 0.1	*Staphylococcus aureus* ATCC 6538P CIP 53.156	A - pH 7.9	32-35 °C
Nystatin	*Nystatin CRS*	*Dimethylformamide R*	pH 6.0 (0.05 M) containing 5 per cent *V/V* of *dimethylformamide R*	*Candida tropicalis* CIP 1433-83 NCYC 1393	F - pH 6.0	30-37 °C
				Saccharomyces cerevisiae NCYC 87 CIP 1432-83 ATCC 9763	F - pH 6.0	30-32 °C
Rifamycin sodium	*Rifamycin sodium CRS*	*Methanol R*	pH 7.0 (0.05 M)	*Micrococcus luteus* NCTC 8340 CIP 53.45 ATCC 9341	A - pH 6.6	35-39 °C

Antibiotic	Reference substance	Solvent to be used in preparing the stock solution	Buffer solution (pH)	Micro-organism	Medium and final pH (± 0.1 pH unit)	Incubation temperature
Spiramycin	*Spiramycin CRS*	*Methanol R*	pH 8.0 (0.05 M)	*Bacillus subtilis* NCTC 10400 CIP 52.62 ATCC 6633	A - pH 7.9	30-32 °C
Streptomycin sulphate	*Streptomycin sulphate CRS*	*Water R*	pH 8.0 (0.05 M)	*Bacillus subtilis* NCTC 8236 CIP 1.83	A - pH 7.9	30-37 °C
				Bacillus subtilis NCTC 10400 CIP 52.62 ATCC 6633	A - pH 7.9	30-37 °C
Tylosin for veterinary use Tylosin tartrate for veterinary use	*Tylosin CRS*	2.5 per cent *V/V* solution of *methanol R* in *0.1 M phosphate buffer solution pH 7.0 R*	A mixture of 40 volumes of *methanol R* and 60 volumes of *0.1 M phosphate buffer solution pH 8.0 R*	*Micrococcus luteus* NCTC 8340 CIP 53.45 ATCC 9341	A - pH 8.0	32-35 °C
Vancomycin hydrochloride	*Vancomycin hydrochloride CRS*	*Water R*	pH 8.0	*Bacillus subtilis* NCTC 8236 CIP 52.62 ATCC 6633	A - pH 8.0	37-39 °C

Arrange the solutions on each Petri dish or on each rectangular dish according to a statistically suitable design, except for small Petri dishes that cannot accommodate more than 6 solutions, arrange the solutions of the antibiotic to be examined and the solutions of the reference substance in an alternate manner to avoid interaction of the more concentrated solutions.

Incubate at a suitable temperature for about 18 h. A period of diffusion prior to incubation, usually 1 h to 4 h, at room temperature or at about 4 °C, as appropriate, may be used to minimise the effects of the variation in time between the application of the solutions and to improve the regression slope.

Measure the diameters with a precision of at least 0.1 mm or the areas of the circular inhibition zones with a corresponding precision and calculate the potency using appropriate statistical methods.

Use in each assay the number of replications per dose sufficient to ensure the required precision. The assay may be repeated and the results combined statistically to obtain the required precision and to ascertain whether the potency of the antibiotic to be examined is not less than the minimum required.

B. TURBIDIMETRIC METHOD

Inoculate a suitable medium with a suspension of the chosen micro-organism having a sensitivity to the antibiotic to be examined such that a sufficiently large inhibition of microbial growth occurs in the conditions of the test. Use a known quantity of the suspension chosen so as to obtain a readily measurable opacity after an incubation period of about 4 h.

Use the inoculated medium immediately after its preparation.

Using the solvent and the buffer solution indicated in Table 2.7.2.-2 prepare solutions of the reference substance and of the antibiotic to be examined having known concentrations presumed to be of equal activity.

In order that the validity of the assay may be assessed, use not fewer than 3 doses of the reference substance and 3 doses of the antibiotic to be examined having the same presumed activity as the doses of the reference substance. It is preferable to use a series of doses in geometric progression. In order to obtain the required linearity, it may be necessary to select from a large number 3 consecutive doses, using corresponding doses for the reference substance and the antibiotic to be examined.

Distribute an equal volume of each of the solutions into identical test-tubes and add to each tube an equal volume of inoculated medium (for example, 1 ml of the solution and 9 ml of the medium). For the assay of tyrothricin add 0.1 ml of the solution to 9.9 ml of inoculated medium.

Prepare at the same time 2 control tubes without antibiotic, both containing the inoculated medium and to one of which is added immediately 0.5 ml of *formaldehyde R*. These tubes are used to set the optical apparatus used to measure the growth.

Place all the tubes, randomly distributed or in a Latin square or randomised block arrangement, in a water-bath or other suitable apparatus fitted with a means of bringing all the tubes rapidly to the appropriate incubation temperature and maintain them at that temperature for 3 h to 4 h, taking precautions to ensure uniformity of temperature and identical incubation time.

After incubation, stop the growth of the micro-organisms by adding 0.5 ml of *formaldehyde R* to each tube or by heat treatment and measure the opacity to 3 significant figures using suitable optical apparatus. Alternatively use a method which allows the opacity of each tube to be measured after exactly the same period of incubation.

Calculate the potency using appropriate statistical methods.

Linearity of the dose-response relationship, transformed or untransformed, is often obtained only over a very limited range. It is this range which must be used in calculating the activity and it must include at least 3 consecutive doses in order to permit linearity to be verified. In routine assays when the linearity of the system has been demonstrated over an adequate number of experiments using a three-point assay, a two-point assay may be sufficient, subject to agreement by the competent authority. However, in all cases of dispute, a three-point assay must be applied.

Use in each assay the number of replications per dose sufficient to ensure the required precision. The assay may be repeated and the results combined statistically to obtain the required precision and to ascertain whether the potency of the antibiotic to be examined is not less than the minimum required.

Table 2.7.2.-2. – *Turbidimetric assay*

Antibiotic	Reference substance	Solvent to be used in preparing the stock solution	Buffer solution (pH)	Micro-organism	Medium and final pH (± 0.1 pH unit)	Incubation temperature
Colistimethate sodium	*Colistimethate sodium CRS*	*Water R*	pH 7.0	*Escherichia coli* NCIB 8666 CIP 2.83 ATCC 9637	C - pH 7.0	35-37 °C
Dihydrostreptomycin sulphate	*Dihydrostreptomycin CRS*	*Water R*	pH 8.0	*Klebsiella pneumoniae* NCTC 7427 CIP 53.153 ATCC 10031	C - pH 7.0	35-37 °C
Erythromycin estolate	*Erythromycin CRS*	*Methanol R* (see the monographs)	pH 8.0	*Klebsiella pneumoniae* NCTC 7427 CIP 53.153 ATCC 10031	D - pH 7.0	35-37 °C
Erythromycin ethylsuccinate				*Staphylococcus aureus* NCTC 7447 CIP 53.156 ATCC 6538 P	C - pH 7.0	35-37 °C
Framycetin sulphate	*Framycetin sulphate CRS*	*Water R*	pH 8.0	*Staphylococcus aureus* NCTC 7447 CIP 53.156 ATCC 6538 P	C - pH 7.0	35-37 °C
Gentamicin sulphate	*Gentamicin sulphate CRS*	*Water R*	pH 7.0	*Staphylococcus aureus* NCTC 7447 CIP 53.156 ATCC 6538 P	C - pH 7.0	35-37 °C
Gramicidin	*Gramicidin CRS*	*Methanol R*	pH 7.0[*]	*Enterococcus hirae* CIP 58.55 ATCC 10541 *Staphylococcus aureus* ATCC 6538 P	C - pH 7.0	35-37 °C
	[*]Addition of a detergent may be necessary to avoid adsorption on the material during the dilutions, for example 0.1 mg/ml of *polysorbate 80 R*					
Josamycin	*Josamycin CRS*	*Methanol R* (see the monograph)	pH 5.6	*Staphylococcus aureus* CIP 53.156 ATCC 6538 P NCTC 7447	C - pH 8.0	35-37 °C
Josamycin propionate	*Josamycin propionate CRS*	*Methanol R* (see the monograph)	pH 5.6	*Staphylococcus aureus* CIP 53.156 ATCC 6538 P NCTC 7447	C - pH 8.0	35-37 °C
Kanamycin monosulphate Kanamycin acid sulphate	*Kanamycin monosulphate CRS*	*Water R*	pH 8.0	*Staphylococcus aureus* NCTC 7447 CIP 53.156 ATCC 6538 P	C - pH 7.0	35-37 °C
Neomycin sulphate	*Neomycin sulphate for microbiological assay CRS*	*Water R*	pH 8.0	*Staphylococcus aureus* NCTC 7447 CIP 53.156 ATCC 6538 P	C - pH 7.0	35-37 °C
Rifamycin sodium	*Rifamycin sodium CRS*	*Methanol R*	pH 7.0	*Escherichia coli* NCIB 8879 CIP 54.127 ATCC 10536	C - pH 7.0	35-37 °C

Antibiotic	Reference substance	Solvent to be used in preparing the stock solution	Buffer solution (pH)	Micro-organism	Medium and final pH (± 0.1 pH unit)	Incubation temperature
Spiramycin	*Spiramycin CRS*	*Methanol R*	pH 7.0	*Staphylococcus aureus* NCTC 7447 CIP 53.156 ATCC 6538 P	C - pH 7.0	35-37 °C
Streptomycin sulphate	*Streptomycin sulphate CRS*	*Water R*	pH 8.0	*Klebsiella pneumoniae* NCTC 7427 CIP 53.153 ATCC 10031	C - pH 7.0	35-37 °C
Tylosin for veterinary use Tylosin tartrate for veterinary use	*Tylosin CRS*	2.5 per cent *V/V* solution of *methanol R* in *0.1 M phosphate buffer solution pH 7.0 R*	pH 7.0	*Staphylococcus aureus* NCTC 6571 ATCC 9144 CIP 53.154	C - pH 7.0	37 °C
Tyrothricin	*Gramicidin CRS*	*Alcohol R*	*Alcohol R*	*Enterococcus hirae* ATCC 10541	C - pH 7.0	37 °C
Vancomycin hydrochloride	*Vancomycin hydrochloride CRS*	*Water R*	pH 8.0	*Staphylococcus aureus* CIP 53.156 ATCC 6538 P	C - pH 7.0	37-39 °C

The following section is published for information.

RECOMMENDED MICRO-ORGANISMS

The following text details the recommended micro-organisms and the conditions of use. Other micro-organisms may be used provided that they are shown to be sensitive to the antibiotic to be examined and are used in appropriate media and appropriate conditions of temperature and pH. The concentrations of the solutions used should be chosen so as to ensure that a linear relationship exists between the logarithm of the dose and the response in the conditions of the test.

Preparation of inocula. *Bacillus cereus* var. *mycoides*; *Bacillus subtilis*; *Bacillus pumilus.* Spore suspensions of the organisms to be used as inocula are prepared as follows.

Grow the organism at 35-37 °C for 7 days on the surface of a suitable medium to which has been added 0.001 g/l of *manganese sulphate R*. Using sterile *water R*, wash off the growth, which consists mainly of spores. Heat the suspension at 70 °C for 30 min and dilute to give an appropriate concentration of spores, usually 10 × 10^6 to 100 × 10^6 per millilitre. The spore suspensions may be stored for long periods at a temperature not exceeding 4 °C.

Alternatively, spore suspensions may be prepared by cultivating the organisms in medium C at 26 °C for 4-6 days, then adding, aseptically, sufficient *manganese sulphate R* to give a concentration of 0.001 g/l and incubating for a further 48 h. Examine the suspension microscopically to ensure that adequate spore formation has taken place (about 80 per cent) and centrifuge. Re-suspend the sediment in sterile *water R* to give a concentration of 10 × 10^6 to 100 × 10^6 spores per millilitre, and then heat to 70 °C for 30 min. Store the suspension at a temperature not exceeding 4 °C.

Bordetella bronchiseptica. Grow the test organism on medium B at 35-37 °C for 16-18 h. Wash off the bacterial growth with sterile *water R* and dilute to a suitable opacity.

Staphylococcus aureus; *Klebsiella pneumoniae*; *Escherichia coli*; *Micrococcus luteus*; *Staphylococcus epidermidis.* Prepare as described above for *B. bronchiseptica* but using medium A and adjusting the opacity to one which has been shown to produce a satisfactory dose-response relationship in the turbidimetric assay, or to produce clearly defined zones of inhibition of convenient diameter in the diffusion assay, as appropriate.

Saccharomyces cerevisiae; *Candida tropicalis.* Grow the test organism on medium F at 30-37 °C for 24 h. Wash off the growth with a sterile 9 g/l solution of *sodium chloride R*. Dilute to a suitable opacity with the same solution.

Buffer solutions. Buffer solutions having a pH between 5.8 and 8.0 are prepared by mixing 50.0 ml of *0.2 M potassium dihydrogen phosphate R* with the quantity of *0.2 M sodium hydroxide* indicated in Table 2.7.2.-3. Dilute with freshly prepared *distilled water R* to produce 200.0 ml.

These buffer solutions are used for all microbiological assays shown in Table 2.7.2.-1 with the exception of bleomycin sulphate and amphotericin B.

For bleomycin sulphate, prepare the buffer solution pH 6.8 as follows: dissolve 6.4 g of *potassium dihydrogen phosphate R* and 18.9 g of *disodium hydrogen phosphate R* in *water R* and dilute to 1000 ml with *water R*.

For amphotericin B, prepare the 0.2 M phosphate buffer solution pH 10.5 as follows: dissolve 35 g of *dipotassium hydrogen phosphate R* in 900 ml of *water R*, add 20 ml of *1 M sodium hydroxide* and dilute to 1000.0 ml with *water R*.

Table 2.7.2.-3.

pH	***0.2 M Sodium hydroxide* (ml)**
5.8	3.72
6.0	5.70
6.2	8.60
6.4	12.60
6.6	17.80
6.8	23.65
7.0	29.63
7.2	35.00
7.4	39.50
7.6	42.80
7.8	45.20
8.0	46.80

Culture media. The following media or equivalent media may be used.

Medium A

Peptone	6 g
Pancreatic digest of casein	4 g
Beef extract	1.5 g
Yeast extract	3 g
Glucose monohydrate	1 g
Agar	15 g
Water to produce	1000 ml

Medium B

Pancreatic digest of casein	17 g
Papaic digest of soya bean	3 g
Sodium chloride	5 g
Dipotassium hydrogen phosphate	2.5 g
Glucose monohydrate	2.5 g
Agar	15 g
Polysorbate 80	10 g
Water to produce	1000 ml

The polysorbate 80 is added to the hot solution of the other ingredients after boiling, and immediately before adjusting to volume.

Medium C

Peptone	6 g
Beef extract	1.5 g
Yeast extract	3 g
Sodium chloride	3.5 g
Glucose monohydrate	1 g
Dipotassium hydrogen phosphate	3.68 g
Potassium dihydrogen phosphate	1.32 g
Water to produce	1000 ml

Medium D

Heart extract	1.5 g
Yeast extract	1.5 g
Peptone-casein	5 g
Glucose monohydrate	1 g
Sodium chloride	3.5 g
Dipotassium hydrogen phosphate	3.68 g
Potassium dihydrogen phosphate	1.32 g
Potassium nitrate	2 g
Water to produce	1000 ml

Medium E

Peptone	5 g
Meat extract	3 g
Disodium hydrogen phosphate,$12H_2O$	26.9 g
Agar	10 g
Water to produce	1000 ml

The disodium hydrogen phosphate is added as a sterile solution after sterilisation of the medium.

Medium F

Peptone	9.4 g
Yeast extract	4.7 g
Beef extract	2.4 g
Sodium chloride	10.0 g
Glucose monohydrate	10.0 g
Agar	23.5 g
Water to produce	1000 ml

Medium G

Glycerol	10 g
Peptone	10 g
Meat extract	10 g
Sodium chloride	3 g
Agar	15 g
Water to produce	1000 ml

pH 7.0 ± 0.1 after sterilisation.

2.7.21. ASSAY OF HUMAN VON WILLEBRAND FACTOR

The potency of human von Willebrand factor is determined by comparing, in given conditions its activity in collagen binding or as ristocetin cofactor with the same activity of a reference preparation calibrated against the International Standard, in International Units where applicable.

The International Unit is the activity of a stated amount of the International Standard for von Willebrand factor in human blood coagulation factor VIII concentrate. The equivalence in International Units of the International Standard is stated by the World Health Organisation.

COLLAGEN-BINDING ASSAY

Collagen-binding is determined by an enzyme-linked immunosorbent assay on collagen-coated microtitre plates. The method is based on the specific binding of von Willebrand factor to collagen fibrils and the subsequent binding of polyclonal anti-von Willebrand factor antibody conjugated to an enzyme, which on addition of a chromogenic substrate yields a product that can be quantitated spectrophotometrically. Under appropriate conditions, there is a linear relationship between von Willebrand factor collagen-binding and absorbance.

MATERIALS

Collagen. Use native equine or human fibrils of collagen type I or III. For the ease of handling, collagen solutions may be used.

Collagen diluent. Dissolve 50 g of *glucose R* in *water R*, adjust to pH 2.7-2.9 with *1 M hydrochloric acid* and dilute to 1000 ml with *water R*.

Phosphate-buffered saline solution (PBS). Dissolve 8.0 g of *sodium chloride R*, 1.05 g of *disodium hydrogen phosphate dihydrate R*, 0.2 g of *sodium dihydrogen phosphate R* and

0.2 g of *potassium chloride R* in *water R*. Adjust to pH 7.2 using *1 M sodium hydroxide* or *1 M hydrochloric acid* and dilute to 1000 ml with *water R*.

Washing buffer. PBS containing 1 g/l of *polysorbate 20 R*.

Blocking reagent. PBS containing 1 g/l of *polysorbate 20 R* and 10 g/l of *bovine serum albumin R*.

Dilution buffer. PBS containing 1 g/l of *polysorbate 20 R* and 50 g/l of *bovine serum albumin R*.

Conjugate. Rabbit anti-human von Willebrand factor serum horse-radish peroxidase conjugate. Use according to the manufacturer's instructions.

Substrate solution. Immediately before use, dissolve a tablet of *o*-phenylenediamine dihydrochloride and a tablet of urea hydrogen peroxide in 20 ml of *water R* or use a suitable volume of hydrogen peroxide. Protect from light.

Microtitre plates. Flat-bottomed polystyrene plates with surface properties optimised for enzyme immunoassay and high protein-binding capacity.

METHOD

Test solutions. Reconstitute the preparation to be examined as stated on the label. Dilute with dilution buffer to produce a solution containing approximately 1 IU of von Willebrand factor. Prepare 2 independent series of not fewer than 3 dilutions using dilution buffer.

Reference solutions. Reconstitute the reference preparation as directed. Dilute with dilution buffer to produce a solution containing approximately 1 IU of von Willebrand factor. Prepare 2 independent series of not fewer than 3 dilutions using dilution buffer.

Allow the solution of collagen to warm to room temperature. Dilute with collagen diluent to obtain a solution containing 30-75 µg/ml of collagen, mix gently to produce a uniform suspension of collagen fibrils. Pipette 100 µl into each well of the microtitre plate. Cover the plate with plastic film and incubate at 37 °C overnight. Empty the wells of the collagen-coated plate by inverting and draining on a paper towel. Add 250 µl of washing buffer. Empty the wells of the plate by inverting and draining on a paper towel. Repeat this operation 3 times. Add 250 µl of blocking reagent to each well, cover the plate with plastic film and incubate at 37 °C for 1 h. Empty the wells of the plate by inverting and draining on a paper towel. Add 250 µl of washing buffer. Empty the wells of the plate by inverting and draining on a paper towel. Repeat this operation 3 times.

Add 100 µl each of the test solutions or reference solutions to the wells. Add 100 µl of dilution buffer to a series of wells to serve as negative control. Cover the plate with plastic film and incubate at 37 °C for 2 h. Empty the wells of the plate by inverting and draining on a paper towel. Add 250 µl of washing buffer. Empty the wells of the plate by inverting and draining on a paper towel. Repeat this operation 3 times.

Prepare a suitable dilution of the conjugate with PBS containing 5 g/l of *bovine serum albumin R* and add 100 µl to each well. Cover the plate with plastic film and incubate at 37 °C for 2 h. Empty the wells of the plate by inverting and draining on a paper towel. Add 250 µl of washing buffer. Empty the wells of the plate by inverting and draining on a paper towel. Repeat this operation 3 times.

Add 100 µl of substrate solution to each of the wells and incubate at room temperature for 20 min in the dark. Add 100 µl of *1 M hydrochloric acid* to each of the wells.

Measure the absorbance at 492 nm. Use the absorbance values to estimate the potency of the preparation to be examined by the usual statistical methods (for example, *5.3*).

The assay is invalid if the absorbances measured for the negative controls are greater than 0.05.

RISTOCETIN COFACTOR ASSAY

Carry out appropriate dilutions of the preparation to be examined and of the reference preparation using as diluent a solution containing 9 g/l of *sodium chloride R* and 10-50 g/l of *human albumin R*. Add to each dilution suitable amounts of a von Willebrand reagent containing stabilised human platelets and ristocetin A. Mix on a glass slide by moving it gently in circles for 1 min. Allow to stand for a further 1 min and read the result against a dark background with side lighting. The last dilution which clearly shows visible agglutination indicates the ristocetin cofactor titre of the sample. Use diluent as a negative control.

2.9. PHARMACEUTICAL TECHNICAL PROCEDURES

2.9.1. DISINTEGRATION OF TABLETS AND CAPSULES

The disintegration test determines whether tablets or capsules disintegrate within the prescribed time when placed in a liquid medium in the experimental conditions prescribed below.

Disintegration is considered to be achieved when:

a) no residue remains on the screen, or

b) if there is a residue, it consists of a soft mass having no palpably firm, unmoistened core, or

c) only fragments of coating (tablets) or only fragments of shell (capsules) remain on the screen; if a disc has been used (capsules), fragments of shell may adhere to the lower surface of the disc.

Use apparatus A for tablets and capsules that are not greater than 18 mm long. For larger tablets or capsules use apparatus B.

TEST A - TABLETS AND CAPSULES OF NORMAL SIZE

Apparatus. The main part of the apparatus (Figure 2.9.1.-1) is a rigid basket-rack assembly supporting 6 cylindrical transparent tubes 77.5 ± 2.5 mm long, 21.5 mm in internal diameter, and with a wall thickness of about 2 mm. Each tube is provided with a cylindrical disc 20.7 ± 0.15 mm in diameter and 9.5 ± 0.15 mm thick, made of transparent plastic with a relative density of 1.18 to 1.20 or weighing 3.0 ± 0.2 g. Each disc is pierced by 5 holes 2 mm in diameter, 1 in the centre and the other 4 spaced equally on a circle of radius 6 mm from the centre of the disc. On the lateral surface of the disc, 4 equally spaced grooves are cut in such a way that at the upper surface of the disc they are 9.5 mm wide and 2.55 mm deep and at the lower surface 1.6 mm square. The tubes are held vertically by 2 separate and superimposed rigid plastic plates 90 mm in diameter and 6 mm thick with 6 holes. The holes are equidistant from the centre of the plate and equally spaced. Attached to the under side of the lower plate is a piece of woven gauze made from stainless steel wire 0.635 mm in diameter and having mesh apertures of 2.00 mm. The plates are held rigidly in position and 77.5 mm apart by vertical metal rods at the periphery, a metal rod is also fixed to the centre of the upper plate to enable the assembly to be attached to a mechanical device capable of raising and lowering it smoothly at a constant frequency between 29 and 32 cycles per minute, through a distance of 50 mm to 60 mm.

The assembly is suspended in the specified liquid in a suitable vessel, preferably a 1 litre beaker. The volume of the liquid is such that when the assembly is in the highest position the wire mesh is at least 15 mm below the surface of the liquid, and when the assembly is in the lowest position the wire mesh is at least 25 mm above the bottom of the

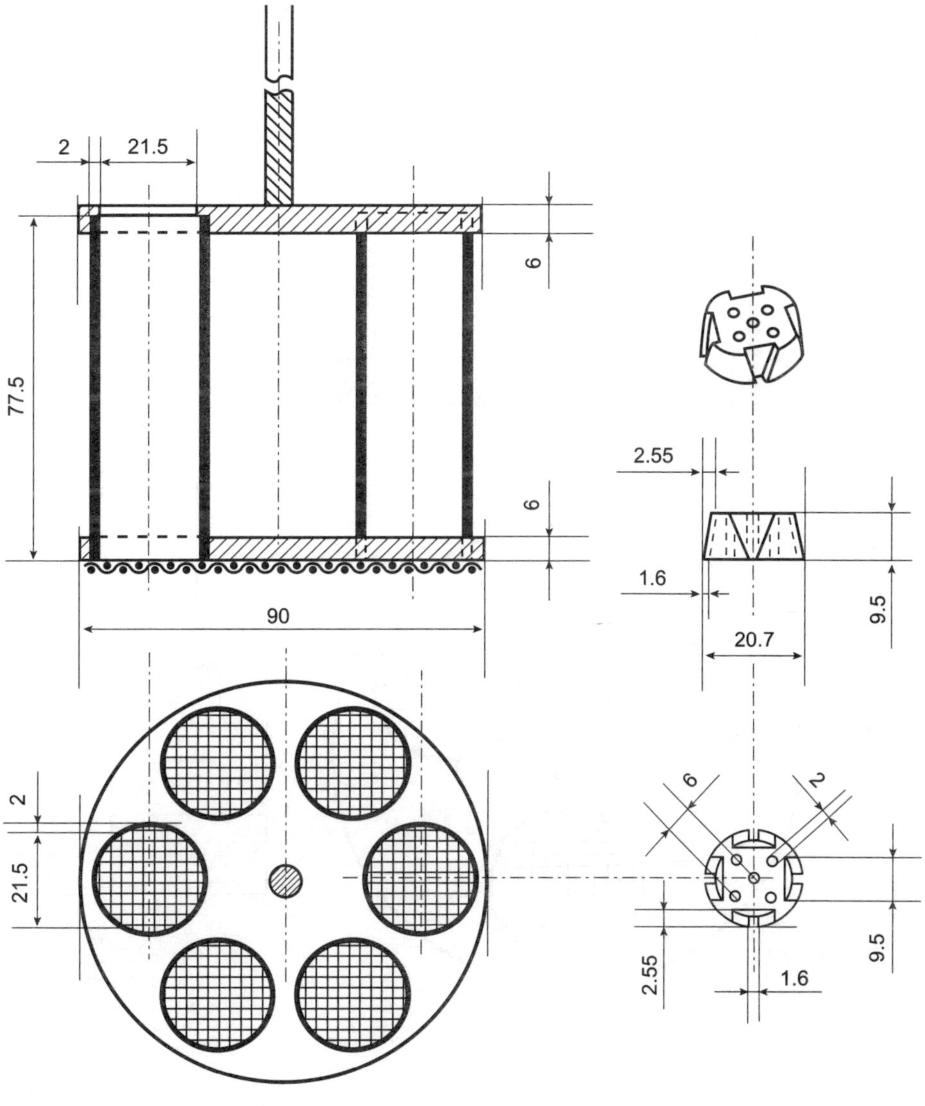

Figure 2.9.1.-1. – Apparatus A
Dimensions in millimetres

beaker and the upper open ends of the tubes remain above the surface of the liquid. A suitable device maintains the temperature of the liquid at 35-39 °C.

The design of the basket-rack assembly may be varied provided the specifications for the tubes and wire mesh are maintained.

Method. In each of the 6 tubes, place one tablet or capsule and, if prescribed, add a disc; suspend the assembly in the beaker containing the specified liquid. Operate the apparatus for the prescribed period, withdraw the assembly and examine the state of the tablets or capsules. To pass the test, all the tablets or capsules must have disintegrated.

TEST B – LARGE TABLETS AND LARGE CAPSULES

Apparatus. The main part of the apparatus (Figure 2.9.1.-2) is a rigid basket-rack assembly supporting 3 cylindrical transparent tubes 77.5 ± 2.5 mm long, 33.0 mm ± 0.5 mm in internal diameter, and with a wall thickness of 2.5 ± 0.5 mm. Each tube is provided with a cylindrical disc 31.4 ± 0.13 mm in diameter and 15.3 ± 0.15 mm thick, made of transparent plastic with a relative density of 1.18 to 1.20 or weighing 13.0 ± 0.2 g. Each disc is pierced by 7 holes, each 3.15 ± 0.1 mm in diameter, 1 in the centre and the other 6 spaced equally on a circle of radius 4.2 mm from the centre of the disc. The tubes are held vertically by 2 separate and superimposed rigid plastic plates 97 mm in diameter and 9 mm thick, with 3 holes. The holes are equidistant from the centre of the plate and equally spaced. Attached to the under side of the lower plate is a piece of woven gauze made from stainless steel wire 0.63 ± 0.03 mm in diameter and having mesh apertures of 2.0 ± 0.2 mm. The plates are held rigidly in position and 77.5 mm apart by vertical metal rods at the periphery, a metal rod is also fixed to the centre of the upper plate to enable the assembly to be attached to a mechanical device capable of raising and lowering it smoothly at constant frequency between 29 and 32 cycles per minute, through a distance of 55 ± 2 mm.

The assembly is suspended in the specified liquid medium in a suitable vessel, preferably a 1 litre beaker. The volume of the liquid is such that when the assembly is in the highest position the wire mesh is at least 15 mm below the surface of the liquid, and when the assembly is in the lowest position the wire mesh is at least 25 mm above the bottom of the

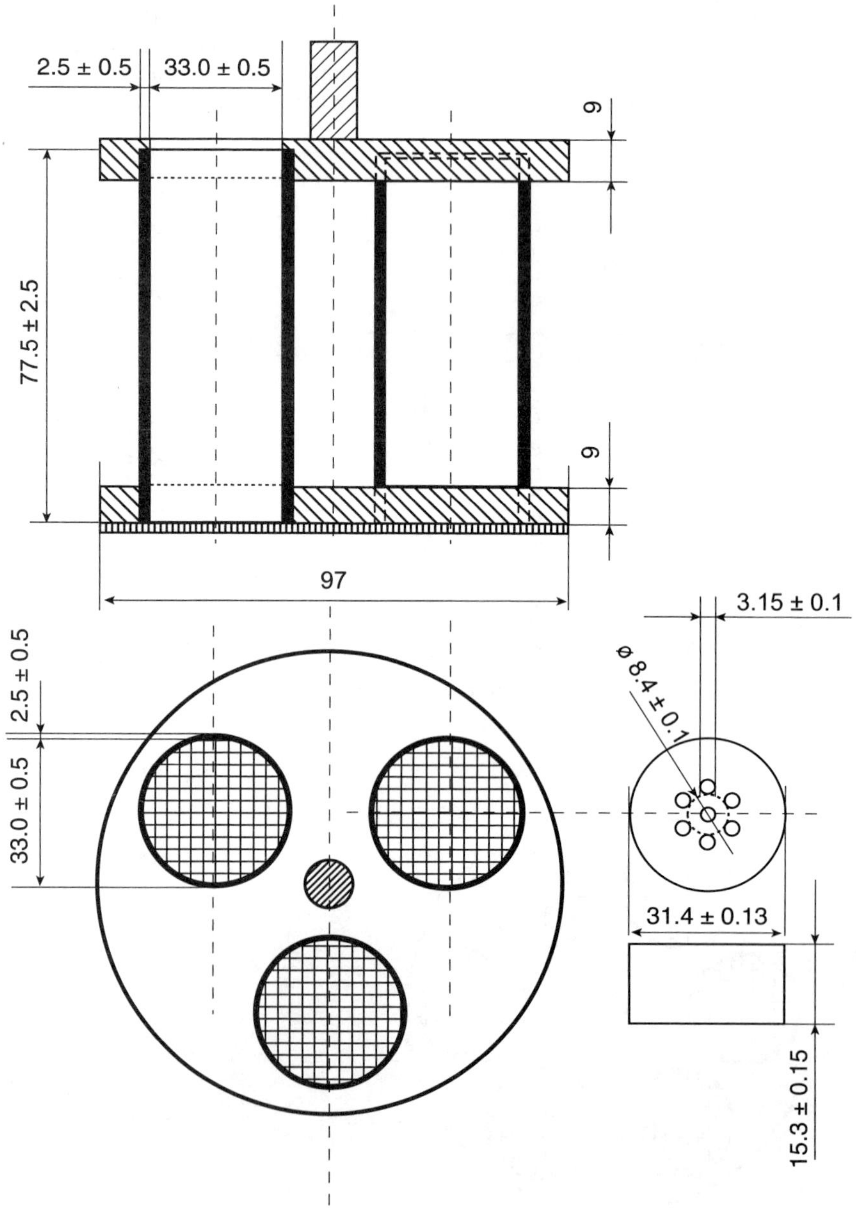

Figure 2.9.1.-2. – Apparatus B
Dimensions in millimetres

beaker and the upper open ends of the tubes remain above the surface of the liquid. A suitable device maintains the temperature of the liquid at 35-39 °C.

The design of the basket-rack assembly may be varied provided the specifications for the tubes and wire mesh are maintained.

Method. Test 6 tablets or capsules either by using 2 basket-rack assemblies in parallel or by repeating the procedure. In each of the 3 tubes, place one tablet or capsule and, if prescribed, add a disc; suspend the assembly in the beaker containing the specified liquid. Operate the apparatus for the prescribed period, withdraw the assembly and examine the state of the tablets or capsules. To pass the test, all 6 of the tablets or capsules must have disintegrated.

2.9.27. UNIFORMITY OF MASS OF DELIVERED DOSES FROM MULTIDOSE CONTAINERS

The following test is intended for oral dosage forms such as granules, powders for oral use and liquids for oral use, which are supplied in multidose containers provided at manufacture with a measuring device.

Weigh individually 20 doses taken at random from one or more containers with the measuring device provided and determine the individual and average masses. Not more than 2 of the individual masses deviate from the average mass by more than 10 per cent and none deviates by more than 20 per cent.

2. Methods of analysis

4. REAGENTS

4.1.1. REAGENTS

Berberine chloride. $C_{20}H_{18}ClNO_4,2H_2O$. (M_r 407.8). *1153400.* [5956-60-5]. 9,10-Dimethoxy-5,6-dihydrobenzo[*g*]-1,3-benzodioxolo[5,6-*a*]quinolizinium chloride.
Yellow crystals, slightly soluble in water, practically insoluble in alcohol.
mp: 204 °C to 206 °C.
Berberine chloride used in liquid chromatography complies with the following additional requirement.

Assay. Examine by liquid chromatography (*2.2.29*) as prescribed in the monograph on *Goldenseal rhizome (1831).* The content is not less than 95 per cent, calculated by the normalisation procedure.

Boric acid. *1011800.*

Boric acid solution, saturated, cold. *1011801.*
To 3 g of *boric acid R* add 50 ml of *water R* and shake for 10 min. Place the solution for 2 h in the refrigerator.

Carbon for chromatography, graphitised R1. *1153500.* Porous spherical carbon particles comprised of flat sheets of hexagonally arranged carbon atoms.

Particle size: 5-7 µm.

Pore volume: 0.7 cm^3/g.

2,3-Dichloro-5,6-dicyanobenzoquinone. $C_8Cl_2N_2O_2$. (M_r 227.0). *1153600.* [84-58-2]. 4,5-Dichloro-3,6-dioxocyclohexa-1,4-diene-1,2-dicarbonitrile.
Yellow or orange crystals, soluble in dioxan and in acetic acid, slightly soluble in methylene chloride. It decomposes in water.
mp: about 214 °C.
Store at a temperature of 2 °C to 8 °C.

Ferric sulphate pentahydrate. $Fe_2(SO_4)_3,5H_2O$. (M_r 489.9). *1153700.* [142906-29-4].
White or yellowish powder.

Flunitrazepam. *1153800.* [1622-62-4].
See *Flunitrazepam (0717).*

Hydrastine hydrochloride. $C_{21}H_{22}ClNO_6$. (M_r 419.9). *1154000.* [5936-28-7]. (3*S*)-6,7-Dimethoxy-3-[(5*R*)-6-methyl-5,6,7,8-tetrahydro-1,3-dioxolo[4,5-*g*]isoquinolin-5-yl]isobenzofuran-1(3*H*)-one hydrochloride.
A white powder, hygroscopic, very soluble in water and in alcohol.
$[\alpha]_D^{17}$: about + 127.
mp: about 116 °C.
Hydrastine hydrochloride used in liquid chromatography complies with the following additional test.

Assay. Examine by liquid chromatography (*2.2.29*) as prescribed in the monograph on *Goldenseal rhizome (1831).* The content is not less than 98 per cent, calculated by the normalisation procedure.

Magnesium nitrate. *1049800.*

Magnesium nitrate solution R1. *1049802.*
Dissolve 20 g of *magnesium nitrate R* ($Mg(NO_3)_2,6H_2O$) in *deionised distilled water R* and dilute to 100 ml with the same solvent. Immediately before use, dilute 10 ml to 100 ml with *deionised distilled water R.* A volume of 5 µl will provide 0.06 mg of Mg $(NO_3)_2$.

Methyl 4-acetylbenzoate. $C_{10}H_{10}O_3$. (M_r 178.2). *1154100.* [3609-53-8].
mp: about 94 °C.

Methyl 4-acetylbenzoate reagent. *1154101.*
Dissolve 0.25 g of *methyl 4-acetylbenzoate R* in a mixture of 5 ml of *sulphuric acid R* and 85 ml of cooled *methanol R.*

Nitric acid. *1058400.*

Nitric acid, lead-free R1. *1058405.*
Nitric acid R containing not more than 1 µg/kg of lead.

Nitric acid, lead-free, dilute. *1058406.*
Dilute 5 g of *lead-free nitric acid R1* to 100 ml with *deionised distilled water R.*

Propidium iodide. $C_{27}H_{34}I_2N_4$. (M_r 668.4). *1154200.* [25535-16-4]. 3,8-Diamino-5-[3(diethylmethylammonio)propyl]-6-phenylphenanthridinium diiodide.
Dark red solid.

Silica gel for chromatography, palmitamidopropylsilyl, end-capped. *1115200.*
A very finely divided (3 µm-10 µm) silica gel, chemically modified at the surface by the bonding of palmitamidopropyl groups and end-capped with acetamidopropyl groups. The particle size is indicated after the name of the reagent in the tests where it is used.

A fine, white, homogeneous powder, practically insoluble in water and in alcohol.

Silica gel for chromatography, phenylhexylsilyl. *1153900.* A very finely divided silica gel, chemically modified at the surface by the bonding of phenylhexyl groups. The particle size is indicated after the name of the reagent in the tests where it is used.

Sodium bromide. *1154300.* [7647-15-6].
See *Sodium bromide (0190).*

Stanolone. $C_{19}H_{30}O_2$. (M_r 290.4). *1154400.* [521-18-6]. 17β-Hydroxy-5α-androstan-3-one.
White or almost white powder.
mp: about 180 °C.

Water. *1095500.*

Water, distilled, deionised. *1095508.*
Deionised *water R* prepared by distillation with a resistivity of not less than 18 Mohm·m.

4.1.2. STANDARD SOLUTIONS FOR LIMIT TESTS

Lead standard solution (0.1 per cent Pb) R1. *5005400.* Dissolve in *dilute lead-free nitric acid R* a quantity of *lead nitrate R* equivalent to 0.400 g of Pb $(NO_3)_2$ and dilute to 250.0 ml with the same solvent.

Lead standard solution (10 ppm Pb) R2. *5005401.*
Dilute *lead standard solution (0.1 per cent Pb) R1* to 100 times its volume with *dilute lead-free nitric acid R.* Use within 1 week.

Lead standard solution (0.5 ppm Pb) R1. *5005402.*
Dilute *lead standard solution (10 ppm Pb) R2* to 20 times its volume with *dilute lead-free nitric acid R.* Use within 1 day.

Sulphite standard solution (80 ppm SO_2). *5005500.*
Dissolve 3.150 g of *anhydrous sodium sulphite R* in freshly prepared *distilled water R* and dilute to 100.0 ml with the same solvent. Dilute 0.5 ml to 100.0 ml with freshly prepared *distilled water R.*

A

07/2004:0576

ALLOPURINOL

Allopurinolum

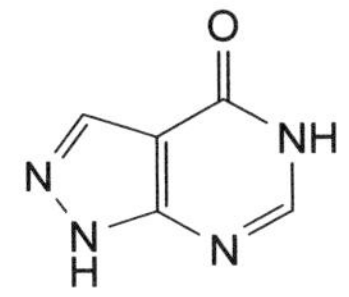

$C_5H_4N_4O$ M_r 136.1

DEFINITION

1,5-Dihydro-4*H*-pyrazolo[3,4-*d*]pyrimidin-4-one.

Content: 98.0 per cent to 102.0 per cent (dried substance).

CHARACTERS

Appearance: white or almost white powder.

Solubility: very slightly soluble in water and in alcohol. It dissolves in dilute solutions of alkali hydroxides.

IDENTIFICATION

First identification: B.

Second identification: A, C, D.

A. Dissolve 10 mg in 1 ml of a 4 g/l solution of *sodium hydroxide R* and dilute to 100.0 ml with a 10.3 g/l solution of *hydrochloric acid R*. Dilute 10.0 ml of this solution to 100.0 ml with a 10.3 g/l solution of *hydrochloric acid R*. Examined between 220 nm and 350 nm (*2.2.25*), the solution shows an absorption maximum at 250 nm and an absorption minimum at 231 nm. The ratio of the absorbance measured at the absorption minimum at 231 nm to that measured at the absorption maximum at 250 nm is 0.52 to 0.62.

B. Infrared absorption spectrophotometry (*2.2.24*).

Preparation: discs.

Comparison: *allopurinol CRS.*

C. Dissolve 0.3 g in 2.5 ml of *dilute sodium hydroxide solution R* and add 50 ml of *water R*. Add slowly and with shaking 5 ml of *silver nitrate solution R1*. A white precipitate is formed which does not dissolve on the addition of 5 ml of *ammonia R*.

D. Thin-layer chromatography (*2.2.27*).

Test solution. Dissolve 20 mg of the substance to be examined in *concentrated ammonia R* and dilute to 10 ml with the same solvent.

Reference solution. Dissolve 20 mg of *allopurinol CRS* in *concentrated ammonia R* and dilute to 10 ml with the same solvent.

Plate: *TLC silica gel F_{254} plate R.*

Mobile phase: *ethanol R, methylene chloride R* (40:60 *V/V*).

Application: 10 µl.

Development: over 2/3 of the plate.

Drying: in air.

Detection: examine in ultraviolet light at 254 nm.

Results: the principal spot in the chromatogram obtained with the test solution is similar in position and size to the principal spot in the chromatogram obtained with the reference solution.

TESTS

Related substances. Liquid chromatography (*2.2.29*).

Prepare the solutions immediately before use. Store them and inject them at 8 °C using a cooled autosampler.

Test solution (a). Dissolve 25.0 mg of the substance to be examined in 2.5 ml of a 4 g/l solution of *sodium hydroxide R* and dilute immediately to 50.0 ml with the mobile phase.

Test solution (b). Dissolve 20.0 mg of the substance to be examined in 5.0 ml of a 4 g/l solution of *sodium hydroxide R* and dilute immediately to 250.0 ml with the mobile phase.

Reference solution (a). Dilute 2.0 ml of test solution (a) to 100.0 ml with the mobile phase. Dilute 5.0 ml of this solution to 100.0 ml with the mobile phase.

Reference solution (b). Dissolve 5.0 mg of *allopurinol impurity A CRS*, 5.0 mg of *allopurinol impurity B CRS* and 5.0 mg of *allopurinol impurity C CRS* in 5.0 ml of a 4 g/l solution of *sodium hydroxide R* and dilute immediately to 100.0 ml with the mobile phase. Dilute 1.0 ml of this solution to 100.0 ml with the mobile phase.

Reference solution (c). Dissolve 20.0 mg of *allopurinol CRS* in 5.0 ml of a 4 g/l solution of *sodium hydroxide R* and dilute immediately to 250.0 ml with the mobile phase.

Column:

– *size*: l = 0.25 m, Ø = 4.6 mm,

– *stationary phase*: *octadecylsilyl silica gel for chromatography R* (5 µm).

Mobile phase: 1.25 g/l solution of *potassium dihydrogen phosphate R.*

Flow rate: 1.4 ml/min.

Detection: spectrophotometer at 230 nm.

Injection: 20 µl of test solution (a) and reference solutions (a) and (b).

Run time: twice the retention time of allopurinol.

Elution order: impurity A, impurity B, impurity C, allopurinol.

Retention time: allopurinol = about 10 min.

System suitability: reference solution (b):

– *resolution*: minimum 1.1 between the peaks due to impurity B and impurity C.

Limits:

– *impurity A*: not more than twice the area of the principal peak in the chromatogram obtained with reference solution (a) (0.2 per cent),

– *impurity B*: not more than the area of the principal peak in the chromatogram obtained with reference solution (a) (0.1 per cent),

– *impurity C*: not more than the area of the corresponding peak in the chromatogram obtained with reference solution (b) (0.1 per cent),

– *any other impurity*: for each impurity, not more than the area of the principal peak in the chromatogram obtained with reference solution (a) (0.1 per cent),

– *total of impurities other than A, B and C*: not more than 3 times the area of the principal peak in the chromatogram obtained with reference solution (a) (0.3 per cent),

– *disregard limit*: 0.5 times the area of the principal peak in the chromatogram obtained with reference solution (a) (0.05 per cent).

Impurities D and E. Liquid chromatography (*2.2.29*).

Prepare the solutions immediately before use. Store them and inject them at 8 °C using a cooled autosampler.

Solution A: 1.25 g/l solution of *potassium dihydrogen phosphate R.*

Test solution. Dissolve 50.0 mg of the substance to be examined in 5.0 ml of a 4 g/l solution of *sodium hydroxide R* and dilute immediately to 100.0 ml with solution A.

Reference solution. Dissolve 5.0 mg of *allopurinol impurity D CRS* and 5.0 mg of *allopurinol impurity E CRS* in 5.0 ml of a 4 g/l solution of *sodium hydroxide R* and dilute immediately to 100.0 ml with solution A. Dilute 1.0 ml of this solution to 100.0 ml with solution A.

Column:

- *size*: *l* = 0.05 m, Ø = 4.6 mm,
- *stationary phase*: *base-deactivated octadecylsilyl silica gel for chromatography R* (3 µm).

Mobile phase: *methanol R*, 1.25 g/l solution of *potassium dihydrogen phosphate R* (10:90 *V/V*).

Flow rate: 2 ml/min.

Detection: spectrophotometer at 230 nm.

Injection: 20 µl.

Run time: 1.5 times the retention time of impurity E.

Retention times: impurity D = about 3.6 min; impurity E = about 4.5 min.

System suitability: reference solution:

- *resolution*: minimum 2.0 between the peaks due to impurity D and impurity E.

Limits:

- *impurity D*: not more than the area of the corresponding peak in the chromatogram obtained with the reference solution (0.1 per cent),
- *impurity E*: not more than the area of the corresponding peak in the chromatogram obtained with the reference solution (0.1 per cent).

Heavy metals (*2.4.8*): maximum 20 ppm.

1.0 g complies with limit test C. Prepare the standard using 2 ml of *lead standard solution (10 ppm Pb) R*.

Loss on drying (*2.2.32*): maximum 0.5 per cent, determined on 1.000 g by drying in an oven at 100-105 °C.

Sulphated ash (*2.4.14*): maximum 0.1 per cent, determined on 1.0 g.

ASSAY

Liquid chromatography (*2.2.29*) as described in the test for related substances with the following modification.

Injection: test solution (b) and reference solution (c).

Calculate the percentage content of $C_5H_4N_4O$ from the areas of the peaks and the declared content of *allopurinol CRS*.

IMPURITIES

Specified impurities (see note for information p. xli): A, B, C, D, E.

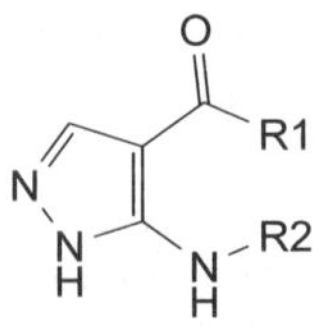

A. R1 = NH_2, R2 = H: 5-amino-1*H*-pyrazole-4-carboxamide,

B. R1 = NH_2, R2 = CHO: 5-(formylamino)-1*H*-pyrazole-4-carboxamide,

D. R1 = O-CH_2-CH_3, R2 = H: ethyl 5-amino-1*H*-pyrazole-4-carboxylate,

E. R1 = O-CH_2-CH_3, R2 = CHO: ethyl 5-(formylamino)-1*H*-pyrazole-4-carboxylate,

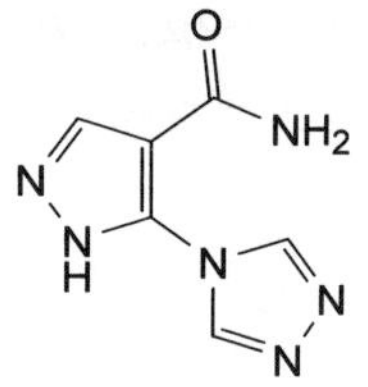

C. 5-(4*H*-1,2,4-triazol-4-yl)-1*H*-pyrazole-4-carboxamide.

07/2004:1664

ALUMINIUM HYDROXIDE, HYDRATED, FOR ADSORPTION

Aluminii hydroxidum hydricum ad adsorptionem

$[AlO(OH)],nH_2O$

DEFINITION

Content: 90.0 per cent to 110.0 per cent of the content of aluminium stated on the label.

NOTE: shake the gel vigorously for at least 30 s immediately before examining.

CHARACTERS

Appearance: white or almost white, translucent, viscous, colloidal gel. A supernatant may be formed upon standing.

Solubility: a clear or almost clear solution is obtained with alkali hydroxide solutions and mineral acids.

IDENTIFICATION

Solution S (see Tests) gives the reaction of aluminium.

To 10 ml of solution S add about 0.5 ml of *dilute hydrochloric acid R* and about 0.5 ml of *thioacetamide reagent R*. No precipitate is formed. Add dropwise 5 ml of *dilute sodium hydroxide solution R*. Allow to stand for 1 h. A gelatinous white precipitate is formed which dissolves upon addition of 5 ml of *dilute sodium hydroxide solution R*. Gradually add 5 ml of *ammonium chloride solution R* and allow to stand for 30 min. The gelatinous white precipitate is re-formed.

TESTS

Solution S. Add 1 g to 4 ml of *hydrochloric acid R*. Heat at 60 °C for 1 h, cool, dilute to 50 ml with *distilled water R* and filter if necessary.

pH (*2.2.3*): 5.5 to 8.5.

Adsorption power. Dilute the substance to be examined with *distilled water R* to obtain an aluminium concentration of 5 mg/ml. Prepare *bovine albumin R* solutions with the following concentrations of bovine albumin: 0.5 mg/ml, 1 mg/ml, 2 mg/ml, 3 mg/ml, 5 mg/ml and 10 mg/ml. If necessary, adjust the gel and the *bovine albumin R* solutions to pH 6.0 with *dilute hydrochloric acid R* or *dilute sodium hydroxide solution R*.

For adsorption, mix 1 part of the diluted gel with 4 parts of each of the solutions of *bovine albumin R* and allow to stand at room temperature for 1 h. During this time shake the mixture vigorously at least 5 times. Centrifuge or filter through a non-protein-retaining filter. Immediately determine the protein content (*2.5.33, Method 2*) of either the supernatant or the filtrate.

It complies with the test if no bovine albumin is detectable in the supernatant or filtrate of the 2 mg/ml *bovine albumin R* solution (maximum level of adsorption) and in the supernatant or filtrate of *bovine albumin R* solutions of lower concentrations. Those containing 3 mg/ml, 5 mg/ml and 10 mg/ml *bovine albumin R* solutions may show bovine albumin in the supernatant or filtrate, proportional to the amount of bovine albumin in the solutions.

Sedimentation. If necessary, adjust the substance to be examined to pH 6.0 using *dilute hydrochloric acid R* or dilute *sodium hydroxide solution R*. Dilute with *distilled water R* to obtain an aluminium concentration of approximately 5 mg/ml. If the aluminium content of the substance to be examined is lower than 5 mg/ml, adjust to pH 6.0 and dilute with a 9 g/l solution of *sodium chloride R* to obtain an aluminium concentration of about 1 mg/ml. After shaking for at least 30 s, place 25 ml of the preparation in a 25 ml graduated cylinder and allow to stand for 24 h.

It complies with the test if the volume of the clear supernatant is less than 5 ml for the gel with an aluminium content of about 5 mg/ml.

It complies with the test if the volume of the clear supernatant is less than 20 ml for the gel with an aluminium content of about 1 mg/ml.

Chlorides (*2.4.4*): maximum 0.33 per cent.

Dissolve 0.5 g in 10 ml of *dilute nitric acid R* and dilute to 500 ml with *water R*.

Nitrates: maximum 100 ppm.

Place 5 g in a test-tube immersed in ice-water, add 0.4 ml of a 100 g/l solution of *potassium chloride R*, 0.1 ml of *diphenylamine solution R* and, dropwise with shaking, 5 ml of *sulphuric acid R*. Transfer the tube to a water-bath at 50 °C. After 15 min, any blue colour in the solution is not more intense than that in a standard prepared at the same time and in the same manner using 5 ml of *nitrate standard solution (100 ppm NO_3) R*.

Sulphates (*2.4.13*): maximum 0.5 per cent.

Dilute 2 ml of solution S to 20 ml with *water R*.

Ammonium (*2.4.1*): maximum 50 ppm.

1.0 g complies with limit test B. Prepare the standard using 0.5 ml of *ammonium standard solution (100 ppm NH_4) R*.

Arsenic (*2.4.2, Method A*): maximum 1 ppm, determined on 1 g.

Iron (*2.4.9*): maximum 10 ppm, determined on 1 g.

Heavy metals (*2.4.8*): maximum 20 ppm.

Dissolve 2.0 g in 10 ml of *dilute nitric acid R* and dilute to 20 ml with *water R*. The solution complies with limit test A. Prepare the standard using *lead standard solution (2 ppm Pb) R*.

Bacterial endotoxins (*2.6.14*): less than 5 IU of endotoxin per milligram of aluminium, if intended for use in the manufacture of an adsorbed product without a further appropriate procedure for the removal of bacterial endotoxins.

ASSAY

Dissolve 10.00 g in 10 ml of *hydrochloric acid R1*, heating on a water-bath. Cool and dilute to 20 ml with *water R*. To 10 ml of the solution, add *dilute ammonia R1* until a precipitate is obtained. Add the smallest quantity of *dilute hydrochloric acid R* needed to dissolve the precipitate and dilute to 20 ml with *water R*. Carry out the complexometric titration of aluminium (*2.5.11*). Carry out a blank titration.

STORAGE

At a temperature not exceeding 30 °C. Do not allow to freeze. If the substance is sterile, store in a sterile, airtight, tamper-proof container.

LABELLING

The label states:

– where applicable, that the substance is free from bacterial endotoxins,
– the declared content of aluminium.

07/2004:0804

ANISE OIL

Anisi aetheroleum

DEFINITION

Essential oil obtained by steam distillation from the dry ripe fruits of *Pimpinella anisum* L.

CHARACTERS

Appearance: clear, colourless or pale yellow liquid.

IDENTIFICATION

First identification: B.

Second identification: A.

A. Thin-layer chromatography (*2.2.27*).

Test solution. Dissolve 1 g of the substance to be examined in *toluene R* and dilute to 10 ml with the same solvent.

Reference solution. Dissolve 10 µl of *linalol R*, 30 µl of *anisaldehyde R* and 200 µl of *anethole R* in *toluene R* and dilute to 15 ml with the same solvent. Dilute 1 ml of this solution to 5 ml with *toluene R*.

Plate: *TLC silica gel F_{254} plate R.*

Mobile phase: *ethyl acetate R, toluene R* (7:93 *V/V*).

Application: 5 µl as bands of 10 mm (for normal TLC plates) or 2 µl as bands of 10 mm (for fine particle size plates).

Development: over a path of 15 cm (for normal TLC plates) or over a path of 6 cm (for fine particle size plates).

Drying: in air.

Detection A: examine in ultraviolet light at 254 nm.

Results A: see below the sequence of zones present in the chromatograms obtained with the reference solution and the test solution. Furthermore, other zones may be present in the chromatogram obtained with the test solution.

Top of the plate	
Anethole: a quenching zone	A very strong quenching zone (anethole)
_______	_______
Anisaldehyde: a quenching zone	A quenching zone
	A quenching zone (anisalaldehyde)
_______	_______
Reference solution	**Test solution**

Detection B: spray with *methyl 4-acetylbenzoate reagent R* and heat at 100-105 °C for 10 min; examine the still hot plate in daylight within 5 min.

Results B: see below the sequence of zones present in the chromatograms obtained with the reference solution and the test solution. Furthermore, other zones may be present in the chromatogram obtained with the test solution.

Top of the plate	
	A violet-brown zone (monoterpene hydrocarbons) (solvent front)
Anethole: a brown zone	A very strong brown zone (anethole), distinctly separated
_______	_______
	A grey zone
Anisaldehyde: a yellow zone	A yellow zone (anisaldehyde)
_______	_______
Linalol: a grey zone	A grey zone (linalol)
	A grey zone
Reference solution	**Test solution**

B. Examine the chromatograms obtained in the test for chromatographic profile.

Results: the characteristic peaks in the chromatogram obtained with the test solution are similar in retention time to those in the chromatogram obtained with the reference solution.

TESTS

Relative density (*2.2.5*): 0.980 to 0.990.

Refractive index (*2.2.6*): 1.552 to 1.561.

Freezing point (*2.2.18*): 15 °C to 19 °C.

Fenchone. Gas chromatography (*2.2.28*) as described in the test for chromatographic profile with the following modifications.

Test solution. Dissolve 400 µl of the substance to be examined in 2.0 ml of *hexane R.*

Reference solution (a). Dilute 10 µl of *fenchone R* to 1.2 g with *hexane R.*

Reference solution (b). Dilute 100 µl of reference solution (a) to 100 ml with *hexane R.*

System suitability: reference solution (b):

– *signal-to-noise ratio*: minimum 10 for the principal peak.

Limit:

– *fenchone*: maximum 0.01 per cent.

Foeniculin. Gas chromatography (*2.2.28*) as described in the test for chromatographic profile with the following modifications.

Test solution. The substance to be examined.

Reference solution (a). Dilute 10 mg of the test solution to 1.000 g with *hexane R.* Dilute 0.5 ml of this solution to 100 ml with *hexane R.*

Reference solution (b). Star anise oil CRS.

System suitability:

– the chromatogram obtained with reference solution (b) is similar to the chromatogram provided with *star anise oil CRS,*

– *signal-to-noise ratio*: minimum 10 for the principal peak in the chromatogram obtained with reference solution (a).

Limit: locate the peak due to foeniculin by comparison with the chromatogram provided with *star anise oil CRS.*

– *foeniculin*: maximum 0.01 per cent.

Fatty oils and resinified essential oils (*2.8.7*). It complies with the test for fatty oils and resinified essential oils.

Chromatographic profile. Gas chromatography (*2.2.28*): use the normalisation procedure.

Test solution. Dissolve 200 µl of the substance to be examined in 1.0 ml of *hexane R.*

Reference solution. To 1.0 ml of *hexane R,* add 20 µl of *linalol R,* 20 µl of *estragole R,* 20 µl of *α-terpineol R,* 60 µl of *anethole R* and 30 µl of *anisaldehyde R.*

Column:

– *material*: fused silica,

– *size*: l = 30 m, Ø = 0.25 mm,

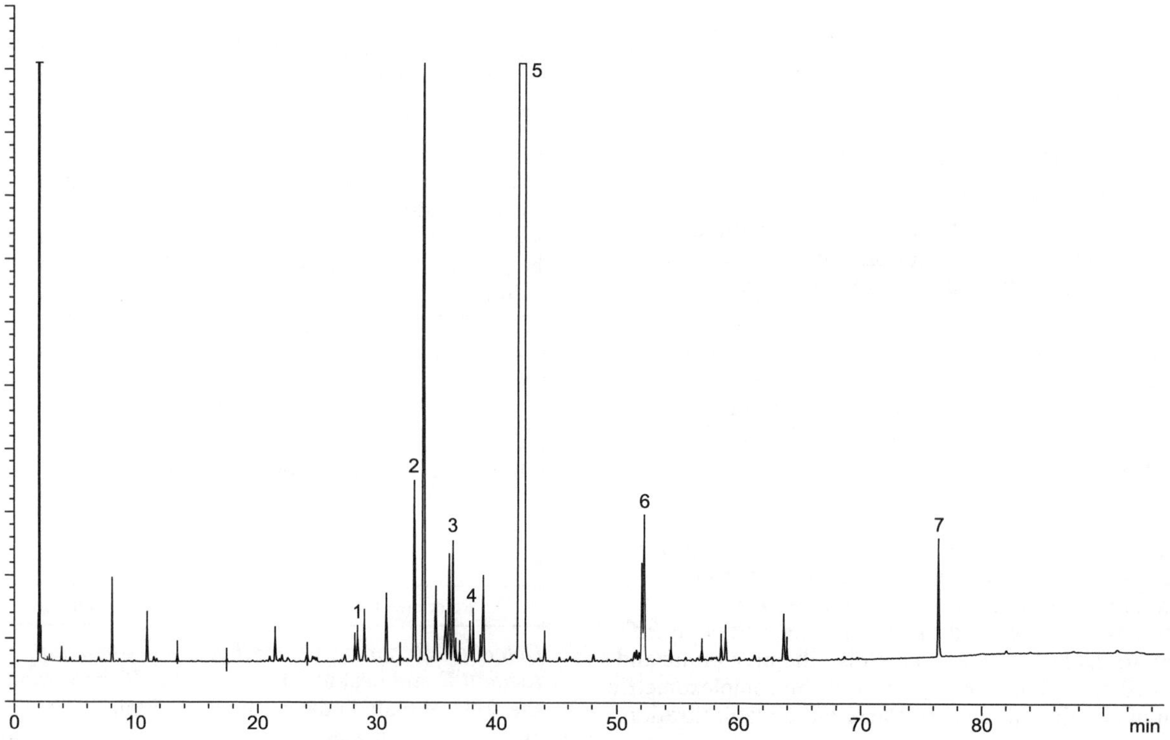

1. linalol
2. estragole
3. α-terpineol
4. *cis*-anethole
5. *trans*-anethole
6. anisaldehyde
7. pseudoisoeugenyl 2-methylbutyrate

Figure 0804.-1. – *Chromatogram for the test for chromatographic profile of anise oil*

Monographs A - C

– *stationary phase*: *macrogol 20 000 R* (film thickness 0.25 µm).

Carrier gas: *helium for chromatography R.*

Flow rate: 1.0 ml/min.

Split ratio: 1:100.

Temperature:

	Time (min)	Temperature (°C)
Column	0 - 5	60
	5 - 80	60 → 210
	80 - 95	210
Injection port		200
Detector		220

Detection: flame ionisation.

Injection: 0.2 µl.

Elution order: order indicated in the composition of the reference solution. Record the retention times of these substances.

System suitability: reference solution:

– *resolution*: minimum 1.5 between the peaks due to estragole and α-terpineol.

Using the retention times determined from the chromatogram obtained with the reference solution, locate the components of the reference solution in the chromatogram obtained with the test solution and locate *cis*-anethole and pseudoisoeugenyl 2-methylbutyrate using the chromatogram shown in Figure 0804.-1 (disregard any peak due to hexane).

Determine the percentage content of these components. The percentages are within the following ranges:

– *linalol*: less than 1.5 per cent,
– *estragole*: 0.5 per cent to 5.0 per cent,
– *α-terpineol*: less than 1.2 per cent,
– *cis-anethole*: 0.1 per cent to 0.4 per cent,
– *trans-anethole*: 87 per cent to 94 per cent,
– *anisaldehyde*: 0.1 per cent to 1.4 per cent,
– *pseudoisoeugenyl 2-methylbutyrate*: 0.3 per cent to 2.0 per cent.

STORAGE

In a well-filled, airtight container, protected from light and at a temperature not exceeding 25 °C.

07/2004:1928

ANTI-T LYMPHOCYTE IMMUNOGLOBULIN FOR HUMAN USE, ANIMAL

Immunoglobulinum anti-T lymphocytorum ex animale ad usum humanum

DEFINITION

Anti-T lymphocyte immunoglobulin for human use is a liquid or freeze-dried preparation containing immunoglobulins, obtained from serum or plasma of animals, mainly rabbits or horses, immunised with human lymphocytic antigens.

The immunoglobulin has the property of diminishing the number and function of immunocompetent cells, in particular T-lymphocytes. The preparation contains principally immunoglobulin G. It may contain antibodies against other lymphocyte subpopulations and against other cells. The preparation is intended for intravenous administration, after dilution with a suitable diluent where applicable.

Applicable provisions of the monograph on *Immunosera for human use, animal (0084)* are stated below.

PRODUCTION

GENERAL PROVISIONS

The production method has been shown to yield consistently immunoglobulins of acceptable safety, potency in man and stability.

Any reagent of biological origin used in production shall be free of contamination with bacteria, fungi and viruses. The method of preparation includes a step or steps that have been shown to remove or inactivate known agents of infection.

During development studies, it shall be demonstrated that the production method yields a product that:

– does not transmit infectious agents,
– is characterised by a defined pattern of immunological activity, notably: antigen binding, complement-dependent and independent cytotoxicity, cytokine release, induction of T-cell activation, cell death,
– does not contain antibodies that cross-react with human tissues to a degree that would impair clinical safety,
– has a defined maximum content of anti-thrombocyte antibody activity,
– has a defined maximum content of haemoglobin.

The product has been shown, by suitable tests in animals and evaluation during clinical trials, to be well tolerated.

Reference preparation. A batch shown to be suitable for checking the validity of the assay and whose efficacy has been demonstrated in clinical trials, or a batch representative thereof.

ANIMALS

The animals used are of a species approved by the competent authority, are healthy and exclusively reserved for production of anti-T lymphocyte immunoglobulin. They are tested and shown to be free from a defined list of infectious agents. The introduction of animals into a closed herd follows specified procedures, including definition of quarantine measures. Where appropriate, tests for additional specific agents are considered depending on the geographical localisation of the establishment used for the breeding and production of the animals. The feed originates from a controlled source and no animal proteins are added. The suppliers of animals are certified by the competent authority.

If the animals are treated with antibiotics, a suitable withdrawal period is allowed before collection of blood or plasma. The animals are not treated with penicillin antibiotics. If a live vaccine is administered, a suitable waiting period is imposed between vaccination and collection of serum or plasma for immunoglobulin production.

The species, origin and identification number of the animals are specified.

IMMUNISATION

The antigens used are identified and characterised, where appropriate. They are identified by their names and a batch number; information on the source and preparation are recorded.

The selected animals are isolated for at least 1 week before being immunised according to a defined schedule with booster injections at suitable intervals. Adjuvants may be used.

Animals are kept under general health surveillance and specific antibody production is controlled at each cycle of immunisation.

Monographs A - C

Animals are thoroughly examined before collection of blood or plasma. If an animal shows any pathological lesion not related to the immunisation process, it is not used, nor are any other of the animals in the group concerned, unless it is evident that their use will not impair the safety of the product.

Human antigens such as continuously growing T-lymphocyte cell lines or thymocytes are used to immunise the animals. Cells may be subjected to a sorting procedure. The immunising antigens are shown to be free from infectious agents by validated methods for relevant blood-borne pathogens, notably hepatitis B virus (HBV), hepatitis C virus (HCV) and human immunodeficiency virus (HIV) and other relevant adventitious agents originating from the preparation of the antigen. The cells used comply with defined requirements for purity of the cell population and freedom from adventitious agents.

COLLECTION OF BLOOD OR PLASMA

Collection of blood is made by venepuncture or plasmapheresis. The puncture area is shaved, cleaned and disinfected. The animals may be anaesthetised under conditions that do not influence the quality of the product.

No antimicrobial preservative is added to the plasma and serum samples. The blood or plasma is collected in such a manner as to maintain sterility of the product. The blood or plasma collection is conducted at a site separate from the area where the animals are kept or bred and the area where the immunoglobulin is purified. If the serum or plasma is stored before further processing, precautions are taken to avoid microbial contamination.

Several single plasma or serum samples may be pooled before purification. The single or pooled samples are tested before purification for the following tests.

Tests for contaminating viruses. Each pool is tested for contaminating viruses by suitable *in vitro* tests including inoculation to cell cultures capable of detecting a wide range of viruses relevant for the particular product. Where applicable, *in vitro* tests for contaminating viruses are carried out on the adsorbed pool, after the last production stage that may introduce viral contaminants.

PURIFICATION AND VIRAL INACTIVATION

The immunoglobulins are concentrated and purified by fractional precipitation, chromatography, immuno-adsorption or by other suitable chemical or physical methods. The methods are selected and validated to avoid contamination at all steps of processing and to avoid formation of protein aggregates that effect immunobiological characteristics of the product.

Unless otherwise justified and authorised, validated procedures are applied for removal and/or inactivation of viruses.

After purification and treatment for removal and/or inactivation of viruses, a stabiliser may be added to the intermediate product, which may be stored for a period defined in the light of stability data.

Only an intermediate product that complies with the following requirements may be used in the preparation of the final bulk.

If the method of preparation includes a step for adsorption of cross-reacting anti-human antibodies using material from human tissues and/or red blood cells, the human materials are submitted to a validated procedure for inactivation of infectious agents, unless otherwise justified and authorised. If erythrocytes are used for adsorption, the donors for such materials comply with the requirements for donors of blood and plasma of the monograph on *Human plasma for fractionation (0853)*. If other human material is used, it is shown by validated methods to be free from relevant blood-borne pathogens, notably HBV, HCV and HIV. If substances are used for inactivation or removal of viruses, it shall have been shown that any residues present in the final product have no adverse effects on the patients treated with the anti-T lymphocyte immunoglobulin.

FINAL BULK

The final bulk is prepared from a single intermediate product or from a pool of intermediate products obtained from animals of the same species. A stabiliser may be added. No antimicrobial preservative is added either during the manufacturing procedure or for preparation of the final bulk solution. During manufacturing, the solution is passed through a bacteria-retentive filter.

FINAL LOT

The final bulk of anti-T-lymphocyte immunoglobulin is distributed aseptically into sterile, tamper-proof containers. The containers are closed as to prevent contamination. Only a final lot that complies with the requirements prescribed below under Identification, Tests and Assay may be released for use.

CHARACTERS

The liquid preparation is clear or slightly opalescent and colourless or pale yellow. The freeze-dried preparation is a white or slightly yellow powder or solid friable mass, which after reconstitution gives a liquid preparation corresponding to the description above.

IDENTIFICATION

A. Using a suitable range of species-specific antisera, carry out precipitation tests on the preparation to be examined. It is recommended that the test be carried out using antisera specific to the plasma proteins of each species of domestic animal commonly used in the preparation of materials of biological origin in the country concerned and antisera specific to human plasma proteins. The preparation is shown to contain proteins originating from the animal used for the anti-T lymphocyte immunoglobulin production.

B. Examine by a suitable immunoelectrophoresis technique. Using antiserum to normal serum of the animal used for production, compare this serum and the preparation to be examined, both diluted to a concentration that will allow a clear gammaglobulin precipitation arc to be obtained on the gel. The main component of the preparation to be examined corresponds to the IgG component of normal serum of the animal used for production.

C. The preparation complies with the assay.

TESTS

Solubility. To a container of the preparation to be examined, add the volume of the liquid for reconstitution stated on the label. The preparation dissolves completely within the time stated on the label.

Extractable volume (*2.9.17*). It complies with the requirement for extractable volume.

pH (*2.2.3*). The pH is within the limits approved for the particular product.

Osmolality (*2.2.35*): minimum 240 mosmol/kg after dilution, where applicable.

Proteins (*2.5.33*): 90 per cent to 110 per cent of the amount stated on the label.

Stabiliser. Determine the amount of stabiliser by a suitable physico-chemical method. The preparation contains not less than 80 per cent and not more than 120 per cent of the quantity stated on the label.

Distribution of molecular size. Size exclusion chromatography (*2.2.30*).

Test solution. Dilute the preparation to be examined with a 9 g/l solution of *sodium chloride R* to a concentration suitable for the chromatographic system used. A concentration in the range 2-20 g/l is usually suitable.

Reference solution. Dilute *human immunoglobulin BRP* with a 9 g/l solution of *sodium chloride R* to the same protein concentration as the test solution.

Column:

- *size*: l = 0.6 m, Ø = 7.5 mm,
- *stationary phase*: *silica gel for size-exclusion chromatography R*, a grade suitable for fractionation of globular proteins in the molecular mass range of 20 000 to 200 000.

Mobile phase: dissolve 4.873 g of *disodium hydrogen phosphate dihydrate R*, 1.741 g of *sodium dihydrogen phosphate monohydrate R* and 11.688 g of *sodium chloride R* in 1 litre of *water R*.

Flow rate: 0.5 ml/min.

Detection: spectrophotometer at 280 nm.

Injection: 50-600 µg of protein.

Retention time: identify the peaks in the chromatogram obtained with the test solution by comparison with the chromatogram obtained with the reference solution; any peak with a retention time shorter than that of dimer corresponds to polymers and aggregates.

System suitability:

- *reference solution*: the principal peak corresponds to IgG monomer and there is a peak corresponding to dimer with a retention time relative to monomer of 0.85 ± 0.05,
- *test solution*: the relative retentions of monomer and dimer are 1 ± 0.05 with reference to the corresponding peaks in the chromatogram obtained with the reference solution.

Limits:

- *total monomer and dimer*: at least 95 per cent of the total area of the peaks,
- *total polymers and aggregates*: maximum 5 per cent of the total area of the peaks.

Purity. Polyacrylamide gel electrophoresis (*2.2.31*), under non-reducing and reducing conditions.

Resolving gel. Non-reducing conditions: 8 per cent acrylamide; reducing conditions: 12 per cent acrylamide.

Test solution. Dilute the preparation to be examined to a protein concentration of 0.5-2 mg/ml.

Reference solution. Dilute the reference preparation to the same protein concentration as the test solution.

Application: 10 µl.

Detection: Coomassie staining.

Results: compared with the electropherogram of the reference solution, no additional bands are found in the electropherogram of the test solution.

Anti-A and anti-B haemagglutinins (*2.6.20*). The 1 to 64 dilution does not show agglutination.

Where applicable, dilute the preparation to be examined as prescribed for use before preparing the dilutions for the test.

Haemolysins. Prepare a 1 to 64 dilution of the preparation to be examined, diluted if necessary as stated on the label. Take 6 aliquots of the 1 to 64 dilution. To 1 volume of 3 of the aliquots, add 1 volume of a 10 per cent *V/V* suspension of group A1, group B and group O erythrocytes in a 9 g/l solution of *sodium chloride R*, respectively. To 1 volume of the remaining 3 aliquots, add 1 volume of a 10 per cent *V/V* suspension of group A1, group B and group O erythrocytes in a 9 g/l solution of *sodium chloride R*, respectively, and to each aliquot 1 volume of fresh group AB serum (as a source of complement). Mix and incubate at 37 °C for 1 h. Examine the supernatant liquids for haemolysis. No signs of haemolysis are present.

Thrombocyte antibodies. Examined by a suitable method, the level of thrombocyte antibodies is shown to be below that approved for the specific product.

Water (*2.5.12*): maximum 3 per cent.

Sterility (*2.6.1*). It complies with the test for sterility.

Pyrogens (*2.6.8*). Unless otherwise justified and authorised, it complies with the test for pyrogens. Unless otherwise prescribed, inject 1 ml per kilogram of the rabbit's body mass.

ASSAY

The biological activity is determined by measuring the complement-dependent cytotoxicity on target cells. Flow cytometry is performed with read-out of dead cells stained using propidium iodide. The activity is expressed as the concentration of anti-T lymphocyte immunoglobulin in milligrams per millilitre which mediates 50 per cent cytotoxicity.

Lymphocyte separation medium. Commercial separation media with low viscosity and a density of 1.077 g/ml.

Complement. Commercial complement is suitable.

Buffered salt solution pH 7.2. Dissolve 8.0 g of *sodium chloride R*, 0.2 g of *potassium chloride R*, 3.18 g of *disodium hydrogen phosphate R* and 0.2 g of *potassium dihydrogen phosphate R* in *water R* and dilute to 1000.0 ml with the same solvent.

Buffer solution for flow cytometry. Add 40 ml of 0.1 per cent *V/V sodium azide R* and 10 ml of foetal calf serum to 440 ml of buffered salt solution pH 7.2. The foetal calf serum is inactivated at 56 °C for 30 min prior to use. Store at 4 °C.

Propidium iodide solution. Dissolve *propidium iodide R* in buffered salt solution pH 7.2, to a concentration of 1 mg/ml. Store this stock solution at 2-8 °C and use within 1 month. For the assay, dilute this solution with buffer solution for flow cytometry, to obtain a concentration of 5 µg/ml. Store at 2-8 °C and use within 3 h.

Microtitre plates. Plates used to prepare immunoglobulin dilutions are U- or V-bottomed polystyrene or poly(vinyl chloride) plates without surface treatment.

Micronic tubes. Suitable for flow cytometry measurement.

Cell suspension. Collect blood in anticoagulant from at least one healthy donor. Immediately isolate the peripheral blood mononuclear cells (PBMC) by gradient centrifugation in lymphocyte separation medium so that the PBMC form a visible clean interface between the plasma and the separation medium. Collect the layer containing the cells and dispense into centrifuge tubes containing buffered salt solution pH 7.2. Centrifuge at 400 *g* at 2-8 °C for 10 min. Discard the supernatant. Suspend the cell pellet in buffer solution for flow cytometry. Repeat the centrifugation and resuspension procedure of the cells twice. After the third centrifugation, resuspend the cell pellet in 1 ml of buffer solution for flow cytometry. Determine the number and vitality of the cells using a haemocytometer. Cell viability of at least 90 per cent is required. Adjust the cell number to 7×10^6/ml by adding buffer solution for flow cytometry. Store the cell suspension at 4 °C and use within 12 h.

If necessary, the first PBMC pellet may be resuspended in buffered salt solution pH 7.2 containing 20 per cent fœtal calf serum and stored overnight at 2 °C. Centrifuge at 400 *g* at 2-8 °C for 10 min. Discard the supernatant. Suspend the

Monographs A - C

cell pellet in buffer solution for flow cytometry. Determine the number and vitality of the cells using a haemocytometer. Cell viability of at least 90 per cent is required. Adjust the cell number to 7 × 10^6/ml by adding buffer solution for flow cytometry.

It is also possible for cells to be immediately frozen and stored in nitrogen using the following method.

Buffer solution for freezing. To 20 ml of cell culture medium, add 25 ml of fœtal calf serum and 5 ml of dimethyl sulphoxide (DMSO). Store this solution at 2-8 °C and use within 3 h.

20 × 10^6 cells per ampoule are frozen. These ampoules are stored in liquid nitrogen.

Buffer solution for thawing. To 450 ml of cell culture medium, add 50 ml of foetal calf serum. Store this solution at 2-8 °C and use within 3 h.

Each ampoule is thawed in a water-bath at 37 °C with shaking. Cell suspension is repeated in a buffer solution for thawing. Centrifuge at 200 *g* at 2-8 °C for 10 min. Discard the supernatant. Suspend the cell pellet in buffer solution for flow cytometry. Repeat the procedure for centrifugation and resuspension of cells once. After the second centrifugation, resuspend the cells pellet in 1 ml of buffer solution for flow cytometry. Determine the number and vitality of the cells using a haemocytometer. Cell viability of at least 90 per cent is required. Adjust the cell number to 7 × 10^6/ml by adding buffer solution for flow cytometry. Store the cell suspension at 4 °C and use within 3 h.

Test solutions. For freeze-dried preparations, reconstitute as stated on the label. Prepare 3 independent series of not fewer than 7 dilutions using buffer solution for flow cytometry as diluent.

Reference solutions. For freeze-dried preparations, reconstitute according to the instructions for use. Prepare 3 independent dilution series of not fewer than 7 dilutions using buffer solution for flow cytometry as diluent.

Distribute 75 µl of each of the dilutions of the test solution or reference solution to each of a series of wells of a microtitre plate. Add 25 µl of the cell suspension of PBMC into each well. Add 25 µl of rabbit complement to each of the wells. Incubate at 37 °C for 30 min.

Centrifuge the plates at 200 *g* at 4 °C for 8 min, discard the supernatant and keep the plate on ice. Preparation for flow cytometry measurement is done step-wise by using a certain number of wells in order to allow labelling with *propidium iodide R* solution and measurement within a defined time period. Resuspend carefully the cell pellet of a certain number of wells with 200 µl of propidium iodide solution. Transfer the suspension into tubes. Incubate at 25 °C for 10 min then place immediately on ice.

Proceed with fluorescence measurement in a flow cytometer. Define a region including all propidium iodide-positive cells on the basis of Forward-Scattered, light (FSC) and flourescence (FL2 or FL3 for propidium iodide). Measure the percentage of propidium iodide-positive cells, without gating but excluding debris. Analyse at least 3000 cells for each of the test and reference solutions.

Use the percentages of dead cells to estimate the potency as the concentration in milligrams per millilitre of the preparation to be examined necessary to induce 50 per cent of cytotoxicity by fitting a sigmoidal dose response curve to the data obtained with the test and the reference preparations and by using a 4-parameter logistic model (see, for example, chapter *5.3*) and suitable software. The test is not valid unless the percentage of propidium iodide-positive cells at the lower asymptote of the curve is less then 15 per cent and the percentage of propidium iodide-positive cells at the upper asymptote of the curve is at least 80 per cent.

The estimated activity is 70 per cent to 130 per cent of the activity approved for the particular product.

The confidence interval (P = 0.95) of the estimated potency is not greater than 80 per cent to 125 per cent.

STORAGE

Protected from light at the temperature stated on the label.

Expiry date. The expiry date is calculated from the beginning of the assay.

LABELLING

The label states:

- for liquid preparations, the volume of the preparation in the container and the protein content,
- for freeze-dried preparations:
  - the name and the volume of the reconstitution liquid to be added,
  - the quantity of protein in the container,
  - that the immunoserum is to be used immediately after reconstitution,
  - the time required for complete dissolution,
- the animal species of origin,
- the name and amount of stabiliser, where applicable,
- the dilution to be made before use of the product.

07/2004:2096

ARGININE ASPARTATE

Arginini aspartas

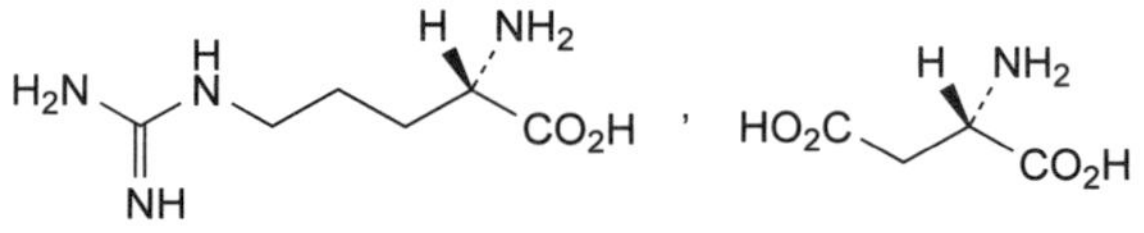

$C_{10}H_{21}N_5O_6$ M_r 307.3

DEFINITION

(2*S*)-2-Amino-5-guanidinopentanoic acid (2*S*)-2-aminobutanedioate.

Content: 99.0 per cent to 101.0 per cent (dried substance).

CHARACTERS

Appearance: white granules or powder.

Solubility: very soluble in water, practically insoluble in alcohol and in methylene chloride.

IDENTIFICATION

A. It complies with the test for specific optical rotation (see Tests).

B. Infrared absorption spectrophotometry (*2.2.24*).
Comparison: *arginine aspartate CRS.*

C. Examine the chromatograms obtained in the test for ninhydrin-positive substances.
Results: the 2 principal spots in the chromatogram obtained with test solution (b) are similar in position, colour and size to the 2 principal spots in the chromatogram obtained with reference solution (a).

TESTS

Solution S. Dissolve 5.0 g in *carbon dioxide-free water R* and dilute to 50 ml with the same solvent.

Appearance of solution. Solution S is clear (*2.2.1*) and not more intensely coloured than reference solution Y_7 (*2.2.2, Method II*).

pH (*2.2.3*): 6.0 to 7.0 for solution S.

Specific optical rotation (*2.2.7*): + 25 to + 27 (dried substance).

Dissolve 2.50 g in *dilute hydrochloric acid R* and dilute to 25.0 ml with the same acid.

Ninhydrin-positive substances. Thin-layer chromatography (*2.2.27*).

Test solution (a). Dissolve 0.20 g of the substance to be examined in *water R* and dilute to 10 ml with the same solvent.

Test solution (b). Dilute 1 ml of test solution (a) to 10 ml with *water R.*

Reference solution (a). Dissolve 25 mg of *arginine R* and 25 mg of *aspartic acid R* in *water R* and dilute to 25 ml with the same solvent.

Reference solution (b). Dilute 2 ml of reference solution (a) to 50 ml with *water R.*

Plate: *TLC silica gel G plate R.*

Mobile phase: *ammonia R, propanol R* (36:64 *V/V*).

Application: 5 µl.

Development: over 2/3 of the plate.

Drying: at 100-105 °C for 10 min.

Detection: spray with *ninhydrin solution R* and heat at 100-105 °C for 10 min.

System suitability: reference solution (b):

- the chromatogram shows 2 clearly separated principal spots.

Limit: test solution (a):

- *any impurity*: any spots, apart from the 2 principal spots, are not more intense than each of the 2 principal spots in the chromatogram obtained with reference solution (b) (0.2 per cent).

Chlorides (*2.4.4*): maximum 200 ppm.

Dilute 2.5 ml of solution S to 15 ml with *water R.*

Sulphates (*2.4.13*): maximum 300 ppm.

To 0.5 g add 2.5 ml of *dilute hydrochloric acid R* and dilute to 15 ml with *distilled water R.* Examine after 30 min.

Ammonium (*2.4.1*): maximum 100 ppm, determined on 100 mg.

Heavy metals (*2.4.8*): maximum 20 ppm.

12 ml of solution S complies with limit test A. Prepare the standard using *lead standard solution (2 ppm Pb) R.*

Loss on drying (*2.2.32*): maximum 0.5 per cent, determined on 1.000 g by drying in an oven at 60 °C for 24 h.

Sulphated ash (*2.4.14*): maximum 0.1 per cent, determined on 1.0 g.

ASSAY

Dissolve 80.0 mg in 2 ml of *anhydrous formic acid R.* Add 50 ml of *anhydrous acetic acid R.* Titrate with *0.1 M perchloric acid,* determining the end-point potentiometrically (*2.2.20*).

1 ml of *0.1 M perchloric acid* is equivalent to 10.24 mg of $C_{10}H_{21}N_5O_6$.

07/2004:2086

ASPARAGINE MONOHYDRATE

Asparaginum monohydricum

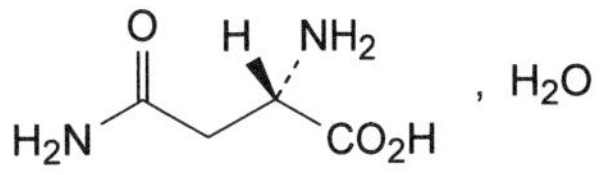

$C_4H_8N_2O_3,H_2O$ M_r 150.1

DEFINITION

(2*S*)-2,4-Diamino-4-oxobutanoic acid monohydrate.

Content: 99.0 per cent to 101.0 per cent (dried substance).

CHARACTERS

Appearance: white, crystalline powder or colourless crystals.

Solubility: slightly soluble in water, practically insoluble in alcohol and in methylene chloride.

IDENTIFICATION

First identification: A, B.

Second identification: A, C.

A. It complies with the test for specific optical rotation (see Tests).

B. Infrared absorption spectrophotometry (*2.2.24*).

Comparison: *asparagine monohydrate CRS.*

C. Examine the chromatograms obtained in the test for ninhydrin-positive substances.

Results: the principal spot in the chromatogram obtained with test solution (b) is similar in position, colour and size to the principal spot in the chromatogram obtained with reference solution (c).

TESTS

Solution S. Dissolve with heating 2.0 g in *carbon dioxide-free water R* and dilute to 100 ml with the same solvent.

Appearance of solution. Solution S is clear (*2.2.1*) and colourless (*2.2.2, Method II*).

pH (*2.2.3*): 4.0 to 6.0 for solution S.

Specific optical rotation (*2.2.7*): + 33.7 to + 36.0 (dried substance).

Dissolve 2.50 g in a 309.0 g/l solution of *hydrochloric acid R* and dilute to 25.0 ml with the same acid.

Ninhydrin-positive substances. Thin-layer chromatography (*2.2.27*).

Test solution (a). Dissolve 0.25 g of the substance to be examined in *water R*, heating to not more than 40 °C, and dilute to 10 ml with the same solvent.

Test solution (b). Dilute 1 ml of test solution (a) to 10 ml with *water R.*

Reference solution (a). Dilute 1.0 ml of test solution (a) to 200 ml with *water R.*

Reference solution (b). Dissolve 25 mg of *glutamic acid R* in *water R*, add 1 ml of test solution (a) and dilute to 10 ml with *water R.*

Reference solution (c). Dissolve 25 mg of *asparagine monohydrate CRS* in *water R* and dilute to 10 ml with the same solvent.

Plate: *TLC silica gel G plate R.*

Mobile phase: *glacial acetic acid R, water R, butanol R* (25:25:50 *V/V/V*).

Application: 5 µl.

Development: over half of the plate.

Drying: at 110 °C for 15 min.

Detection: spray with *ninhydrin solution R* and heat at 110 °C for 10 min.

System suitability: reference solution (b):

- the chromatogram shows 2 clearly separated principal spots.

Limit: test solution (a):

- *any impurity*: any spot, apart from the principal spot, is not more intense than the principal spot in the chromatogram obtained with reference solution (a) (0.5 per cent).

Chlorides (*2.4.4*): maximum 200 ppm.

Dilute 12.5 ml of solution S to 15 ml with *water R*.

Sulphates (*2.4.13*): maximum 200 ppm.

To 0.75 g add 2.5 ml of *dilute hydrochloric acid R* and dilute to 15 ml with *distilled water R*. Examine after 30 min.

Ammonium (*2.4.1, Method B*): maximum 0.1 per cent, determined on 10 mg.

Iron (*2.4.9*): maximum 10 ppm.

Dissolve 1.0 g in *dilute hydrochloric acid R* and dilute to 10 ml with the same acid. Shake 3 times with 10 ml of *methyl isobutyl ketone R1* for 3 min. Wash the combined organic phases with 10 ml of *water R* for 3 min. The aqueous phase complies with the limit test for iron.

Heavy metals (*2.4.8*): maximum 10 ppm.

Dissolve 2.0 g in a mixture of 3 ml of *dilute hydrochloric acid R* and 15 ml of *water R* with gentle warming if necessary. Dilute to 20 ml with *water R*. 12 ml of the solution complies with limit test A. Prepare the standard using *lead standard solution (1 ppm Pb) R*.

Loss on drying (*2.2.32*): 10.5 per cent to 12.5 per cent, determined on 1.000 g by drying in an oven at 60 °C for 24 h.

Sulphated ash (*2.4.14*): maximum 0.1 per cent, determined on 1.0 g.

ASSAY

Dissolve 0.110 g in 5 ml of *anhydrous formic acid R*. Add 50 ml of *anhydrous acetic acid R*. Titrate with *0.1 M perchloric acid*, determining the end-point potentiometrically (*2.2.20*).

1 ml of *0.1 M perchloric acid* is equivalent to 13.21 mg of $C_4H_8N_2O_3$.

IMPURITIES

Specified impurities (see note for information p. xli): A, B.

A. aspartic acid,

B. glutamic acid.

07/2004:1633

AZELASTINE HYDROCHLORIDE

Azelastini hydrochloridum

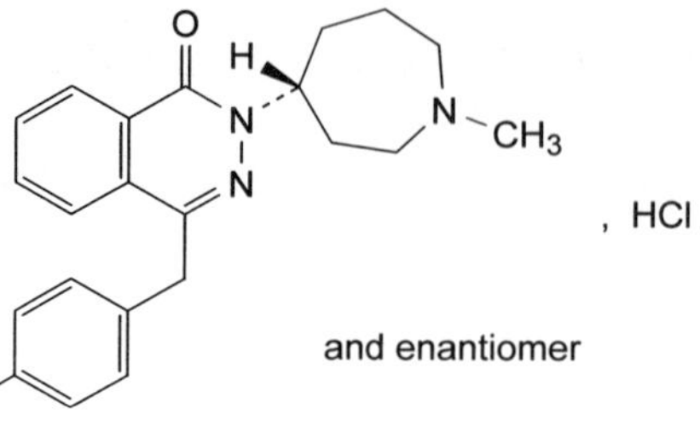

$C_{22}H_{25}Cl_2N_3O$ M_r 418.4

DEFINITION

4-(4-Chlorobenzyl)-2-[(4*RS*)-1-methylhexahydro-1*H*-azepin-4-yl]phthalazin-1(2*H*)-one hydrochloride.

Content: 99.0 per cent to 101.0 per cent (dried substance).

CHARACTERS

Appearance: white or almost white, crystalline powder.

Solubility: sparingly soluble in water, soluble in ethanol and in methylene chloride.

IDENTIFICATION

A. Infrared absorption spectrophotometry (*2.2.24*).
Comparison: *azelastine hydrochloride CRS.*

B. Solution S (see Tests) gives reaction (a) of chlorides (*2.3.1*).

TESTS

Solution S. Dissolve 1.0 g in *carbon dioxide-free water R* and dilute to 100 ml with the same solvent.

Appearance of solution. Solution S is clear (*2.2.1*) and colourless (*2.2.2, Method II*).

Acidity or alkalinity. To 10 ml of solution S add 0.2 ml of *bromothymol blue solution R1*. Not more than 0.1 ml of *0.01 M hydrochloric acid* or *0.01 M sodium hydroxide* is required to change the colour of the solution.

Related substances. Liquid chromatography (*2.2.29*).

Solvent mixture: *acetonitrile R, water R* (45:55 *V/V*).

Test solution. Dissolve 0.125 g of the substance to be examined in the solvent mixture and dilute to 50.0 ml with the solvent mixture.

Reference solution (a). Dilute 1.0 ml of the test solution to 100.0 ml with the solvent mixture. Dilute 1.0 ml of this solution to 10.0 ml with the solvent mixture.

Reference solution (b). Dissolve 1 mg of *azelastine impurity B CRS*, 1 mg of *azelastine impurity D CRS* and 1 mg of *azelastine impurity E CRS* in the test solution and dilute to 20 ml with the test solution.

Column:

- *size*: l = 0.25 m, Ø = 4.6 mm,
- *stationary phase*: *nitrile silica gel for chromatography R* (10 µm),
- *temperature*: 30°C.

Mobile phase: dissolve 2.16 g of *sodium octanesulphonate R* and 0.68 g of *potassium dihydrogen phosphate R* in 740 ml of *water for chromatography R*, adjust to pH 3.0-3.1 with *dilute phosphoric acid R*, add 260 ml of *acetonitrile R* and mix.

Flow rate: 2.0 ml/min.

Detection: spectrophotometer at 210 nm.

Injection: 10 μl.

Run time: twice the retention time of azelastine.

Relative retention with reference to azelastine (retention time = about 8-9 min): impurity A = about 0.2; impurity B = about 0.3; impurity C = about 0.4; impurity D = about 0.6; impurity E = about 1.4.

System suitability: reference solution (b):

- *resolution*: minimum 4.0 between the peaks due to impurity B and impurity D,
- the peaks due to impurity D and impurity E are baseline separated from the principal peak.

Limits:

- *correction factors*: for the calculation of contents, multiply the peak areas of the following impurities by the corresponding correction factor: impurity B = 3.6; impurity D = 0.7; impurity E = 2.1;
- *impurities A, B, C, D, E*: for each impurity, not more than the area of the principal peak in the chromatogram obtained with reference solution (a) (0.1 per cent);
- *any other impurity*: for each impurity, not more than the area of the principal peak in the chromatogram obtained with reference solution (a) (0.1 per cent);
- *total*: not more than twice the area of the principal peak in the chromatogram obtained with reference solution (a) (0.2 per cent);
- *disregard limit*: 0.5 times the area of the principal peak in the chromatogram obtained with reference solution (a) (0.05 per cent).

Loss on drying (*2.2.32*): maximum 0.5 per cent, determined on 1.000 g by drying in an oven at 100-105 °C.

ASSAY

In order to avoid overheating in the reaction medium, mix thoroughly throughout and stop the titration immediately after the end-point has been reached.

Dissolve 0.300 g in 5 ml of *anhydrous formic acid R*. Add 30 ml of *acetic anhydride R*. Titrate quickly with *0.1 M perchloric acid*, determining the end-point potentiometrically (*2.2.20*).

1.0 ml of *0.1 M perchloric acid* is equivalent to 41.84 mg of $C_{22}H_{25}Cl_2N_3O$.

IMPURITIES

Specified impurities (see note for information p. xli): A, B, C, D, E.

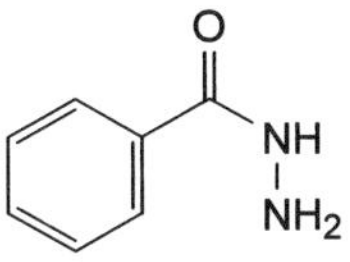

A. benzoyldiazane (benzohydrazide),

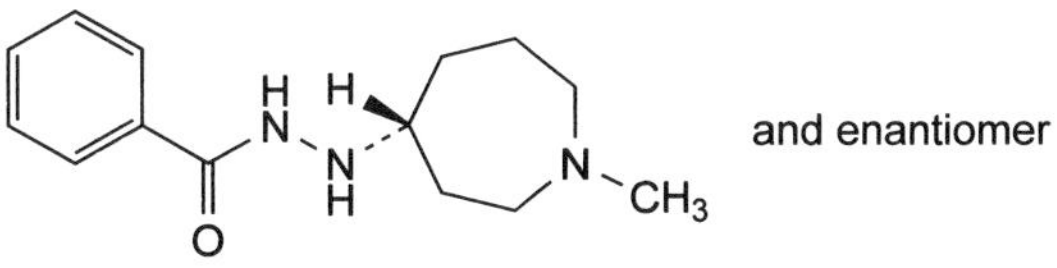

B. 1-benzoyl-2-[(4*RS*)-1-methylhexahydro-1*H*-azepin-4-yl]diazane,

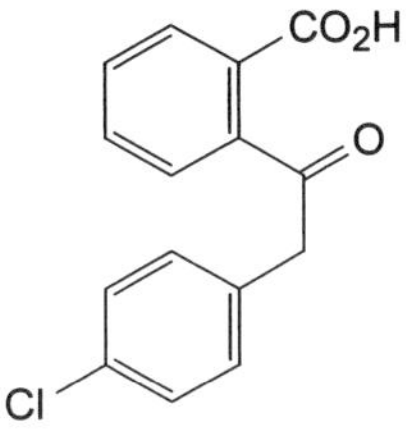

C. 2-[(4-chlorophenyl)acetyl]benzoic acid,

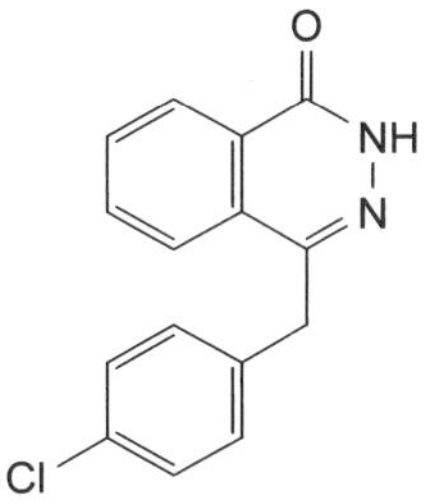

D. 4-(4-chlorobenzyl)phthalazin-1(2*H*)-one,

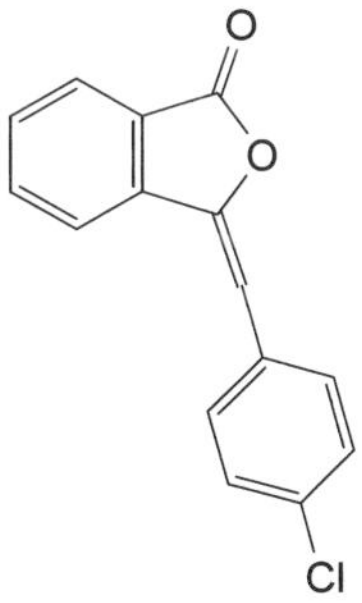

E. 3-(4-chlorobenzylidene)isobenzofuran-1(3*H*)-one.

B

07/2004:0706

BROMHEXINE HYDROCHLORIDE

Bromhexini hydrochloridum

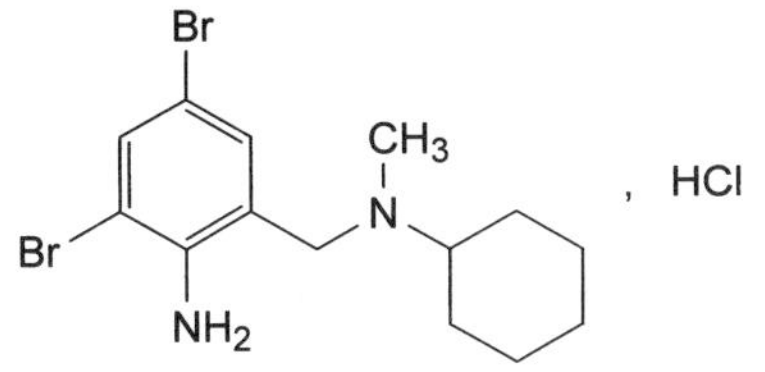

$C_{14}H_{21}Br_2ClN_2$ M_r 412.6

DEFINITION

N-(2-Amino-3,5-dibromobenzyl)-*N*-methylcyclohexanamine hydrochloride.

Content: 98.5 per cent to 101.5 per cent (dried substance).

CHARACTERS

Appearance: white or almost white, crystalline powder.

Solubility: very slightly soluble in water, slightly soluble in alcohol and in methylene chloride.

It shows polymorphism.

IDENTIFICATION

First identification: A, E.

Second identification: B, C, D, E.

A. Infrared absorption spectrophotometry (*2.2.24*).

Comparison: *bromhexine hydrochloride CRS.*

If the spectra obtained in the solid state show differences, dissolve the substance to be examined and the reference substance separately in *methanol R*, evaporate to dryness and record new spectra using the residues.

B. Thin-layer chromatography (*2.2.27*).

Test solution. Dissolve 20 mg of the substance to be examined in *methanol R* and dilute to 10 ml with the same solvent.

Reference solution. Dissolve 20 mg of *bromhexine hydrochloride CRS* in *methanol R* and dilute to 10 ml with the same solvent.

Plate: *TLC silica gel F_{254} plate R.*

Mobile phase: *glacial acetic acid R, water R, butanol R* (17:17:66 *V/V/V*).

Application: 20 µl.

Development: over 3/4 of the plate.

Drying: in air.

Detection: examine in ultraviolet light at 254 nm.

Results: the principal spot in the chromatogram obtained with the test solution is similar in position and size to the principal spot in the chromatogram obtained with the reference solution.

C. Dissolve about 25 mg in a mixture of 1 ml of *dilute sulphuric acid R* and 50 ml of *water R*. Add 2 ml of *methylene chloride R* and 5 ml of *chloramine solution R* and shake. A brownish-yellow colour develops in the lower layer.

D. Dissolve about 1 mg in 3 ml of *0.1 M hydrochloric acid.* The solution gives the reaction of primary aromatic amines (*2.3.1*).

E. Dissolve about 20 mg in 1 ml of *methanol R* and add 1 ml of *water R*. The solution gives reaction (a) of chlorides (*2.3.1*).

TESTS

Appearance of solution. The solution is clear (*2.2.1*) and not more intensely coloured than reference solution Y_6 (*2.2.2, Method II*).

Dissolve 0.6 g in *methanol R* and dilute to 20 ml with the same solvent.

Related substances. Liquid chromatography (*2.2.29*).

Test solution. Dissolve 50 mg of the substance to be examined in *methanol R* and dilute to 10.0 ml with the same solvent.

Reference solution (a). Dissolve 5 mg of *bromhexine impurity C CRS* in *methanol R*, add 1.0 ml of the test solution and dilute to 10.0 ml with the same solvent.

Reference solution (b). Dilute 1.0 ml of the test solution to 100.0 ml with *methanol R*. Dilute 1.0 ml of this solution to 10.0 ml with *methanol R.*

Column:

- *size*: l = 0.12 m, Ø = 4.6 mm,
- *stationary phase*: *end-capped octadecylsilyl silica gel for chromatography R* (3 µm).

Mobile phase: mix 0.50 ml of *phosphoric acid R* in 950 ml of *water R*, adjust to pH 7.0 with *triethylamine R* (about 1.5 ml) and dilute to 1000 ml with *water R*; mix 20 volumes of this solution with 80 volumes of *acetonitrile R.*

Flow rate: 1.0 ml/min.

Detection: spectrophotometer at 248 nm.

Injection: 10 µl.

Run time: 2.5 times the retention time of bromhexine.

Relative retention with reference to bromhexine (retention time = about 11 min): impurity A = about 0.1; impurity B = about 0.2; impurity C = about 0.4; impurity D = about 0.5.

System suitability: reference solution (a):

- *resolution*: minimum 12.0 between the peaks due to impurity C and bromhexine.

Limits:

- *any impurity*: not more than twice the area of the principal peak in the chromatogram obtained with reference solution (b) (0.2 per cent), and not more than 1 such peak has an area greater than the area of the principal peak in the chromatogram obtained with reference solution (b) (0.1 per cent),
- *total*: not more than 3 times the area of the principal peak in the chromatogram obtained with reference solution (b) (0.3 per cent),
- *disregard limit*: 0.5 times the area of the principal peak in the chromatogram obtained with reference solution (b) (0.05 per cent).

Loss on drying (*2.2.32*): maximum 1.0 per cent, determined on 1.000 g by drying in an oven at 100-105 °C.

Sulphated ash (*2.4.14*): maximum 0.1 per cent, determined on 1.0 g.

ASSAY

Dissolve 0.300 g in 70 ml of *alcohol R* and add 1 ml of *0.1 M hydrochloric acid.* Carry out a potentiometric titration (*2.2.20*), using *0.1 M sodium hydroxide.* Read the volume between the 2 points of inflexion.

1 ml of *0.1 M sodium hydroxide* is equivalent to 41.26 mg of $C_{14}H_{21}Br_2ClN_2$.

STORAGE

Protected from light.

Monographs A - C

IMPURITIES

Specified impurities (see note for information p. xli): A, B, C, D.

Other detectable impurities: E.

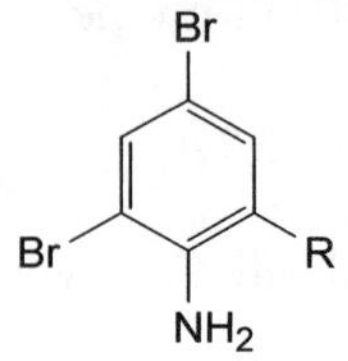

A. R = CH_2OH: (2-amino-3,5-dibromophenyl)methanol,

B. R = CHO: 2-amino-3,5-dibromobenzaldehyde,

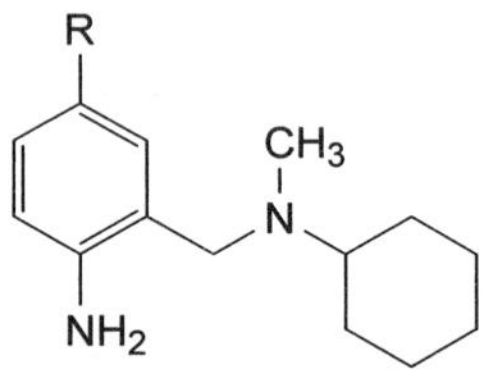

C. R = H: *N*-(2-aminobenzyl)-*N*-methylcyclohexanamine,

D. R = Br: *N*-(2-amino-5-bromobenzyl)-*N*-methylcyclohexanamine,

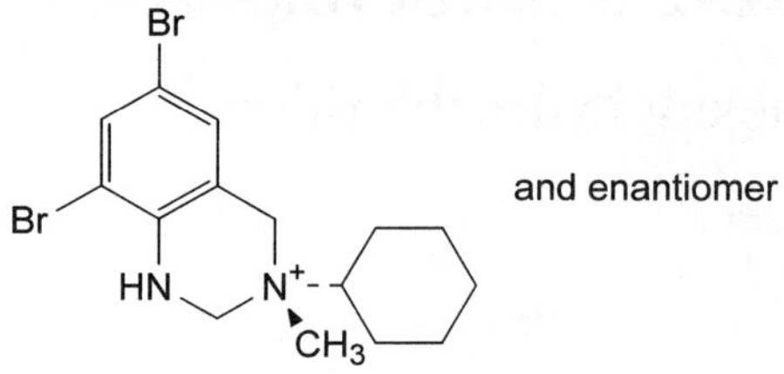

E. (3*RS*)-6,8-dibromo-3-cyclohexyl-3-methyl-1,2,3,4-tetrahydroquinazolin-3-ium.

C

01/2004:1632
corrected

CELIPROLOL HYDROCHLORIDE

Celiprololi hydrochloridum

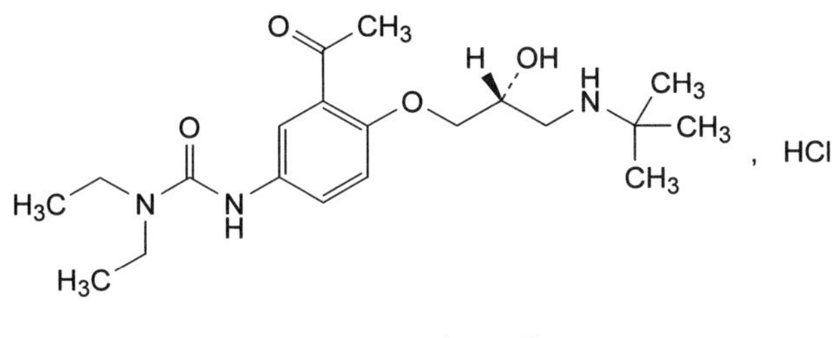

and enantiomer

$C_{20}H_{34}ClN_3O_4$ M_r 416.0

DEFINITION

3-[3-Acetyl-4-[(2*RS*)-3-[(1,1-dimethylethyl)amino]-2-hydroxypropoxy]phenyl]-1,1-diethylurea hydrochloride.

Content: 99.0 per cent to 101.0 per cent (dried substance).

CHARACTERS

Appearance: white or very slightly yellow, crystalline powder.

Solubility: freely soluble in water and in methanol, soluble in alcohol, very slightly soluble in methylene chloride.

It shows polymorphism.

IDENTIFICATION

A. Infrared absorption spectrophotometry (*2.2.24*).

Comparison: *celiprolol hydrochloride CRS.*

If the spectra obtained in the solid state show differences, dissolve the substance to be examined and the reference substance separately in *methanol R*, evaporate to dryness and record new spectra using the residues.

B. It gives reaction (a) of chlorides (*2.3.1*).

TESTS

Optical rotation (*2.2.7*): − 0.10° to + 0.10°.

Dissolve 1.0 g in *water R* and dilute to 10.0 ml with the same solvent.

Related substances. Liquid chromatography (*2.2.29*).

Prepare the solutions immediately before use.

Test solution. Dissolve 0.100 g of the substance to be examined in mobile phase A and dilute to 20.0 ml with mobile phase A.

Reference solution (a). Dissolve 2 mg of the substance to be examined and 2 mg of *acebutolol hydrochloride R* in mobile phase A and dilute to 50.0 ml with mobile phase A.

Reference solution (b). Dissolve 10 mg of the substance to be examined in 2 ml of mobile phase A and allow to stand for 24 h (for identification of impurity A).

Reference solution (c). Dilute 1.0 ml of the test solution to 100.0 ml with mobile phase A. Dilute 1.0 ml of this solution to 10.0 ml with mobile phase A.

Reference solution (d). Dissolve 10 mg of *celiprolol for peak identification CRS* in mobile phase A and dilute to 2 ml with mobile phase A.

Reference solution (e). This solution is only prepared if required (see below) and is used to determine the identity of impurity I which co-elutes with impurity H (the 2 impurities originate from different synthesis routes). Dissolve 2 mg of *celiprolol impurity I CRS* in mobile phase A and dilute to 20 ml with mobile phase A. Dilute 1.0 ml of the solution to 10.0 ml with mobile phase A.

Column:

- *size*: *l* = 0.15 m, Ø = 4.6 mm,
- *stationary phase*: *octylsilyl silica gel for chromatography R* (5 µm),
- *temperature*: 30 °C.

Mobile phase:

- *mobile phase A*: mix 91 ml of *tetrahydrofuran R,* 63 ml of *acetonitrile R1,* 0.6 ml of *pentafluoropropanoic acid R* and 0.2 ml of *trifluoroacetic acid R*; dilute to 1000 ml with *water R*;
- *mobile phase B*: *acetonitrile R1*;

Time (min)	Mobile phase A (per cent *V/V*)	Mobile phase B (per cent *V/V*)
0 - 50	100 → 80	0 → 20
50 - 51	80 → 100	20 → 0
51 - 65	100	0

Flow rate: 1.4 ml/min.

Detection: spectrophotometer at 232 nm.

Injection: 10 µl.

Relative retention with reference to celiprolol (retention time = about 10 min): impurity A = about 0.3; impurity D = about 0.7; impurity G = about 1.2; impurity B = about 1.4; impurity F = about 1.6; impurity C = about 2.2; impurity H or I = about 2.5; impurity E = about 3.9.

System suitability: reference solution (a):

- *resolution*: minimum 4.0 between the peaks due to celiprolol and acebutolol.

Limits: use the chromatogram supplied with *celiprolol for peak identification CRS* and the chromatogram obtained with reference solution (d) to identify the peaks due to impurities B, E and F:

- *correction factors*: for the calculation of contents, multiply the peak areas of the following impurities by the corresponding correction factor: impurity A = 4.0; impurity B = 1.5; impurity E = 2.3; impurity F = 0.5; impurity I = 1.7;
- *any impurity*: not more than twice the area of the principal peak in the chromatogram obtained with reference solution (c) (0.2 per cent), and not more than 1 such peak has an area greater than the area of the principal peak in the chromatogram obtained with reference solution (c) (0.1 per cent);
- *total*: not more than 5 times the area of the principal peak in the chromatogram obtained with reference solution (c) (0.5 per cent);
- if any of the above limits are exceeded and if a peak occurs with a relative retention of about 2.5 (impurity H or I), the identity of this peak has to be clarified by use of a UV spectrum recorded with a diode array detector; if this spectrum is different from the one obtained with reference solution (e), no correction factor is applied;
- *disregard limit*: 0.5 times the area of the principal peak in the chromatogram obtained with reference solution (c) (0.05 per cent).

Loss on drying (*2.2.32*): maximum 0.5 per cent, determined on 1.000 g by drying in an oven at 100-105 °C for 3 h.

Monographs A - C

ASSAY

Dissolve 0.350 g under an atmosphere of nitrogen in 50 ml of *alcohol R* and add 1.0 ml of *0.1 M hydrochloric acid.* Carry out a potentiometric titration (*2.2.20*), using *0.1 M sodium hydroxide*. Read the volume added between the 2 points of inflexion.

1 ml of *0.1 M sodium hydroxide* is equivalent to 41.60 mg of $C_{20}H_{34}ClN_3O_4$.

STORAGE

Protected from light.

IMPURITIES

Specified impurities (see note for information p. xli): A, B, C, D, E, F, G, H, I.

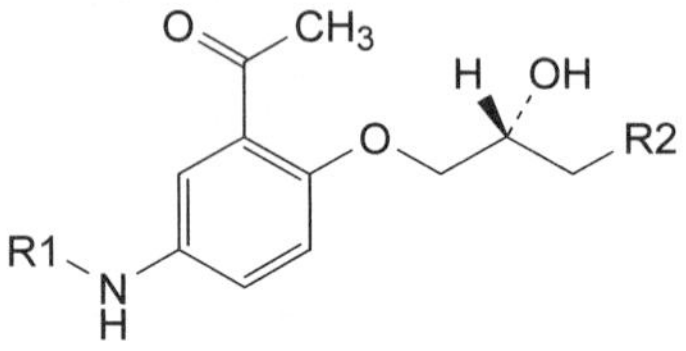

and enantiomer

A. R1 = H, R2 = NH-C$(CH_3)_3$: 1-[5-amino-2-[(2*RS*)-3-[(1,1-dimethylethyl)amino]-2-hydroxypropoxy]phenyl]ethanone,

C. R1 = CO-NH-C$(CH_3)_3$, R2 = NH-C$(CH_3)_3$: 1-[3-acetyl-4-[(2*RS*)-3-[(1,1-dimethylethyl)amino]-2-hydroxypropoxy]phenyl]-3-(1,1-dimethylethyl)urea,

D. R1 = CO-N$(C_2H_5)_2$, R2 = N$(C_2H_5)_2$: 3-[3-acetyl-4-[(2*RS*)-3-(diethylamino)-2-hydroxypropoxy]phenyl]-1,1-diethylurea,

H. R1 = CO-N$(C_2H_5)_2$, R2 = Br: 3-[3-acetyl-4-[(2*RS*)-3-bromo-2-hydroxypropoxy]phenyl]-1,1-diethylurea (bromhydrin compound),

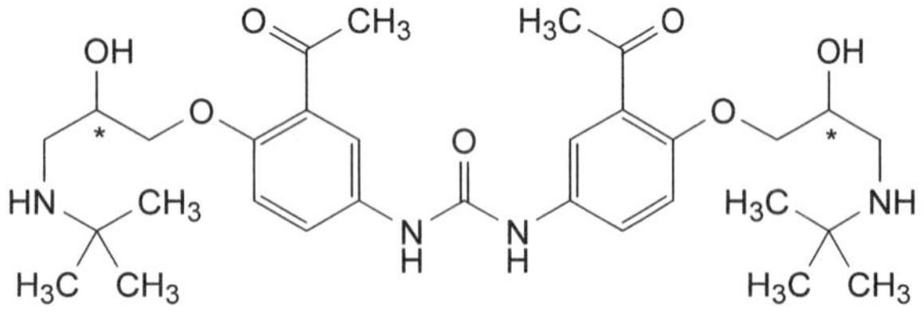

B. 1,3-bis[3-acetyl-4-[3-[(1,1-dimethylethyl)amino]-2-hydroxypropoxy]phenyl]urea,

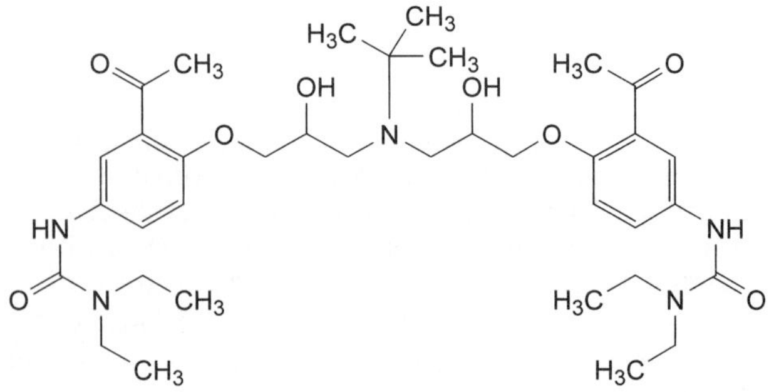

E. 1,1′-[[(1,1-dimethylethyl)imino]bis[(2-hydroxypropane-1,3-diyl)oxy(3-acetyl-1,4-phenylene)]]bis(3,3-diethylurea),

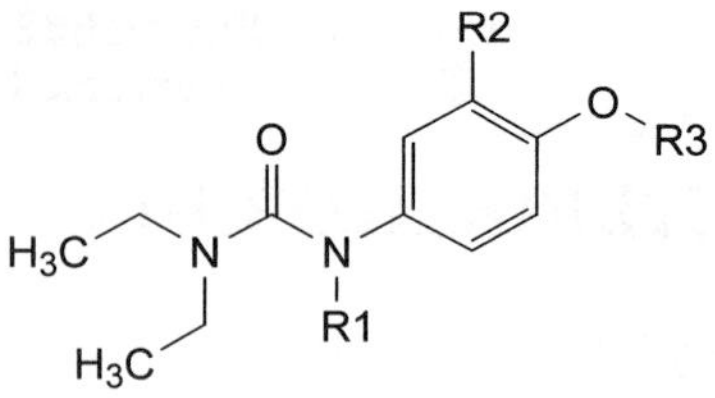

F. R1 = R3 = H, R2 = CO-CH_3: 3-(3-acetyl-4-hydroxyphenyl)-1,1-diethylurea,

I. R1 = CO-CH_3, R2 = H, R3 = C_2H_5: 1-acetyl-1-(4-ethoxyphenyl)-3,3-diethylurea,

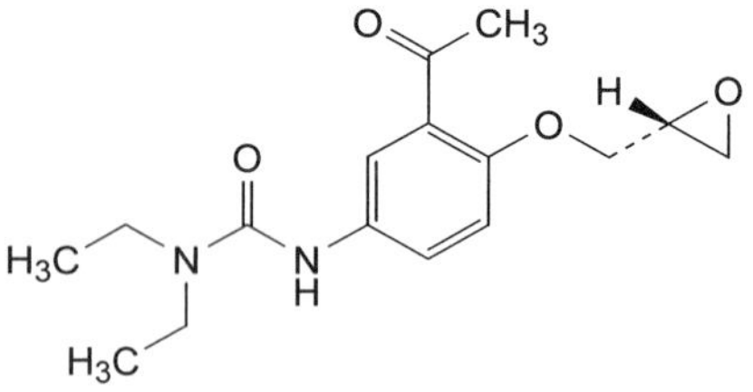

and enantiomer

G. 3-[3-acetyl-4-[[(*RS*)-oxiranyl]methoxy]phenyl]-1,1-diethylurea.

01/2002:0994
corrected

CICLOSPORIN

Ciclosporinum

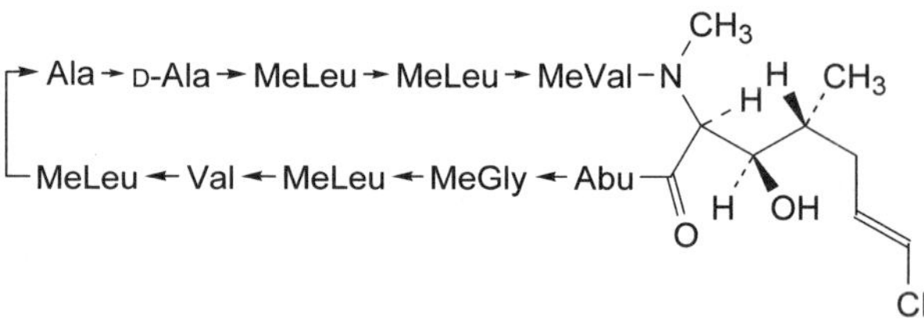

$C_{62}H_{111}N_{11}O_{12}$ M_r 1203

DEFINITION

Ciclosporin contains not less than 98.5 per cent and not more than the equivalent of 101.5 per cent of cyclo[[(2*S*,3*R*,4*R*,6*E*)-3-hydroxy-4-methyl-2-(methylamino)oct-6-enoyl]-L-2-aminobutanoyl-*N*-methylglycyl-*N*-methyl-L-leucyl-L-valyl-*N*-methyl-L-leucyl-L-alanyl-D-alanyl-*N*-methyl-L-leucyl-*N*-methyl-L-leucyl-*N*-methyl-L-valyl], calculated with reference to the dried substance. Ciclosporin is a substance produced by *Beauveria nivea (Tolypocladium inflatum Gams)* or obtained by any other means.

CHARACTERS

A white or almost white powder, practically insoluble in water, freely soluble in ethanol and in methylene chloride.

IDENTIFICATION

A. Examine by infrared absorption spectrophotometry (*2.2.24*), comparing with the spectrum obtained with *ciclosporin CRS*.

B. Examine the chromatograms obtained in the assay. The principal peak in the chromatogram obtained with the test solution is similar in retention time to the principal peak in the chromatogram obtained with reference solution (a).

TESTS

Appearance of solution. Dissolve 1.5 g in *ethanol R* and dilute to 15 ml with the same solvent. The solution is clear (*2.2.1*) and not more intensely coloured than reference solution Y_5, BY_5 or R_7 (*2.2.2, Method II*).

Specific optical rotation (*2.2.7*). Dissolve 0.125 g in *methanol R* and dilute to 25.0 ml with the same solvent. The specific optical rotation is − 185 to − 193, calculated with reference to the dried substance.

Related substances. Examine by liquid chromatography (*2.2.29*) as prescribed under Assay. Inject separately the test solution and reference solution (b). Continue the chromatography for 1.7 times the retention time of the principal peak. In the chromatogram obtained with the test solution: the area of any peak, apart from the principal peak, is not greater than 0.7 times the area of the principal peak in the chromatogram obtained with reference solution (b) (0.7 per cent); the sum of the areas of all the peaks, apart from the principal peak, is not greater than 1.5 times the area of the principal peak in the chromatogram obtained with reference solution (b) (1.5 per cent). Disregard any peak due to the solvent and any peak with an area less than 0.05 times that of the principal peak in the chromatogram with reference solution (b).

Heavy metals (*2.4.8*). The residue obtained in the test for loss on drying complies with limit test C for heavy metals (20 ppm). Prepare the standard using 2 ml of *lead standard solution (10 ppm Pb) R*.

Loss on drying (*2.2.32*). Not more than 2.0 per cent, determined on 1.000 g at 60 °C at a pressure not exceeding 15 Pa for 3 h.

Sterility (*2.6.1*). If intended for use in the manufacture of parenteral dosage forms without a further appropriate sterilisation procedure, it complies with the test for sterility.

Bacterial endotoxins (*2.6.14*): less than 0.84 IU/mg, if intended for use in the manufacture of parenteral dosage forms without a further appropriate procedure for the removal of bacterial endotoxins. Dissolve 50 mg of the substance to be examined in a mixture of 280 mg of *alcohol R* and 650 mg of *polyoxyethylated castor oil R* and dilute to the required concentration using water LAL.

ASSAY

Examine by liquid chromatography (*2.2.29*).

Test solution. Dissolve 30.0 mg of the substance to be examined in a mixture of equal volumes of *acetonitrile R* and *water R* and dilute to 25.0 ml with the same mixture of solvents.

Reference solution (a). Dissolve 30.0 mg of *ciclosporin CRS* in a mixture of equal volumes of *acetonitrile R* and *water R* and dilute to 25.0 ml with the same mixture of solvents.

Reference solution (b). Dilute 2.0 ml of reference solution (a) to 200.0 ml with a mixture of equal volumes of *acetonitrile R* and *water R*.

Reference solution (c). Dissolve the contents of a vial of *cyclosporin U CRS* in 1.0 ml of a mixture of equal volumes of *acetonitrile R* and *water R*. Add 1.0 ml of reference solution (a).

The chromatographic procedure may be carried out using:

- a stainless steel column 0.25 m long and 4 mm in internal diameter packed with *octadecylsilyl silica gel for chromatography R* (3 µm to 5 µm); the column is connected to the injection port by a steel capillary tube about 1 m long and having an internal diameter of 0.25 mm,
- as mobile phase at a flow rate of about 1.5 ml per minute a mixture of 1 volume of *phosphoric acid R*, 50 volumes of *1,1-dimethylethyl methyl ether R*, 430 volumes of *acetonitrile R* and 520 volumes of *water R*,
- as detector a spectrophotometer set at 210 nm,
- a 20 µl loop injector,

maintaining the temperature of the column and of the steel capillary tube at 80 °C.

Inject reference solution (c). The test is not valid unless the resolution between the 2 principal peaks is 1.0 to 1.8. Adjust the ratio of 1,1 dimethylethylmethyl ether to acetonitrile, if necessary. The test is not valid unless the retention time of the principal peak is 25 min to 30 min. Adjust the ratio of acetonitrile to water, if necessary. Inject reference solution (a) 6 times. The test is not valid unless the relative standard deviation of the area of the principal peak is at most 1.0 per cent. Inject alternately the test solution and reference solution (a).

Calculate the percentage content of ciclosporin.

STORAGE

Store in an airtight container, protected from light. If the substance is sterile, store in a sterile, airtight, tamper-proof container.

LABELLING

The label states:

- where applicable, that the substance is sterile,
- where applicable, that the substance is free from bacterial endotoxins.

IMPURITIES

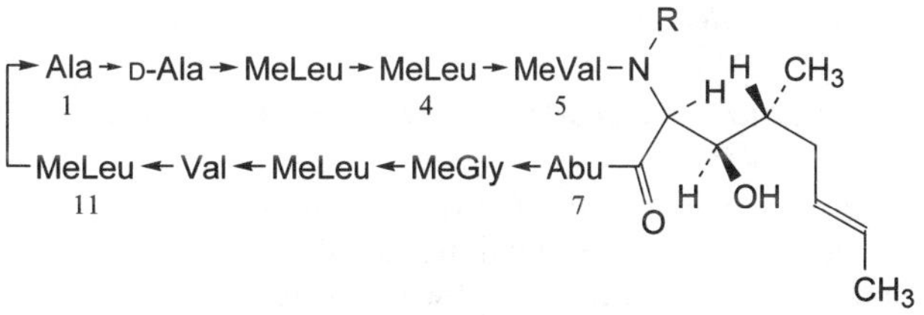

A. different cyclosporins [difference with ciclosporin ($R = CH_3$: cyclosporin A)]: cyclosporin B [7-L-Ala]; cyclosporin C [7-L-Thr]; cyclosporin D [7-L-Val]; cyclosporin E [5-L-Val]; cyclosporin G [7-(L-2-aminopentanoyl)]; cyclosporin H [5-D-MeVal]; cyclosporin L [R = H]; cyclosporin T [4-L-Leu]; cyclosporin U [11-L-Leu]; cyclosporin V [1-L-Abu],

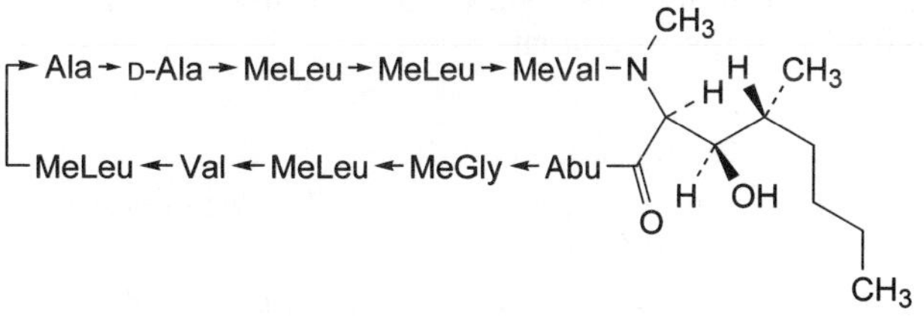

B. [6-[(2*S*,3*R*,4*R*)-3-hydroxy-4-methyl-2-(methylamino)octanoic acid]]cyclosporin A,

C. isocyclosporin A.

07/2004:0890

CLONAZEPAM

Clonazepamum

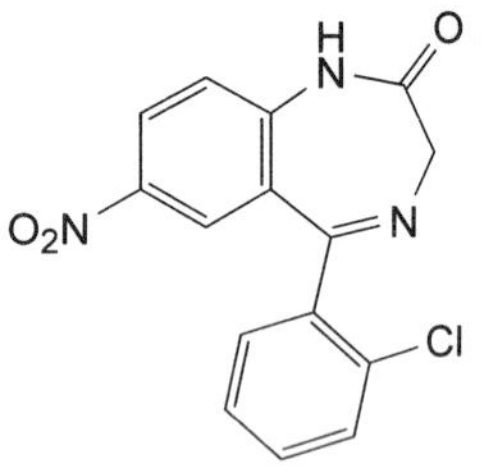

$C_{15}H_{10}ClN_3O_3$ M_r 315.7

DEFINITION

5-(2-Chlorophenyl)-7-nitro-1,3-dihydro-2*H*-1,4-benzodiazepin-2-one.

Content: 99.0 per cent to 101.0 per cent (dried substance).

CHARACTERS

Appearance: slightly yellowish, crystalline powder.

Solubility: practically insoluble in water, slightly soluble in alcohol and in methanol.

mp: about 239 °C.

IDENTIFICATION

Infrared absorption spectrophotometry (*2.2.24*).

Comparison: *Ph. Eur. reference spectrum of clonazepam.*

TESTS

Related substances. Liquid chromatography (*2.2.29*). *Carry out the test protected from light and prepare the solutions immediately before use.*

Solvent mixture: *tetrahydrofuran R, methanol R, water R* (10:42:48 *V/V/V*).

Test solution. Dissolve 0.100 g of the substance to be examined in *methanol R* and dilute to 20.0 ml with the same solvent. Dilute 1.0 ml to 10.0 ml with the solvent mixture.

Reference solution (a). Dilute 1.0 ml of the test solution to 100.0 ml with the solvent mixture. Dilute 1.0 ml of the solution to 10.0 ml with the solvent mixture.

Reference solution (b). Dissolve 5 mg of the substance to be examined and 5 mg of *flunitrazepam R* in the solvent mixture and dilute to 100.0 ml with the solvent mixture.

Reference solution (c). Dissolve 1.0 mg of *clonazepam impurity B CRS* in the solvent mixture and dilute to 20.0 ml with the solvent mixture. Dilute 1.0 ml of the solution to 100.0 ml with the solvent mixture.

Column:

- *size*: *l* = 0.15 m, Ø = 4.6 mm,
- *stationary phase*: *end-capped octylsilyl silica gel for chromatography R* (5 µm).

Mobile phase: mix 10 volumes of *tetrahydrofuran R*, 42 volumes of *methanol R* and 48 volumes of a 6.6 g/l solution of *ammonium phosphate R* previously adjusted to pH 8.0 with a 40 g/l solution of *sodium hydroxide R* or *dilute phosphoric acid R.*

Flow rate: 1.0 ml/min.

Detection: spectrophotometer at 254 nm.

Injection: 10 µl.

Run time: 3 times the retention time of clonazepam.

Relative retention with reference to clonazepam (retention time = about 7 min): impurity B = about 2.1; impurity A = about 2.4.

System suitability: reference solution (b):

- *resolution*: minimum 1.8 between the peaks due to flunitrazepam and to clonazepam.

Limits:

- *impurity A*: not more than the area of the principal peak in the chromatogram obtained with reference solution (a) (0.1 per cent),
- *impurity B*: not more than the area of the principal peak in the chromatogram obtained with reference solution (c) (0.1 per cent)
- *any other impurity*: for each impurity, not more than the area of the principal peak in the chromatogram obtained with reference solution (a) (0.1 per cent),
- *total*: not more than twice the area of the principal peak in the chromatogram obtained with reference solution (a) (0.2 per cent),
- *disregard limit*: 0.5 times the area of the principal peak in the chromatogram obtained with reference solution (a) (0.05 per cent).

Loss on drying (*2.2.32*): maximum 0.5 per cent, determined on 1.000 g by drying in an oven at 100-105 °C for 4 h.

Sulphated ash (*2.4.14*): maximum 0.1 per cent, determined on 1.0 g.

ASSAY

Dissolve 0.275 g in 50 ml of *acetic anhydride R.* Titrate with *0.1 M perchloric acid,* determining the end-point potentiometrically (*2.2.20*).

1 ml of *0.1 M perchloric acid* is equivalent to 31.57 mg of $C_{15}H_{10}ClN_3O_3$.

STORAGE

Protected from light.

IMPURITIES

Specified impurities (see note for information p. xli): A, B.

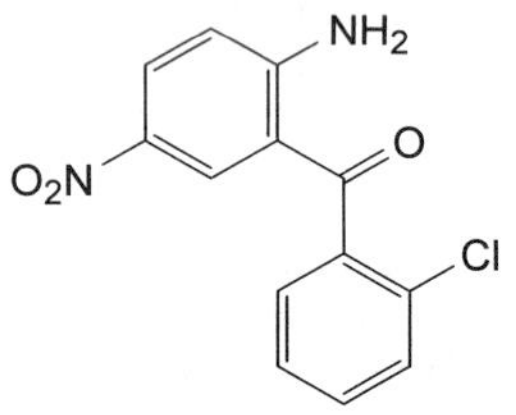

A. (2-amino-5-nitrophenyl)(2-chlorophenyl)methanone,

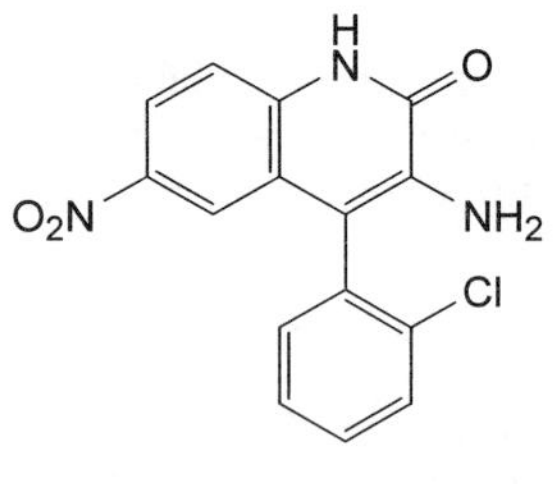

B. 3-amino-4-(2-chlorophenyl)-6-nitroquinolin-2(1*H*)-one.

04/2003:1192
corrected

COD-LIVER OIL (TYPE A)

Iecoris aselli oleum A

DEFINITION

Purified fatty oil obtained from the fresh livers of *Gadus morhua* L. and other species of *Gadidae*, solid substances being removed by cooling and filtering. A suitable antioxidant may be added.

Content: 600 IU (180 µg) to 2500 IU (750 µg) of vitamin A per gram and 60 IU (1.5 µg) to 250 IU (6.25 µg) of vitamin D_3 per gram.

CHARACTERS

Appearance: clear, yellowish, viscous liquid.

Solubility: practically insoluble in water, slightly soluble in alcohol, miscible with light petroleum.

IDENTIFICATION

First identification: A, B, C.

Second identification: C, D.

A. In the assay for vitamin A using method A, the test solution shows an absorption maximum (*2.2.25*) at 325 ± 2 nm. In the assay for vitamin A using method B, the chromatogram obtained with the test solution shows a peak corresponding to the peak of all-*trans*-retinol in the chromatogram obtained with the reference solution.

B. In the assay for vitamin D_3, the chromatogram obtained with test solution (a) shows a peak corresponding to the peak of cholecalciferol in the chromatogram obtained with reference solution (b).

C. It complies with the test for composition of fatty acids (see Tests).

D. To 0.1 g add 0.5 ml of *methylene chloride R* and 1 ml of *antimony trichloride solution R*. Mix. A deep blue colour develops in about 10 s.

TESTS

Colour: not more intensely coloured than a reference solution prepared as follows: to 3.0 ml of red primary solution add 25.0 ml of yellow primary solution and dilute to 50.0 ml with a 10 g/l solution of *hydrochloric acid R* (*2.2.2, Method II*).

Relative density (*2.2.5*): 0.917 to 0.930.

Refractive index (*2.2.6*): 1.477 to 1.484.

Acid value (*2.5.1*): maximum 2.0.

Anisidine value (*2.5.36*): maximum 30.0.

Iodine value (*2.5.4, Method B*): 150 to 180.

Use *starch solution R2.*

Peroxide value (*2.5.5, Method B*): maximum 10.0.

Unsaponifiable matter (*2.5.7*): maximum 1.5 per cent, determined on 2.0 g, and extracting with 3 quantities, each of 50 ml, of *peroxide-free ether R.*

Stearin. 10 ml remains clear after cooling in iced water for 3 h.

Composition of fatty acids. Gas chromatography (*2.2.28*).

Trivial name of fatty acid	Nomenclature	Lower limit area (per cent)	Upper limit area (per cent)
Saturated fatty acids:			
Myristic acid	14:0	2.0	6.0
Palmitic acid	16:0	7.0	14.0
Stearic acid	18:0	1.0	4.0
Mono-unsaturated fatty acids:			
Palmitoleic acid	16:1 n-7	4.5	11.5
cis-Vaccenic acid	18:1 n-7	2.0	7.0
Oleic acid	18:1 n-9	12.0	21.0
Gadoleic acid	20:1 n-11	1.0	5.5
Gondoic acid	20:1 n-9	5.0	17.0
Erucic acid	22:1 n-9	0	1.5
Cetoleic acid (22:1 n-11)	22:1 n-11+13	5.0	12.0
Poly-unsaturated fatty acids:			
Linoleic acid	18:2 n-6	0.5	3.0
α-Linolenic acid	18:3 n-3	0	2.0
Moroctic acid	18:4 n-3	0.5	4.5
Timnodonic (eicosapentaenoic) acid (EPA)	20:5 n-3	7.0	16.0
Cervonic (docosahexaenoic) acid (DHA)	22:6 n-3	6.0	18.0

Test solution. Introduce about 0.45 g of the substance to be examined into a 10 ml volumetric flask, dissolve in *hexane R* containing 50 mg of *butylhydroxytoluene R* per litre and dilute to 10.0 ml with the same solvent. Transfer 2.0 ml of the solution into a quartz tube and evaporate the solvent with a gentle current of *nitrogen R.* Add 1.5 ml of a 20 g/l solution of *sodium hydroxide R* in *methanol R,* cover with *nitrogen R,* cap tightly with a polytetrafluoroethylene lined cap, mix and heat in a water-bath for 7 min. Cool, add 2 ml of *boron trichloride-methanol solution R,* cover with *nitrogen R,* cap tightly, mix and heat in a water-bath for 30 min. Cool to 40-50 °C, add 1 ml of *trimethylpentane R,* cap and vortex or shake vigorously for at least 30 s. Immediately add 5 ml of *saturated sodium chloride solution R,* cover with *nitrogen R,* cap and vortex or shake thoroughly for at least 15 s. Allow the upper layer to become clear and transfer to a separate tube. Shake the methanol layer once more with 1 ml of *trimethylpentane R* and combine the trimethylpentane extracts. Wash the combined extracts with 2 quantities, each of 1 ml, of *water R* and dry over *anhydrous sodium sulphate R.* Prepare 2 solutions for each sample.

Column:

– *material*: fused silica,

– *size*: l = 30 m, Ø = 0.25 mm,

– *stationary phase*: *macrogol 20 000 R* (film thickness 0.25 µm).

Carrier gas: *hydrogen for chromatography R* or *helium for chromatography R,* where oxygen scrubber is applied.

Split ratio: 1:200.

Monographs A - C

Temperature:

	Time (min)	Temperature (°C)
Column	0 - 55	170 → 225
	55 - 75	225
Injection port		250
Detection		280

Detection: flame ionisation.

Injection: 1 µl, twice.

System suitability:

– the 15 fatty acids to be tested are satisfactorily identified from the chromatogram shown in Figure 1192.-1,

– injection of a mixture of equal amounts of *methyl palmitate R, methyl stearate R, methyl arachidate R* and *methyl behenate R* give area percentages of 24.4, 24.8, 25.2 and 25.6 (± 0.5 per cent), respectively,

– *resolution*: minimum of 1.3 between the peaks due to methyl oleate and methyl *cis*-vaccenate; the resolution between the pair due to methyl gadoleate and methyl gondoate is sufficient for purposes of identification and area measurement.

Calculate the area per cent for each fatty acid methyl ester from the expression:

$$\frac{A_x}{A_t} \times 100$$

A_x = peak area of fatty acid *x*,

A_t = sum of the peak areas (up to C22:6 n-3).

The calculation is not valid unless:

– the total area is based only on peaks due to solely fatty acids methyl esters,

– the number of fatty acid methyl ester peaks exceeding 0.05 per cent of the total area is at least 24,

– the 24 largest peaks of the methyl esters account for more than 90 per cent of the total area. (These correspond to, in common elution order: 14:0, 15:0, 16:0, 16:1 n-7, 16:4 n-1, 18:0, 18:1 n-9, 18:1 n-7, 18:2 n-6, 18:3 n-3, 18:4 n-3, 20:1 n-11, 20:1 n-9, 20:1 n-7, 20:2 n-6, 20:4 n-6, 20:3 n-3, 20:4 n-3, 20:5 n-3, 22:1 n-11, 22:1 n-9, 21:5 n-3, 22:5 n-3, 22:6 n-3).

ASSAY

Vitamin A. *Carry out the test as rapidly as possible, avoiding exposure to actinic light and air, oxidising agents, oxidation catalysts (for example, copper and iron) and acids.*

Use method A. If method A is found not to be valid, use method B.

METHOD A

Ultraviolet absorption spectrophotometry (*2.2.25*).

Test solution. To 1.00 g in a round-bottomed flask, add 3 ml of a freshly prepared 50 per cent *m/m* solution of *potassium hydroxide R* and 30 ml of *ethanol R*. Boil under reflux in a current of *nitrogen R* for 30 min. Cool rapidly and add 30 ml of *water R*. Extract with 50 ml of *ether R*. Repeat the extraction 3 times and discard the lower layer after complete separation. Wash the combined upper layers with 4 quantities, each of 50 ml, of *water R* and evaporate to dryness under a gentle current of *nitrogen R* at a temperature not exceeding 30 °C or in a rotary evaporator at a temperature not exceeding 30 °C under reduced pressure (water ejector). Dissolve the residue in sufficient *2-propanol R1* to give an expected concentration of vitamin A equivalent to 10-15 IU/ml.

Measure the absorbances of the solution at 300 nm, 310 nm, 325 nm and 334 nm and at the wavelength of maximum absorption with a suitable spectrophotometer in 1 cm specially matched cells, using *2-propanol R1* as the compensation liquid.

Calculate the content of vitamin A, as all-*trans*-retinol, in International Units per gram from the expression:

$$A_{325} \times \frac{1830}{100m} \times V$$

A_{325} = absorbance at 325 nm,

m = mass of the substance to be examined, in grams,

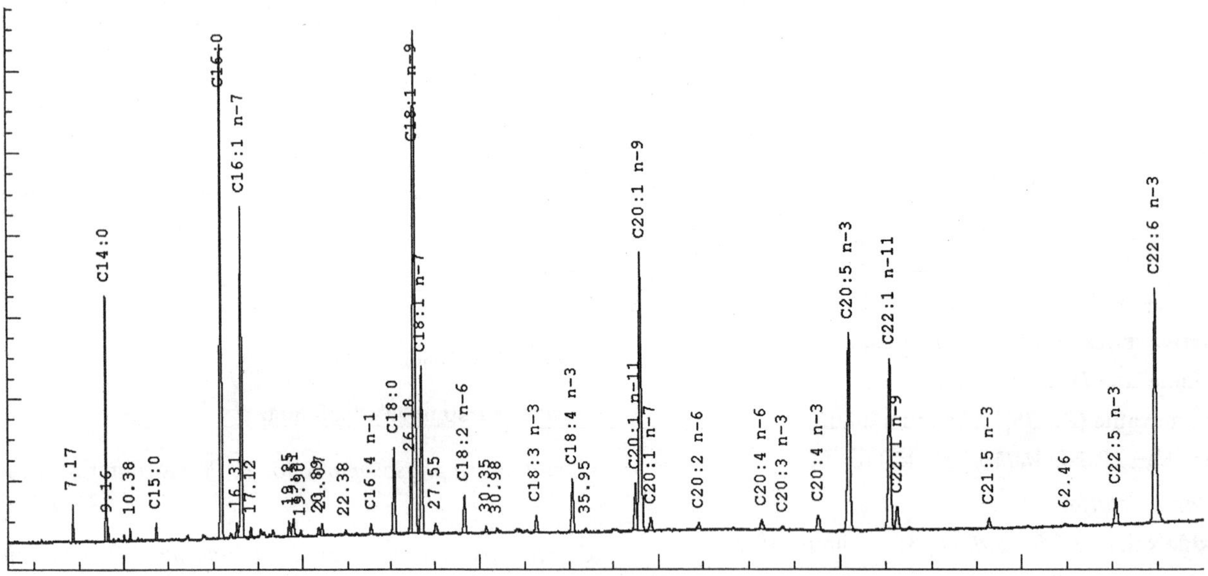

Figure 1192.-1. – *Chromatogram of cod-liver oil (type A) for the test for composition of fatty acids*

V = total volume of solution containing 10-15 IU of vitamin A per millilitre,

1830 = conversion factor for the specific absorbance of all-*trans*-retinol, in International Units.

The above expression can be used only if A_{325} has a value of not greater than $A_{325,corr}/0.970$ where $A_{325,corr}$ is the corrected absorbance at 325 nm and is given by the equation:

$$A_{325,\,corr} = 6.815A_{325} - 2.555A_{310} - 4.260A_{334}$$

A designates the absorbance at the wavelength indicated by the subscript.

If A_{325} has a value greater than $A_{325,corr}/0.970$, calculate the content of vitamin A from the following expression:

$$A_{325,\,corr} \times \frac{1830}{100m} \times V$$

The assay is not valid unless:

- the wavelength of maximum absorption lies between 323 nm and 327 nm,
- the absorbance at 300 nm relative to that at 325 nm is at most 0.73.

METHOD B

Liquid chromatography (*2.2.29*).

Test solution. To 2.00 g in a round-bottomed flask, add 5 ml of a freshly prepared 100 g/l solution of *ascorbic acid R* and 10 ml of a freshly prepared 800 g/l solution of *potassium hydroxide R* and 100 ml of *ethanol R*. Boil under a reflux condenser on a water-bath for 15 min. Add 100 ml of a 10 g/l solution of *sodium chloride R* and cool. Transfer the solution to a 500 ml separating funnel rinsing the round-bottomed flask with about 75 ml of a 10 g/l solution of *sodium chloride R* and then with 150 ml of a mixture of equal volumes of *light petroleum R1* and *ether R*. Shake for 1 min. When the layers have separated completely, discard the lower layer and wash the upper layer, first with 50 ml of a 30 g/l solution of *potassium hydroxide R* in a 10 per cent *V/V* solution of *ethanol R* and then with 3 quantities, each of 50 ml, of a 10 g/l solution of *sodium chloride R*. Filter the upper layer through 5 g of *anhydrous sodium sulphate R* on a fast filter paper into a 250 ml flask suitable for a rotary evaporator. Wash the funnel with 10 ml of fresh extraction mixture, filter and combine the upper layers. Distil them at a temperature not exceeding 30 °C under reduced pressure (water ejector) and fill with *nitrogen R* when evaporation is completed. Alternatively evaporate the solvent under a gentle current of *nitrogen R* at a temperature not exceeding 30 °C. Dissolve the residue in *2-propanol R*, transfer to a 25 ml volumetric flask and dilute to 25 ml with *2-propanol R*. Gentle heating in an ultrasonic bath may be required. (A large fraction of the white residue is cholesterol, constituting approximately 50 per cent of the unsaponifiable matter of cod-liver oil).

Reference solution (a). Prepare a solution of *retinyl acetate CRS* in *2-propanol R1* so that 1 ml contains about 1000 IU of all-*trans*-retinol.

The exact concentration of reference solution (a) is assessed by ultraviolet absorption spectrophotometry (*2.2.25*). Dilute reference solution (a) with *2-propanol R1* to a presumed concentration of 10-15 IU/ml and measure the absorbance at 326 nm in matched 1 cm cells using *2-propanol R1* as the compensation liquid.

Calculate the content of vitamin A in International Units per millilitre of reference solution (a) from the following expression, taking into account the assigned content of *retinyl acetate CRS*:

$$A_{326} \times \frac{1900 \times V_2}{100 \times V_1}$$

A_{326} = absorbance at 326 nm,

V_1 = volume of reference solution (a) used,

V_2 = volume of the diluted solution,

1900 = conversion factor for the specific absorbance of *retinyl acetate CRS*, in International Units.

Reference solution (b). Proceed as described for the test solution but using 2.00 ml of reference solution (a) in place of the substance to be examined.

The exact concentration of reference solution (b) is assessed by ultraviolet absorption spectrophotometry (*2.2.25*). Dilute reference solution (b) with *2-propanol R1* to a presumed concentration of 10-15 IU/ml of all-*trans*-retinol and measure the absorbance at 325 nm in matched 1 cm cells using *2-propanol R1* as the compensation liquid.

Calculate the content of all-*trans*-retinol in International Units per millilitre of reference solution (b) from the expression:

$$A_{325} \times \frac{1830 \times V_3}{100 \times V_4}$$

A_{325} = absorbance at 325 nm,

V_3 = volume of the diluted solution,

V_4 = volume of reference solution (b) used,

1830 = conversion factor for the specific absorbance of all-*trans*-retinol, in International Units.

Column:

- *size*: l = 0.25 m, Ø = 4.6 mm,
- *stationary phase*: *octadecylsilyl silica gel for chromatography R* (film thickness 5-10 μm).

Mobile phase: *water R, methanol R* (3:97 *V/V*).

Flow rate: 1 ml/min.

Detection: spectrophotometer at 325 nm.

Injection: 10 μl; inject in triplicate the test solution and reference solution (b).

Retention time: all-*trans*-retinol = 5 ± 1 min.

System suitability:

- the chromatogram obtained with the test solution shows a peak due to that of all-*trans*-retinol in the chromatogram obtained with reference solution (b),
- when using the method of standard additions to the test solution there is greater than 95 per cent recovery of the added *retinyl acetate CRS*,
- the recovery of all-*trans*-retinol in reference solution (b) as assessed by direct absorption spectrophotometry is greater than 95 per cent.

Monographs A - C

Calculate the content of vitamin A using the following expression:

$$A_1 \times \frac{C \times V}{A_2} \times \frac{1}{m}$$

A_1 = area of the peak due to all-*trans*-retinol in the chromatogram obtained with the test solution,

A_2 = area of the peak due to all-*trans*-retinol in the chromatogram obtained with reference solution (b),

C = concentration of *retinyl acetate CRS* in reference solution (a) as assessed prior to the saponification, in International Units per millilitre (= 1000 IU/ml),

V = volume of reference solution (a) treated (2.00 ml),

m = mass of the substance to be examined in the test solution (2.00 g).

Vitamin D_3. Liquid chromatography (*2.2.29*). *Carry out the assay as rapidly as possible, avoiding exposure to actinic light and air.*

Internal standard solution. Dissolve 0.50 mg of *ergocalciferol CRS* in 100 ml of *ethanol R*.

Test solution (a). To 4.00 g in a round-bottomed flask, add 5 ml of a freshly prepared 100 g/l solution of *ascorbic acid R*, 10 ml of a freshly prepared 800 g/l solution of *potassium hydroxide R* and 100 ml of *ethanol R*. Boil under a reflux condenser on a water-bath for 30 min. Add 100 ml of a 10 g/l solution of *sodium chloride R* and cool the solution to room temperature. Transfer the solution to a 500 ml separating funnel rinsing the round-bottomed flask with about 75 ml of a 10 g/l solution of *sodium chloride R* and then with 150 ml of a mixture of equal volumes of *light petroleum R1* and *ether R*. Shake for 1 min. When the layers have separated completely, discard the lower layer and wash the upper layer, first with 50 ml of a 30 g/l solution of *potassium hydroxide R* in a 10 per cent *V/V* solution of *ethanol R*, and then with 3 quantities, each of 50 ml, of a 10 g/l solution of *sodium chloride R*. Filter the upper layer through 5 g of *anhydrous sodium sulphate R* on a fast filter paper into a 250 ml flask suitable for a rotary evaporator. Wash the funnel with 10 ml of fresh extraction mixture, filter and combine the upper layers. Distil them at a temperature not exceeding 30 °C under reduced pressure (water ejector) and fill with *nitrogen R* when evaporation is completed. Alternatively evaporate the solvent under a gentle current of *nitrogen R* at a temperature not exceeding 30 °C. Dissolve the residue in 1.5 ml of the mobile phase described under Purification. Gentle heating in an ultrasonic bath may be required. (A large fraction of the white residue is cholesterol, constituting approximately 50 per cent *m/m* of the unsaponifiable matter of cod-liver oil).

Test solution (b). To 4.00 g add 2.0 ml of the internal standard solution and proceed as described for test solution (a).

Reference solution (a). Dissolve 0.50 mg of *cholecalciferol CRS* in 100.0 ml of *ethanol R*.

Reference solution (b). In a round-bottomed flask, add 2.0 ml of reference solution (a) and 2.0 ml of the internal standard solution and proceed as described for test solution (a).

PURIFICATION

Column:

- *size*: l = 0.25 m, Ø = 4.6 mm,
- *stationary phase*: *nitrile silica gel for chromatography R* (film thickness 10 µm).

Mobile phase: *isoamyl alcohol R, hexane R* (1.6:98.4 *V/V*).

Flow rate: 1.1 ml/min.

Detection: spectrophotometer at 265 nm.

Inject 350 µl of reference solution (b). Collect the eluate from 2 min before until 2 min after the retention time of cholecalciferol, in a ground-glass-stoppered tube containing 1 ml of a 1 g/l solution of *butylhydroxytoluene R* in *hexane R*. Repeat the procedure with test solutions (a) and (b). Evaporate the eluates obtained from reference solution (b) and from test solutions (a) and (b), separately, to dryness at a temperature not exceeding 30 °C under a gentle current of *nitrogen R*. Dissolve each residue in 1.5 ml of *acetonitrile R*.

DETERMINATION

Column:

- *size*: l = 0.15 m, Ø = 4.6 mm,
- *stationary phase*: *octadecylsilyl silica gel for chromatography R* (film thickness 5 µm).

Mobile phase: *phosphoric acid R*, 96 per cent *V/V* solution of *acetonitrile R* (0.2:99.8 *V/V*).

Flow rate: 1.0 ml/min.

Detection: spectrophotometer at 265 nm.

Injection: 2 quantities not exceeding 200 µl of each of the 3 solutions obtained under Purification.

System suitability:

- *resolution*: minimum 1.4 between the peaks corresponding to ergocalciferol and cholecalciferol in the chromatogram obtained with reference solution (b),
- when using the method of standard additions to test solution (a) there is greater than 95 per cent recovery of the added *cholecalciferol CRS* when due consideration has been given to correction by the internal standard.

Calculate the content of vitamin D_3 in International Units per gram using the following expression, taking into account the assigned content of *cholecalciferol CRS*:

$$\frac{A_2}{A_6} \times \frac{A_3}{A_4 - \left[\frac{A_5}{A_1}\right] \times A_2} \times \frac{m_2}{m_1} \times \frac{V_2}{V_1} \times 40$$

m_1 = mass of the sample in test solution (b) in grams,

m_2 = total mass of *cholecalciferol CRS* used for the preparation of reference solution (a) in micrograms (500 µg),

A_1 = area (or height) of the peak due to cholecalciferol in the chromatogram obtained with test solution (a),

A_2 = area (or height) of the peak due to cholecalciferol in the chromatogram obtained with test solution (b),

A_3 = area (or height) of the peak due to ergocalciferol in the chromatogram obtained with reference solution (b),

A_4 = area (or height) of the peak due to ergocalciferol in the chromatogram obtained with test solution (b),

A_5 = area (or height) of a possible peak in the chromatogram obtained with test solution (a) with the same retention time as the peak co-eluting with ergocalciferol in test solution (b),

A_6 = area (or height) of the peak due to cholecalciferol in the chromatogram obtained with reference solution (b),

Monographs A - C

V_1 = total volume of reference solution (a) (100 ml),

V_2 = volume of reference solution (a) used for preparing reference solution (b) (2.0 ml).

STORAGE

In an airtight and well-filled container, protected from light. If no antioxidant is added, store under an inert gas.

Once the container has been opened, its contents are used as soon as possible and any part of the contents not used at once is protected by an atmosphere of inert gas.

LABELLING

The label states:

- the number of International Units of vitamin A,
- the number of International Units of vitamin D_3,
- the name and concentration of any added antioxidant.

04/2003:1193 corrected

COD-LIVER OIL (TYPE B)

Iecoris aselli oleum B

DEFINITION

Purified fatty oil obtained from the fresh livers of *Gadus morhua* L. and other species of *Gadidae*, solid substances being removed by cooling and filtering. A suitable antioxidant may be added.

Content: 600 IU (180 µg) to 2500 IU (750 µg) of vitamin A per gram and 60 IU (1.5 µg) to 250 IU (6.25 µg) of vitamin D_3 per gram.

CHARACTERS

Appearance: clear, yellowish, viscous liquid.

Solubility: practically insoluble in water, slightly soluble in alcohol, miscible with light petroleum.

IDENTIFICATION

First identification: A, B, C.

Second identification: C, D.

A. In the assay for vitamin A using method A, the test solution shows an absorption maximum (*2.2.25*) at 325 ± 2 nm. In the assay for vitamin A using method B, the chromatogram obtained with the test solution shows a peak corresponding to the peak of all-*trans*-retinol in the chromatogram obtained with the reference solution.

B. In the assay for vitamin D_3, the chromatogram obtained with test solution (a) shows a peak corresponding to the peak of cholecalciferol in the chromatogram obtained with reference solution (b).

C. It complies with the test for composition of fatty acids (see Tests).

D. To 0.1 g add 0.5 ml of *methylene chloride R* and 1 ml of *antimony trichloride solution R*. Mix. A deep blue colour develops in about 10 s.

TESTS

Colour: not more intensely coloured than a reference solution prepared as follows: to 3.0 ml of red primary solution add 25.0 ml of yellow primary solution and dilute to 50.0 ml with a 10 g/l solution of *hydrochloric acid R* (*2.2.2, Method II*).

Relative density (*2.2.5*): 0.917 to 0.930.

Refractive index (*2.2.6*): 1.477 to 1.484.

Acid value (*2.5.1*): maximum 2.0.

Iodine value (*2.5.4, Method B*): 150 to 180.

Use *starch solution R2*.

Peroxide value (*2.5.5, Method B*): maximum 10.0.

Unsaponifiable matter (*2.5.7*): maximum 1.5 per cent, determined on 2.0 g and extracting with 3 quantities, each of 50 ml, of *peroxide-free ether R*.

Stearin. 10 ml remains clear after cooling in iced water for 3 h.

Composition of fatty acids. Gas chromatography (*2.2.28*).

Trivial name of fatty acid	Nomenclature	Lower limit area (per cent)	Upper limit area (per cent)
Saturated fatty acids:			
Myristic acid	14:0	2.0	6.0
Palmitic acid	16:0	7.0	14.0
Stearic acid	18:0	1.0	4.0
Mono-unsaturated fatty acids:			
Palmitoleic acid	16:1 n-7	4.5	11.5
cis-Vaccenic acid	18:1 n-7	2.0	7.0
Oleic acid	18:1 n-9	12.0	21.0
Gadoleic acid	20:1 n-11	1.0	5.5
Gondoic acid	20:1 n-9	5.0	17.0
Erucic acid	22:1 n-9	0	1.5
Cetoleic acid (22:1 n-11)	22:1 n-11+13	5.0	12.0
Poly-unsaturated fatty acids:			
Linoleic acid	18:2 n-6	0.5	3.0
α-Linolenic acid	18:3 n-3	0	2.0
Moroctic acid	18:4 n-3	0.5	4.5
Timnodonic (eicosapentaenoic) acid (EPA)	20:5 n-3	7.0	16.0
Cervonic (docosahexaenoic) acid (DHA)	22:6 n-3	6.0	18.0

Test solution. Introduce about 0.45 g of the substance to be examined into a 10 ml volumetric flask, dissolve in *hexane R* containing 50 mg of *butylhydroxytoluene R* per litre and dilute to 10.0 ml with the same solvent. Transfer 2.0 ml of the solution into a quartz tube and evaporate the solvent with a gentle current of *nitrogen R*. Add 1.5 ml of a 20 g/l solution of *sodium hydroxide R* in *methanol R*, cover with *nitrogen R*, cap tightly with a polytetrafluoroethylene lined cap, mix and heat in a water-bath for 7 min. Cool, add 2 ml of *boron trichloride-methanol solution R*, cover with *nitrogen R*, cap tightly, mix and heat in a water-bath for 30 min. Cool to 40-50 °C, add 1 ml of *trimethylpentane R*, cap and vortex or shake vigorously for at least 30 s. Immediately add 5 ml of *saturated sodium chloride solution R*, cover with *nitrogen R*, cap and vortex or shake thoroughly for at least 15 s. Allow the upper layer to become clear and transfer to a separate tube. Shake the methanol layer once more with 1 ml of *trimethylpentane R* and combine the trimethylpentane extracts. Wash the combined extracts with 2 quantities, each of 1 ml, of *water R* and dry over *anhydrous sodium sulphate R*. Prepare 2 solutions for each sample.

Column:

- *material*: fused silica,
- *size*: l = 30 m, Ø = 0.25 mm,
- *stationary phase*: *macrogol 20 000 R* (film thickness 0.25 µm).

Carrier gas: *hydrogen for chromatography R* or *helium for chromatography R*, where oxygen scrubber is applied.

Monographs A - C

Split ratio: 1:200.

Temperature:

	Time (min)	Temperature (°C)
Column	0 - 55	170 → 225
	55 - 75	225
Injection port		250
Detector		280

Detection: flame ionisation.

Injection: 1 μl, twice.

System suitability:

- the 15 fatty acids to be tested are satisfactorily identified from the chromatogram shown in Figure 1193.-1.
- injection of a mixture of equal amounts of *methyl palmitate R, methyl stearate R, methyl arachidate R*, and *methyl behenate R* give area percentages of 24.4, 24.8, 25.2 and 25.6 (± 0.5 per cent), respectively,
- *resolution*: minimum of 1.3 between the peaks due to methyl oleate and methyl *cis*-vaccenate; the resolution between the pair due to methyl gadoleate and methyl gondoate is sufficient for purposes of identification and area measurement.

Calculate the area per cent for each fatty acid methyl ester from the expression:

$$\frac{A_x}{A_t} \times 100$$

A_x = peak area of fatty acid *x*,

A_t = sum of the peak areas (up to C22:6 n-3).

The calculation is not valid unless:

- the total area is based only on peaks due to solely fatty acids methyl esters,
- the number of fatty acid methyl ester peaks exceeding 0.05 per cent of the total area is at least 24,
- the 24 largest peaks of the methyl esters account for more than 90 per cent of the total area. (These correspond to, in common elution order: 14:0, 15:0, 16:0, 16:1 n-7, 16:4 n-1, 18:0, 18:1 n-9, 18:1 n-7, 18:2 n-6, 18:3 n-3, 18:4 n-3, 20:1 n-11, 20:1 n-9, 20:1 n-7, 20:2 n-6, 20:4 n-6, 20:3 n-3, 20:4 n-3, 20:5 n-3, 22:1 n-11, 22:1 n-9, 21:5 n-3, 22:5 n-3, 22:6 n-3).

ASSAY

Vitamin A. *Carry out the test as rapidly as possible, avoiding exposure to actinic light and air, oxidising agents, oxidation catalysts (for example, copper and iron) and acids.*

Use method A. If method A is found not to be valid, use method B.

METHOD A

Ultraviolet absorption spectrophotometry (*2.2.25*).

Test solution. To 1.00 g in a round-bottomed flask, add 3 ml of a freshly prepared 50 per cent *m/m* solution of *potassium hydroxide R* and 30 ml of *ethanol R*. Boil under reflux in a current of *nitrogen R* for 30 min. Cool rapidly and add 30 ml of *water R*. Extract with 50 ml of *ether R*. Repeat the extraction 3 times and discard the lower layer after complete separation. Wash the combined upper layers with 4 quantities, each of 50 ml, of *water R* and evaporate to dryness under a gentle current of *nitrogen R* at a temperature not exceeding 30 °C or in a rotary evaporator at a temperature not exceeding 30 °C under reduced pressure (water ejector). Dissolve the residue in sufficient *2-propanol R1* to give an expected concentration of vitamin A equivalent to 10-15 IU/ml.

Measure the absorbances of the solution at 300 nm, 310 nm, 325 nm and 334 nm and at the wavelength of maximum absorption with a suitable spectrophotometer in 1 cm specially matched cells, using *2-propanol R1* as the compensation liquid.

Calculate the content of vitamin A, as all-*trans*-retinol, in International Units per gram from the expression:

$$A_{325} \times \frac{1830}{100m} \times V$$

A_{325} = absorbance at 325 nm,

m = mass of the substance to be examined, in grams,

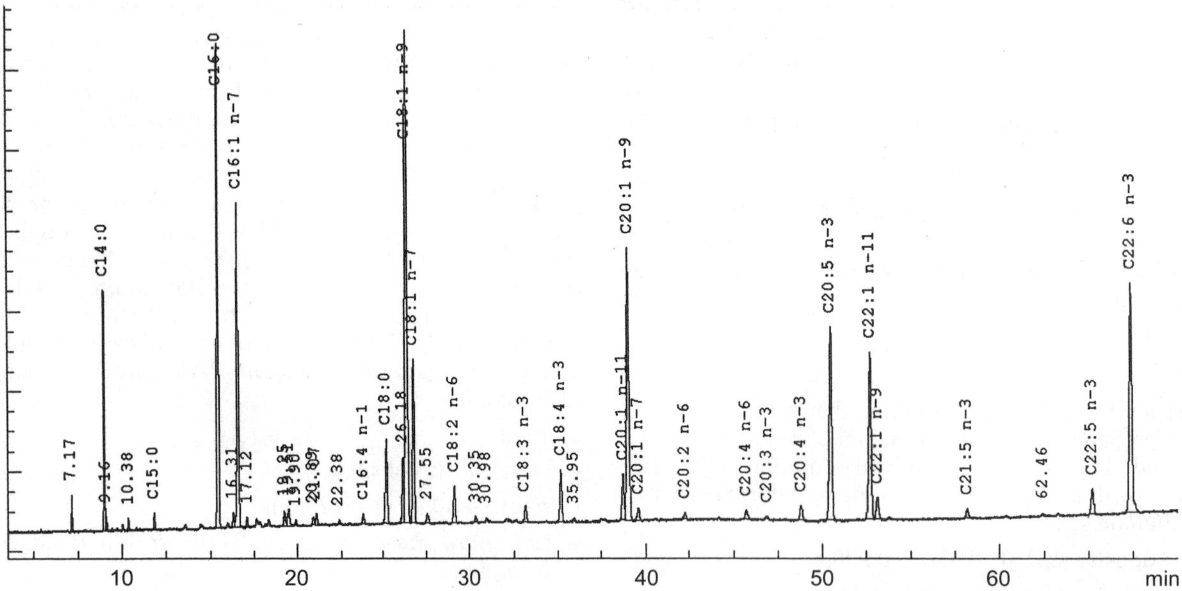

Figure 1193.-1. – *Chromatogram of cod-liver oil (type B) for the test for composition of fatty acids*

V = total volume of solution containing 10-15 IU of vitamin A per millilitre,

1830 = conversion factor for the specific absorbance of all-*trans*-retinol, in International Units.

The above expression can be used only if A_{325} has a value of not greater than $A_{325,corr}/0.970$ where $A_{325,corr}$ is the corrected absorbance at 325 nm and is given by the equation:

$$A_{325,\,corr} = 6.815A_{325} - 2.555A_{310} - 4.260A_{334}$$

A designates the absorbance at the wavelength indicated by the subscript.

If A_{325} has a value greater than $A_{325,corr}/0.970$, calculate the content of vitamin A from the expression:

$$A_{325,\,corr} \times \frac{1830}{100m} \times V$$

The assay is not valid unless:

- the wavelength of maximum absorption lies between 323 nm and 327 nm,
- the absorbance at 300 nm relative to that at 325 nm is at most 0.73.

METHOD B

Liquid chromatography (*2.2.29*).

Test solution. To 2.00 g in a round-bottomed flask, add 5 ml of a freshly prepared 100 g/l solution of *ascorbic acid R* and 10 ml of a freshly prepared 800 g/l solution of *potassium hydroxide R* and 100 ml of *ethanol R*. Boil under a reflux condenser on a water-bath for 15 min. Add 100 ml of a 10 g/l solution of *sodium chloride R* and cool. Transfer the solution to a 500 ml separating funnel rinsing the round-bottomed flask with about 75 ml of a 10 g/l solution of *sodium chloride R* and then with 150 ml of a mixture of equal volumes of *light petroleum R1* and *ether R*. Shake for 1 min. When the layers have separated completely, discard the lower layer and wash the upper layer, first with 50 ml of a 30 g/l solution of *potassium hydroxide R* in a 10 per cent *V/V* solution of *ethanol R* and then with 3 quantities, each of 50 ml, of a 10 g/l solution of *sodium chloride R*. Filter the upper layer through 5 g of *anhydrous sodium sulphate R* on a fast filter paper into a 250 ml flask suitable for a rotary evaporator. Wash the funnel with 10 ml of fresh extraction mixture, filter and combine the upper layers. Distil them at a temperature not exceeding 30 °C under reduced pressure (water ejector) and fill with *nitrogen R* when evaporation is completed. Alternatively evaporate the solvent under a gentle current of *nitrogen R* at a temperature not exceeding 30 °C. Dissolve the residue in *2-propanol R*, transfer to a 25 ml volumetric flask and dilute to 25 ml with *2-propanol R*. Gentle heating in an ultrasonic bath may be required. (A large fraction of the white residue is cholesterol, constituting approximately 50 per cent of the unsaponifiable matter of cod-liver oil).

Reference solution (a). Prepare a solution of *retinyl acetate CRS* in *2-propanol R1* so that 1 ml contains about 1000 IU of all-*trans*-retinol.

The exact concentration of reference solution (a) is assessed by ultraviolet absorption spectrophotometry (*2.2.25*). Dilute reference solution (a) with *2-propanol R1* to a presumed concentration of 10-15 IU/ml and measure the absorbance at 326 nm in matched 1 cm cells using *2-propanol R1* as the compensation liquid.

Calculate the content of vitamin A in International Units per millilitre of reference solution (a) using the following expression, taking into account the assigned content of *retinyl acetate CRS*:

$$A_{326} \times \frac{1900 \times V_2}{100 \times V_1}$$

A_{326} = absorbance at 326 nm,

V_1 = volume of reference solution (a) used,

V_2 = volume of the diluted solution,

1900 = conversion factor for the specific absorbance of *retinyl acetate CRS*, in International Units.

Reference solution (b). Proceed as described for the test solution but using 2.00 ml of reference solution (a) in place of the substance to be examined.

The exact concentration of reference solution (b) is assessed by ultraviolet absorption spectrophotometry (*2.2.25*). Dilute reference solution (b) with *2-propanol R1* to a presumed concentration of 10-15 IU/ml of all-*trans*-retinol and measure the absorbance at 325 nm in matched 1 cm cells using *2-propanol R1* as the compensation liquid.

Calculate the content of all-*trans*-retinol in International Units per millilitre of reference solution (b) from the expression:

$$A_{325} \times \frac{1830 \times V_3}{100 \times V_4}$$

A_{325} = absorbance at 325 nm,

V_3 = volume of the diluted solution,

V_4 = volume of reference solution (b) used,

1830 = conversion factor for the specific absorbance of all-*trans*-retinol, in International Units.

Column:

- *size*: l = 0.25 m, Ø = 4.6 mm,
- *stationary phase*: *octadecylsilyl silica gel for chromatography R* (film thickness 5-10 µm).

Mobile phase: *water R, methanol R* (3:97 *V/V*).

Flow rate: 1 ml/min.

Detection: spectrophotometer at 325 nm.

Injection: 10 µl; inject in triplicate the test solution and reference solution (b).

Retention time: all-*trans*-retinol = 5 ± 1 min.

System suitability:

- the chromatogram obtained with the test solution shows a peak due to that of all-*trans*-retinol in the chromatogram obtained with reference solution (b),
- when using the method of standard additions to the test solution there is greater than 95 per cent recovery of the added *retinyl acetate CRS*,
- the recovery of all-*trans*-retinol in reference solution (b) as assessed by direct absorption spectrophotometry is greater than 95 per cent.

Monographs A - C

Calculate the content of vitamin A using the following expression:

$$A_1 \times \frac{C \times V}{A_2} \times \frac{1}{m}$$

A_1 = area of the peak due to all-*trans*-retinol in the chromatogram obtained with the test solution,

A_2 = area of the peak due to all-*trans*-retinol in the chromatogram obtained with reference solution (b),

C = concentration of *retinyl acetate CRS* in reference solution (a) as assessed prior to the saponification, in International Units per millilitre (= 1000 IU/ml),

V = volume of reference solution (a) treated (2.00 ml),

m = mass of the substance to be examined in the test solution (2.00 g).

Vitamin D_3. Liquid chromatography (*2.2.29*). *Carry out the assay as rapidly as possible, avoiding exposure to actinic light and air.*

Internal standard solution. Dissolve 0.50 mg of *ergocalciferol CRS* in 100 ml of *ethanol R*.

Test solution (a). To 4.00 g in a round-bottomed flask, add 5 ml of a freshly prepared 100 g/l solution of *ascorbic acid R*, 10 ml of a freshly prepared 800 g/l solution of *potassium hydroxide R* and 100 ml of *ethanol R*. Boil under a reflux condenser on a water-bath for 30 min. Add 100 ml of a 10 g/l solution of *sodium chloride R* and cool the solution to room temperature. Transfer the solution to a 500 ml separating funnel rinsing the round-bottomed flask with about 75 ml of a 10 g/l solution of *sodium chloride R* and then with 150 ml of a mixture of equal volumes of *light petroleum R1* and *ether R*. Shake for 1 min. When the layers have separated completely, discard the lower layer and wash the upper layer, first with 50 ml of a 30 g/l solution of *potassium hydroxide R* in a 10 per cent *V/V* solution of *ethanol R*, and then with 3 quantities, each of 50 ml, of a 10 g/l solution of *sodium chloride R*. Filter the upper layer through 5 g of *anhydrous sodium sulphate R* on a fast filter paper into a 250 ml flask suitable for a rotary evaporator. Wash the funnel with 10 ml of fresh extraction mixture, filter and combine the upper layers. Distil them at a temperature not exceeding 30 °C under reduced pressure (water ejector) and fill with *nitrogen R* when evaporation is completed. Alternatively evaporate the solvent under a gentle current of *nitrogen R* at a temperature not exceeding 30 °C. Dissolve the residue in 1.5 ml of the mobile phase described under Purification. Gentle heating in an ultrasonic bath may be required. (A large fraction of the white residue is cholesterol, constituting approximately 50 per cent *m/m* of the unsaponifiable matter of cod-liver oil).

Test solution (b). To 4.00 g add 2.0 ml of the internal standard solution and proceed as described for test solution (a).

Reference solution (a). Dissolve 0.50 mg of *cholecalciferol CRS* in 100.0 ml of *ethanol R*.

Reference solution (b). In a round-bottomed flask, add 2.0 ml of reference solution (a) and 2.0 ml of the internal standard solution and proceed as described for test solution (a).

PURIFICATION

Column:

- *size*: l = 0.25 m, Ø = 4.6 mm,
- *stationary phase*: *nitrile silica gel for chromatography R* (film thickness 10 µm).

Mobile phase: *isoamyl alcohol R*, *hexane R* (1.6:98.4 *V/V*).

Flow rate: 1.1 ml/min.

Detection: spectrophotometer at 265 nm.

Inject 350 µl of reference solution (b). Collect the eluate from 2 min before until 2 min after the retention time of cholecalciferol, in a ground-glass-stoppered tube containing 1 ml of a 1 g/l solution of *butylhydroxytoluene R* in *hexane R*. Repeat the procedure with test solutions (a) and (b). Evaporate the eluates obtained from reference solution (b) and from test solutions (a) and (b), separately, to dryness at a temperature not exceeding 30 °C under a gentle current of *nitrogen R*. Dissolve each residue in 1.5 ml of *acetonitrile R*.

DETERMINATION

Column:

- *size*: l = 0.15 m, Ø = 4.6 mm,
- *stationary phase*: *octadecylsilyl silica gel for chromatography R* (film thickness 5 µm).

Mobile phase: *phosphoric acid R*, a 96 per cent *V/V* solution of *acetonitrile R* (0.2:99.8 *V/V*).

Flow rate: 1.0 ml/min.

Detection: spectrophotometer at 265 nm.

Injection: 2 quantities not exceeding 200 µl of each of the 3 solutions obtained under Purification.

System suitability:

- *resolution*: minimum 1.4 between the peaks due to ergocalciferol and cholecalciferol in the chromatogram obtained with reference solution (b),
- when using the method of standard additions to test solution (a) there is greater than 95 per cent recovery of the added *cholecalciferol CRS* when due consideration has been given to correction by the internal standard.

Calculate the content of vitamin D_3 in International Units per gram using the following expression, taking into account the assigned content of *cholecalciferol CRS*:

$$\frac{A_2}{A_6} \times \frac{A_3}{A_4 - \left[\frac{A_5}{A_1}\right] \times A_2} \times \frac{m_2}{m_1} \times \frac{V_2}{V_1} \times 40$$

m_1 = mass of the sample in test solution (b) in grams,

m_2 = total mass of *cholecalciferol CRS* used for the preparation of reference solution (a) in micrograms (500 µg),

A_1 = area (or height) of the peak due to cholecalciferol in the chromatogram obtained with test solution (a),

A_2 = area (or height) of the peak due to cholecalciferol in the chromatogram obtained with test solution (b),

A_3 = area (or height) of the peak due to ergocalciferol in the chromatogram obtained with reference solution (b),

A_4 = area (or height) of the peak due to ergocalciferol in the chromatogram obtained with test solution (b),

A_5 = area (or height) of a possible peak in the chromatogram obtained with test solution (a) with the same retention time as the peak co-eluting with ergocalciferol in test solution (b),

A_6 = area (or height) of the peak due to cholecalciferol in the chromatogram obtained with reference solution (b),

V_1 = total volume of reference solution (a) (100 ml),

V_2 = volume of reference solution (a) used for preparing reference solution (b) (2.0 ml).

STORAGE

In an airtight and well-filled container, protected from light. If no antioxidant is added, store under an inert gas.

Once the container has been opened, its contents are used as soon as possible and any part of the contents not used at once is protected by an atmosphere of inert gas.

LABELLING

The label states:

- the number of International Units of vitamin A,
- the number of International Units of vitamin D_3,
- the name and concentration of any added antioxidant.

07/2004:0076

CODEINE

Codeinum

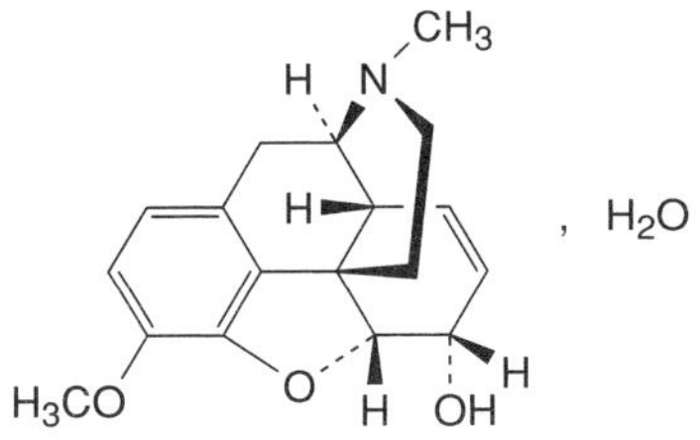

$C_{18}H_{21}NO_3,H_2O$ M_r 317.4

DEFINITION

7,8-Didehydro-4,5α-epoxy-3-methoxy-17-methylmorphinan-6α-ol.

Content: 99.0 per cent to 101.0 per cent (dried substance).

CHARACTERS

Appearance: white or almost white, crystalline powder or colourless crystals.

Solubility: soluble in boiling water, freely soluble in alcohol.

IDENTIFICATION

First identification: A, C.

Second identification: A, B, D, E.

A. Melting point (*2.2.14*): 155 °C to 159 °C.

B. To 2.0 ml of solution S (see Tests) add 50 ml of *water R* then 10 ml of *1 M sodium hydroxide* and dilute to 100.0 ml with *water R*. Examined between 250 nm and 350 nm (*2.2.25*), the solution shows only 1 absorption maximum at 284 nm. The specific absorbance at the absorption maximum is about 50 (dried substance).

C. Infrared absorption spectrophotometry (*2.2.24*).

Preparation: dried substance prepared as a disc of *potassium bromide R*.

Comparison: *Ph. Eur. reference spectrum of codeine*.

D. To about 10 mg add 1 ml of *sulphuric acid R* and 0.05 ml of *ferric chloride solution R2* and heat on a water-bath. A blue colour develops. Add 0.05 ml of *nitric acid R*. The colour changes to red.

E. It gives the reaction of alkaloids (*2.3.1*).

TESTS

Solution S. Dissolve 50 mg in *carbon dioxide-free water R* and dilute to 10.0 ml with the same solvent.

Appearance of solution. Solution S is clear (*2.2.1*) and colourless (*2.2.2, Method II*).

Specific optical rotation (*2.2.7*): − 142 to − 146 (dried substance).

Dissolve 0.50 g in *alcohol R* and dilute to 25.0 ml with the same solvent.

Related substances. Liquid chromatography (*2.2.29*).

Test solution. Dissolve 0.100 g of the substance to be examined and 0.100 g of *sodium octanesulphonate R* in the mobile phase and dilute to 10.0 ml with the mobile phase.

Reference solution (a). Dissolve 5.0 mg of *codeine impurity A CRS* in the mobile phase and dilute to 5.0 ml with the mobile phase.

Reference solution (b). Dilute 1.0 ml of reference solution (a) to 20.0 ml with the mobile phase.

Reference solution (c). Dilute 1.0 ml of the test solution to 50.0 ml with the mobile phase. Dilute 5.0 ml of this solution to 100.0 ml with the mobile phase.

Reference solution (d). Dilute 0.5 ml of the test solution to 5.0 ml with reference solution (a).

Column:

- *size*: *l* = 0.25 m, Ø = 4.6 mm,
- *stationary phase*: *end-capped octylsilyl silica gel for chromatography R* (5 µm).

Mobile phase: dissolve 1.08 g of *sodium octanesulphonate R* in a mixture of 20 ml of *glacial acetic acid R* and 250 ml of *acetonitrile R* and dilute to 1000 ml with *water R*.

Flow rate: 2 ml/min.

Detection: spectrophotometer at 245 nm.

Injection: 10 µl.

Run time: 10 times the retention time of codeine.

Relative retention with reference to codeine (retention time = about 6 min): impurity B = about 0.6; impurity E = about 0.7; impurity A = about 2.0; impurity C = about 2.3; impurity D = about 3.6.

System suitability: reference solution (d):

- *resolution*: minimum 3 between the peaks due to codeine and impurity A.

Limits:

- *correction factor*: for the calculation of content, multiply the peak area of impurity C by 0.25,
- *impurity A*: not more than twice the area of the principal peak in the chromatogram obtained with reference solution (b) (1.0 per cent),
- *impurities B, C, D, E*: for each impurity, not more than twice the area of the principal peak in the chromatogram obtained with reference solution (c) (0.2 per cent),
- *any other impurity*: for each impurity, not more than the area of the principal peak in the chromatogram obtained with reference solution (c) (0.1 per cent),
- *total of impurities other than A*: not more than 10 times the area of the principal peak in the chromatogram obtained with reference solution (c) (1.0 per cent),
- *disregard limit*: 0.5 times the area of the principal peak in the chromatogram obtained with reference solution (c) (0.05 per cent).

Loss on drying (*2.2.32*): 4.0 per cent to 6.0 per cent, determined on 1.000 g by drying in an oven at 100-105 °C.

Sulphated ash (*2.4.14*): maximum 0.1 per cent, determined on 1.0 g.

ASSAY

Dissolve 0.250 g in 10 ml of *anhydrous acetic acid R*. Add 20 ml of *dioxan R*. Titrate with *0.1 M perchloric acid* using 0.05 ml of *crystal violet solution R* as indicator.

1 ml of *0.1 M perchloric acid* is equivalent to 29.94 mg of $C_{18}H_{21}NO_3$.

STORAGE

Protected from light.

IMPURITIES

Specified impurities (see note for information p. xli): A, B, C, D, E.

Other detectable impurities: F, G.

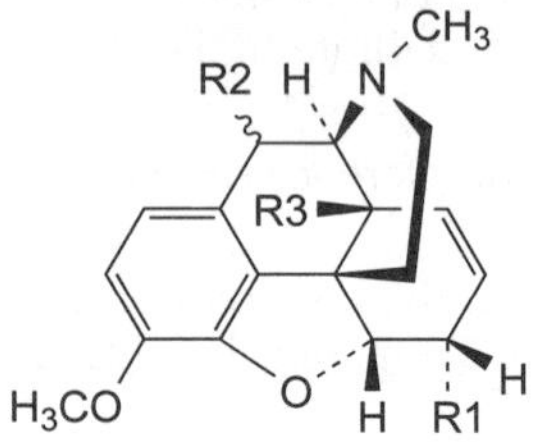

A. R1 = OCH_3, R2 = R3 = H: 7,8-didehydro-4,5α-epoxy-3,6α-dimethoxy-17-methylmorphinan (methylcodeine),

E. R1 = R2 = OH, R3 = H: 7,8-didehydro-4,5α-epoxy-3-methoxy-17-methylmorphinan-6α,10-diol,

F. R1 = R3 = OH, R2 = H: 7,8-didehydro-4,5α-epoxy-3-methoxy-17-methylmorphinan-6α,14-diol,

B. morphine,

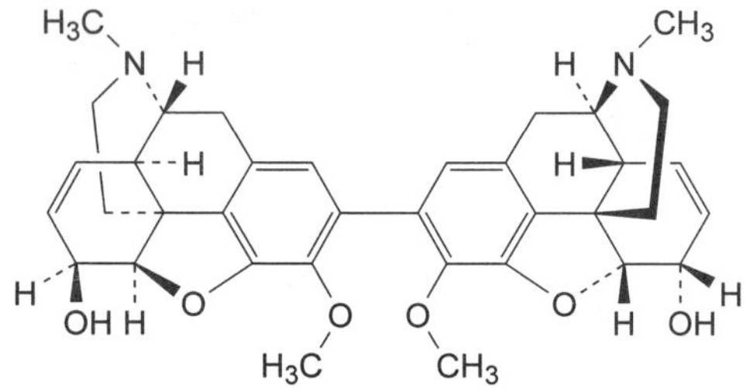

C. 7,7′,8,8′-tetradehydro-4,5α:4′,5′α-diepoxy-3,3′-dimethoxy-17,17′-dimethyl-2,2′-bimorphinanyl-6α,6′α-diol (codeine dimer),

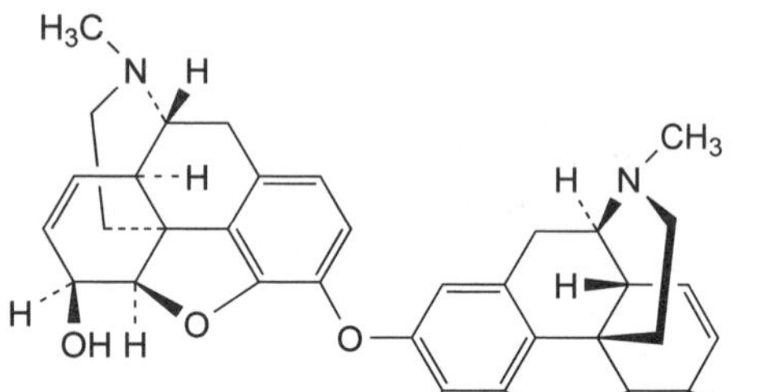

D. 7,8-didehydro-2-[(7,8-didehydro-4,5α-epoxy-6α-hydroxy-17-methylmorphinan-3-yl)oxy]-4,5α-epoxy-3-methoxy-17-methylmorphinan-6α-ol (3-*O*-(codein-2-yl)morphine),

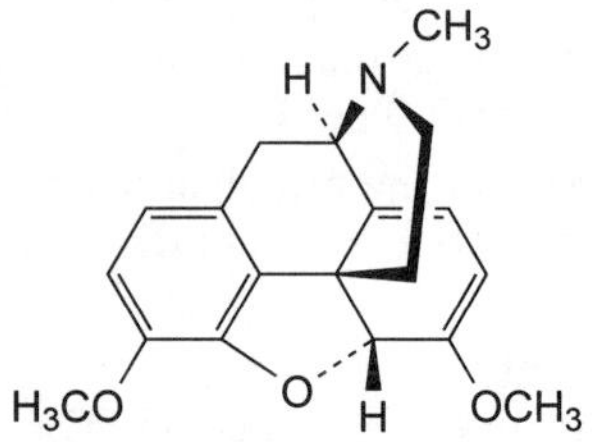

G. 6,7,8,14-tetradehydro-4,5α-epoxy-3,6-dimethoxy-17-methylmorphinan (thebaine).

07/2004:1412

CODEINE HYDROCHLORIDE DIHYDRATE

Codeini hydrochloridum dihydricum

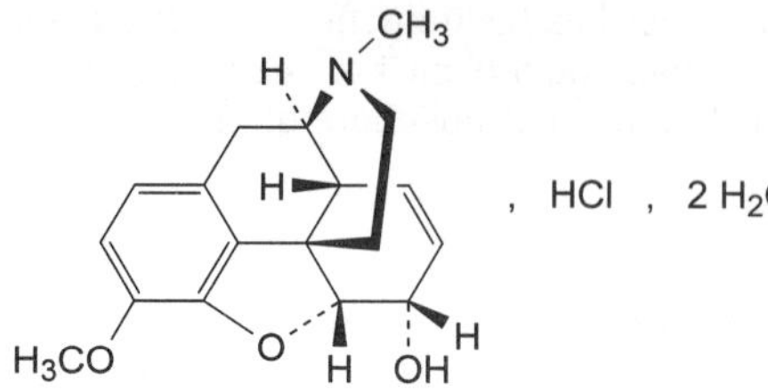

$C_{18}H_{22}ClNO_3,2H_2O$ M_r 371.9

DEFINITION

7,8-Didehydro-4,5α-epoxy-3-methoxy-17-methylmorphinan-6α-ol hydrochloride dihydrate.

Content: 99.0 per cent to 101.0 per cent (anhydrous substance).

CHARACTERS

Appearance: white or almost white, crystalline powder or small, colourless crystals.

Solubility: soluble in water, slightly soluble in ethanol, practically insoluble in cyclohexane.

IDENTIFICATION

First identification: A, D.

Second identification: B, C, D, E.

A. Infrared absorption spectrophotometry (*2.2.24*).

Comparison: *Ph. Eur. reference spectrum of codeine hydrochloride dihydrate.*

B. To 5 ml of solution S (see Tests) add 1 ml of a mixture of equal volumes of *strong sodium hydroxide solution R* and *water R* and initiate crystallisation, if necessary, by scratching the wall of the tube with a glass rod and cooling in iced water. Wash the precipitate with *water R* and dry at 100-105 °C. It melts (*2.2.15*) at 155 °C to 159 °C.

C. To about 10 mg add 1 ml of *sulphuric acid R* and 0.05 ml of *ferric chloride solution R2* and heat on a water-bath. A blue colour develops. Add 0.05 ml of *nitric acid R*. The colour changes to red.

D. Solution S gives reaction (a) of chlorides (*2.3.1*).

E. It gives the reaction of alkaloids (*2.3.1*).

TESTS

Solution S. Dissolve 2.00 g in *carbon dioxide-free water R* prepared from *distilled water R* and dilute to 50.0 ml with the same solvent.

Appearance of solution. Solution S is clear (*2.2.1*) and not more intensely coloured than reference solution Y_6 (*2.2.2, Method II*).

Acidity or alkalinity. To 5 ml of solution S add 5 ml of *carbon dioxide-free water R*. Add 0.05 ml of *methyl red solution R* and 0.2 ml of *0.02 M hydrochloric acid*; the solution is red. Add 0.4 ml of *0.02 M sodium hydroxide*; the solution becomes yellow.

Specific optical rotation (*2.2.7*): − 117 to − 121 (anhydrous substance).

Dilute 5.0 ml of solution S to 10.0 ml with *water R*.

Related substances. Liquid chromatography (*2.2.29*).

Test solution. Dissolve 0.100 g of the substance to be examined and 0.100 g of *sodium octanesulphonate R* in the mobile phase and dilute to 10.0 ml with the mobile phase.

Reference solution (a). Dissolve 5.0 mg of *codeine impurity A CRS* in the mobile phase and dilute to 5.0 ml with the mobile phase.

Reference solution (b). Dilute 1.0 ml of reference solution (a) to 20.0 ml with the mobile phase.

Reference solution (c). Dilute 1.0 ml of the test solution to 50.0 ml with the mobile phase. Dilute 5.0 ml of this solution to 100.0 ml with the mobile phase.

Reference solution (d). Dilute 0.5 ml of the test solution to 5.0 ml with reference solution (a).

Column:

- *size*: l = 0.25 m, Ø = 4.6 mm,
- *stationary phase*: *end-capped octylsilyl silica gel for chromatography R* (5 µm).

Mobile phase: dissolve 1.08 g of *sodium octanesulphonate R* in a mixture of 20 ml of *glacial acetic acid R* and 250 ml of *acetonitrile R* and dilute to 1000 ml with *water R*.

Flow rate: 2 ml/min.

Detection: spectrophotometer at 245 nm.

Injection: 10 µl.

Run time: 10 times the retention time of codeine.

Relative retention with reference to codeine (retention time = about 6 min): impurity B = about 0.6; impurity E = about 0.7; impurity A = about 2.0; impurity C = about 2.3; impurity D = about 3.6.

System suitability: reference solution (d):

- *resolution*: minimum 3 between the peaks due to codeine and impurity A.

Limits:

- *correction factor*: for the calculation of content, multiply the peak area of impurity C by 0.25,
- *impurity A*: not more than twice the area of the principal peak in the chromatogram obtained with reference solution (b) (1.0 per cent),
- *impurities B, C, D, E*: for each impurity, not more than twice the area of the principal peak in the chromatogram obtained with reference solution (c) (0.2 per cent),
- *any other impurity*: for each impurity, not more than the area of the principal peak in the chromatogram obtained with reference solution (c) (0.1 per cent),
- *total of impurities other than A*: not more than 10 times the area of the principal peak in the chromatogram obtained with reference solution (c) (1.0 per cent),
- *disregard limit*: 0.5 times the area of the principal peak in the chromatogram obtained with reference solution (c) (0.05 per cent).

Sulphates (*2.4.13*): maximum 0.1 per cent.

Dilute 5 ml of solution S to 20 ml with *distilled water R*. 15 ml of the solution complies with the limit test for sulphates.

Water (*2.5.12*): 8.0 per cent to 10.5 per cent, determined on 0.250 g.

ASSAY

Dissolve 0.300 g in a mixture of 5 ml of *0.01 M hydrochloric acid R* and 30 ml of *alcohol R*. Carry out a potentiometric titration (*2.2.20*), using *0.1 M sodium hydroxide*. Read the volume added between the 2 points of inflexion.

1 ml of *0.1 M sodium hydroxide* is equivalent to 33.59 mg of $C_{18}H_{22}ClNO_3$.

STORAGE

Protected from light.

IMPURITIES

Specified impurities (see note for information p. xli): A, B, C, D, E.

Other detectable impurities: F, G.

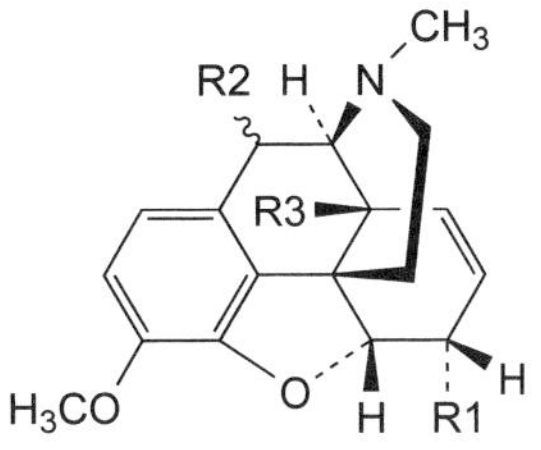

A. R1 = OCH_3, R2 = R3 = H: 7,8-didehydro-4,5α-epoxy-3,6α-dimethoxy-17-methylmorphinan (methylcodeine),

E. R1 = R2 = OH, R3 = H: 7,8-didehydro-4,5α-epoxy-3-methoxy-17-methylmorphinan-6α,10-diol,

F. R1 = R3 = OH, R2 = H: 7,8-didehydro-4,5α-epoxy-3-methoxy-17-methylmorphinan-6α,14-diol,

B. morphine,

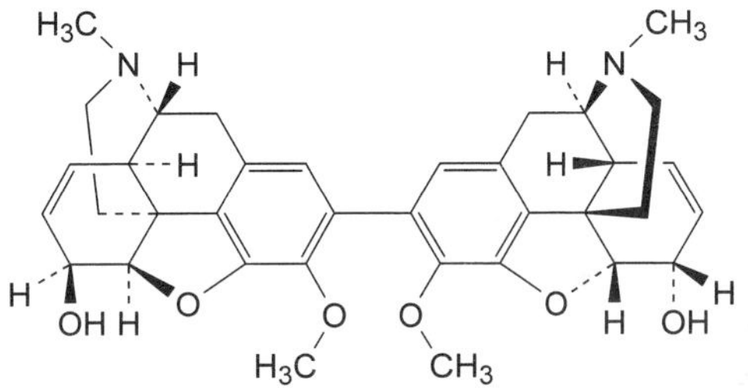

C. 7,7′,8,8′-tetradehydro-4,5α:4′,5′α-diepoxy-3,3′-dimethoxy-17,17′-dimethyl-2,2′-bimorphinanyl-6α,6′α-diol (codeine dimer),

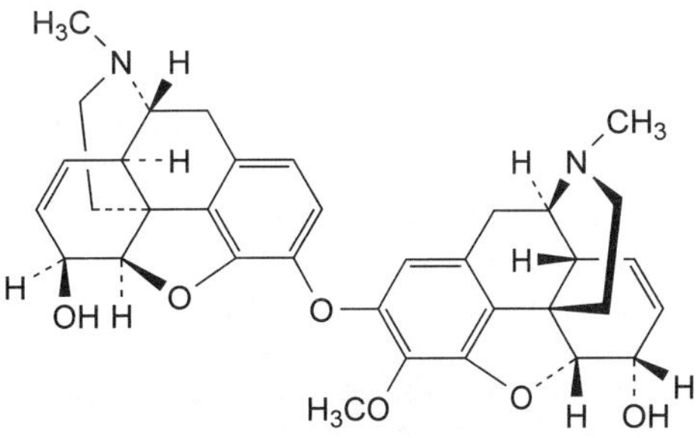

D. 7,8-didehydro-2-[(7,8-didehydro-4,5α-epoxy-6α-hydroxy-17-methylmorphinan-3-yl)oxy]-4,5α-epoxy-3-methoxy-17-methylmorphinan-6α-ol (3-*O*-(codein-2-yl)morphine),

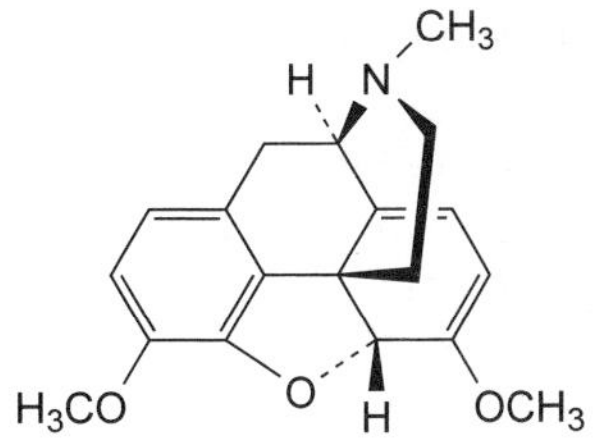

G. 6,7,8,14-tetradehydro-4,5α-epoxy-3,6-dimethoxy-17-methylmorphinan (thebaine).

07/2004:0074

CODEINE PHOSPHATE HEMIHYDRATE

Codeini phosphas hemihydricus

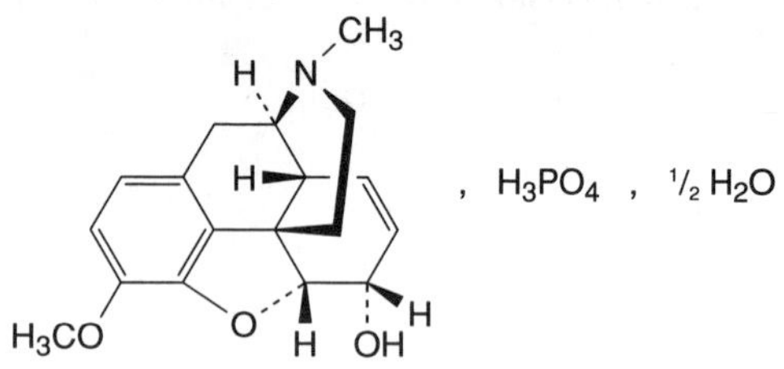

$C_{18}H_{24}NO_7P,{}^1/_2H_2O$ M_r 406.4

DEFINITION

7,8-Didehydro-4,5α-epoxy-3-methoxy-17-methylmorphinan-6α-ol phosphate hemihydrate.

Content: 98.5 per cent to 101.0 per cent (dried substance).

CHARACTERS

Appearance: white or almost white, crystalline powder or small, colourless crystals.

Solubility: freely soluble in water, slightly soluble or very slightly soluble in alcohol.

IDENTIFICATION

First identification: B, E, F.

Second identification: A, C, D, E, F, G.

A. Dilute 1.0 ml of solution S (see Tests) to 100.0 ml with *water R*. To 25.0 ml of this solution add 25 ml of *water R* then 10 ml of *1 M sodium hydroxide* and dilute to 100.0 ml with *water R*. Examined between 250 nm and 350 nm (*2.2.25*), the solution shows only 1 absorption maximum, at 284 nm. The specific absorbance at the absorption maximum is about 38 (dried substance).

B. Infrared absorption spectrophotometry (*2.2.24*).

Preparation: dissolve 0.20 g in 4 ml of *water R*. Add 1 ml of a mixture of equal volumes of *strong sodium hydroxide solution R* and *water R* and initiate crystallisation, if necessary, by scratching the wall of the tube with a glass rod and cooling in iced water. Wash the precipitate with *water R* and dry at 100-105 °C. Examine the dried precipitate prepared as discs using *potassium bromide R*.

Comparison: *Ph. Eur. reference spectrum of codeine.*

C. Dissolve 0.20 g in 4 ml of *water R*. Add 1 ml of a mixture of equal volumes of *strong sodium hydroxide solution R* and *water R* and initiate crystallisation, if necessary, by scratching the wall of the tube with a glass rod and cooling in iced water. The precipitate, washed with *water R* and dried at 100-105 °C, melts (*2.2.14*) at 155 °C to 159 °C.

D. To about 10 mg add 1 ml of *sulphuric acid R* and 0.05 ml of *ferric chloride solution R2* and heat on a water-bath. A blue colour develops. Add 0.05 ml of *nitric acid R*. The colour changes to red.

E. It complies with the test for loss on drying (see Tests).

F. Solution S gives reaction (a) of phosphates (*2.3.1*).

G. It gives the reaction of alkaloids (*2.3.1*).

TESTS

Solution S. Dissolve 1.00 g in *carbon dioxide-free water R* prepared from *distilled water R* and dilute to 25.0 ml with the same solvent.

pH (*2.2.3*): 4.0 to 5.0 for solution S.

Specific optical rotation (*2.2.7*): − 98 to − 102 (dried substance).

Dilute 5.0 ml of solution S to 10.0 ml with *water R*.

Related substances. Liquid chromatography (*2.2.29*).

Test solution. Dissolve 0.100 g of the substance to be examined and 0.100 g of *sodium octanesulphonate R* in the mobile phase and dilute to 10.0 ml with the mobile phase.

Reference solution (a). Dissolve 5.0 mg of *codeine impurity A CRS* in the mobile phase and dilute to 5.0 ml with the mobile phase.

Reference solution (b). Dilute 1.0 ml of reference solution (a) to 20.0 ml with the mobile phase.

Reference solution (c). Dilute 1.0 ml of the test solution to 50.0 ml with the mobile phase. Dilute 5.0 ml of this solution to 100.0 ml with the mobile phase.

Reference solution (d). Dilute 0.5 ml of the test solution to 5.0 ml with reference solution (a).

Column:

- *size*: l = 0.25 m, Ø = 4.6 mm,
- *stationary phase*: *end-capped octylsilyl silica gel for chromatography R* (5 µm).

Mobile phase: dissolve 1.08 g of *sodium octanesulphonate R* in a mixture of 20 ml of *glacial acetic acid R* and 250 ml of *acetonitrile R* and dilute to 1000 ml with *water R*.

Flow rate: 2 ml/min.

Detection: spectrophotometer at 245 nm.

Injection: 10 µl.

Run time: 10 times the retention time of codeine.

Relative retention with reference to codeine (retention time = about 6 min): impurity B = about 0.6; impurity E = about 0.7; impurity A = about 2.0; impurity C = about 2.3; impurity D = about 3.6.

System suitability: reference solution (d):

- *resolution*: minimum 3 between the peaks due to codeine and impurity A.

Limits:

- *correction factor*: for the calculation of content, multiply the peak area of impurity C by 0.25,
- *impurity A*: not more than twice the area of the principal peak in the chromatogram obtained with reference solution (b) (1.0 per cent),
- *impurities B, C, D, E*: for each impurity, not more than twice the area of the principal peak in the chromatogram obtained with reference solution (c) (0.2 per cent),
- *any other impurity*: for each impurity, not more than the area of the principal peak in the chromatogram obtained with reference solution (c) (0.1 per cent),
- *total of impurities other than A*: not more than 10 times the area of the principal peak in the chromatogram obtained with reference solution (c) (1.0 per cent),
- *disregard limit*: 0.5 times the area of the principal peak in the chromatogram obtained with reference solution (c) (0.05 per cent).

Sulphates (*2.4.13*): maximum 0.1 per cent.

Dilute 5 ml of solution S to 20 ml with *distilled water R*. 15 ml of the solution complies with the limit test for sulphates.

Loss on drying (*2.2.32*): 1.5 per cent to 3.0 per cent, determined on 1.000 g by drying in an oven at 100-105 °C.

ASSAY

Dissolve 0.350 g in a mixture of 10 ml of *anhydrous acetic acid R* and 20 ml of *dioxan R*. Titrate with *0.1 M perchloric acid* using 0.05 ml of *crystal violet solution R* as indicator.

1 ml of *0.1 M perchloric acid* is equivalent to 39.74 mg of $C_{18}H_{24}NO_7P$.

STORAGE

Protected from light.

IMPURITIES

Specified impurities (see note for information p. xli): A, B, C, D, E.

Other detectable impurities: F, G.

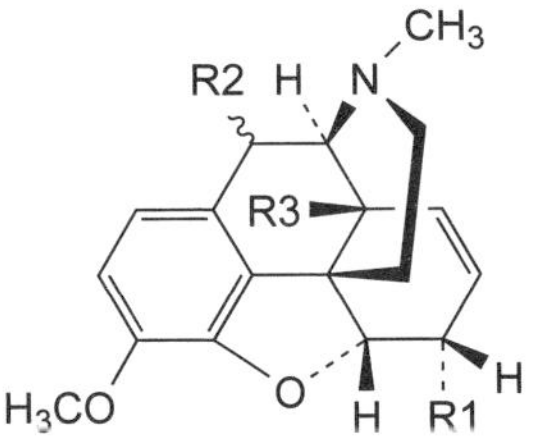

A. R1 = OCH_3, R2 = R3 = H: 7,8-didehydro-4,5α-epoxy-3,6α-dimethoxy-17-methylmorphinan (methylcodeine),

E. R1 = R2 = OH, R3 = H: 7,8-didehydro-4,5α-epoxy-3-methoxy-17-methylmorphinan-6α,10-diol,

F. R1 = R3 = OH, R2 = H: 7,8-didehydro-4,5α-epoxy-3-methoxy-17-methylmorphinan-6α,14-diol,

B. morphine,

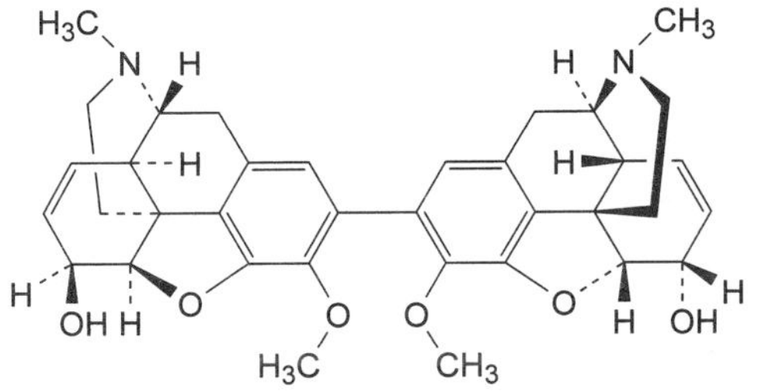

C. 7,7′,8,8′-tetradehydro-4,5α:4′,5′α-diepoxy-3,3′-dimethoxy-17,17′-dimethyl-2,2′-bimorphinanyl-6α,6′α-diol (codeine dimer),

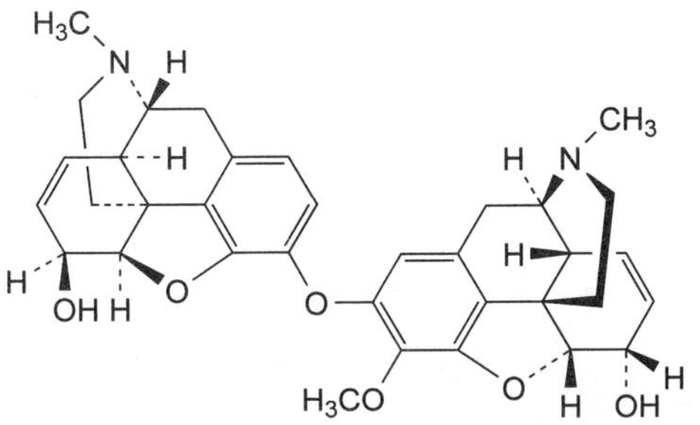

D. 7,8-didehydro-2-[(7,8-didehydro-4,5α-epoxy-6α-hydroxy-17-methylmorphinan-3-yl)oxy]-4,5α-epoxy-3-methoxy-17-methylmorphinan-6α-ol (3-*O*-(codein-2-yl)morphine),

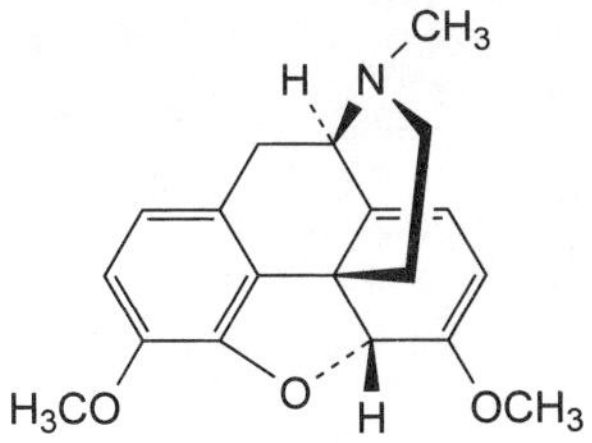

G. 6,7,8,14-tetradehydro-4,5α-epoxy-3,6-dimethoxy-17-methylmorphinan (thebaine).

07/2004:0075

CODEINE PHOSPHATE SESQUIHYDRATE

Codeini phosphas sesquihydricus

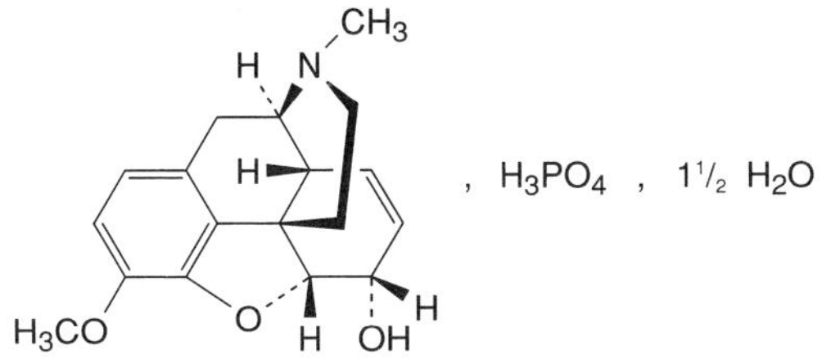

$C_{18}H_{24}NO_7P,1^1/_2H_2O$ M_r 424.4

DEFINITION

7,8-Didehydro-4,5α-epoxy-3-methoxy-17-methylmorphinan-6α-ol phosphate sesquihydrate.

Content: 98.5 per cent to 101.0 per cent (dried substance).

CHARACTERS

Appearance: white or almost white, crystalline powder or small, colourless crystals.

Solubility: freely soluble in water, slightly soluble in alcohol.

IDENTIFICATION

First identification: B, E, F.

Second identification: A, C, D, E, F, G.

A. Dilute 1.0 ml of solution S (see Tests) to 100.0 ml with *water R*. To 25.0 ml of this solution add 25 ml of *water R* then 10 ml of *1 M sodium hydroxide* and dilute to 100.0 ml with *water R*. Examined between 250 nm and 350 nm (*2.2.25*), the solution shows only 1 absorption maximum, at 284 nm. The specific absorbance at the absorption maximum is about 38 (dried substance).

B. Infrared absorption spectrophotometry (*2.2.24*).

Preparation: dissolve 0.20 g in 4 ml of *water R*. Add 1 ml of a mixture of equal volumes of *strong sodium hydroxide solution R* and *water R* and initiate crystallisation, if necessary, by scratching the wall of the tube with a glass rod and cooling in iced water. Wash the precipitate with *water R* and dry at 100-105 °C. Examine the dried precipitate prepared as discs using *potassium bromide R*.

Comparison: *Ph. Eur. reference spectrum of codeine.*

C. Dissolve 0.20 g in 4 ml of *water R*. Add 1 ml of a mixture of equal volumes of *strong sodium hydroxide solution R* and *water R* and initiate crystallisation, if necessary, by scratching the wall of the tube with a glass rod and cooling in iced water. The precipitate, washed with *water R* and dried at 100-105 °C, melts (*2.2.14*) at 155 °C to 159 °C.

D. To about 10 mg add 1 ml of *sulphuric acid R* and 0.05 ml of *ferric chloride solution R2* and heat on a water-bath. A blue colour develops. Add 0.05 ml of *nitric acid R*. The colour changes to red.

E. It complies with the test for loss on drying (see Tests).

F. Solution S gives reaction (a) of phosphates (*2.3.1*).

G. It gives the reaction of alkaloids (*2.3.1*).

TESTS

Solution S. Dissolve 1.00 g in *carbon dioxide-free water R* prepared from *distilled water R* and dilute to 25.0 ml with the same solvent.

pH (*2.2.3*): 4.0 to 5.0 for solution S.

Specific optical rotation (*2.2.7*): − 98 to − 102 (dried substance).

Dilute 5.0 ml of solution S to 10.0 ml with *water R*.

Related substances. Liquid chromatography (*2.2.29*).

Test solution. Dissolve 0.100 g of the substance to be examined and 0.100 g of *sodium octanesulphonate R* in the mobile phase and dilute to 10.0 ml with the mobile phase.

Reference solution (a). Dissolve 5.0 mg of *codeine impurity A CRS* in the mobile phase and dilute to 5.0 ml with the mobile phase.

Reference solution (b). Dilute 1.0 ml of reference solution (a) to 20.0 ml with the mobile phase.

Reference solution (c). Dilute 1.0 ml of the test solution to 50.0 ml with the mobile phase. Dilute 5.0 ml of this solution to 100.0 ml with the mobile phase.

Reference solution (d). Dilute 0.5 ml of the test solution to 5.0 ml with reference solution (a).

Column:

– *size*: *l* = 0.25 m, Ø = 4.6 mm,
– *stationary phase*: *end-capped octylsilyl silica gel for chromatography R* (5 µm).

Mobile phase: dissolve 1.08 g of *sodium octanesulphonate R* in a mixture of 20 ml of *glacial acetic acid R* and 250 ml of *acetonitrile R* and dilute to 1000 ml with *water R*.

Flow rate: 2 ml/min.

Detection: spectrophotometer at 245 nm.

Injection: 10 µl.

Run time: 10 times the retention time of codeine.

Relative retention with reference to codeine (retention time = about 6 min): impurity B = about 0.6; impurity E = about 0.7; impurity A = about 2.0; impurity C = about 2.3; impurity D = about 3.6.

System suitability: reference solution (d):

– *resolution*: minimum 3 between the peaks due to codeine and impurity A.

Limits:

– *correction factor*: for the calculation of content, multiply the peak area of impurity C by 0.25,
– *impurity A*: not more than twice the area of the principal peak in the chromatogram obtained with reference solution (b) (1.0 per cent),
– *impurities B, C, D, E*: for each impurity, not more than twice the area of the principal peak in the chromatogram obtained with reference solution (c) (0.2 per cent),
– *any other impurity*: for each impurity, not more than the area of the principal peak in the chromatogram obtained with reference solution (c) (0.1 per cent),
– *total of impurities other than A*: not more than 10 times the area of the principal peak in the chromatogram obtained with reference solution (c) (1.0 per cent),
– *disregard limit*: 0.5 times the area of the principal peak in the chromatogram obtained with reference solution (c) (0.05 per cent).

Sulphates (*2.4.13*): maximum 0.1 per cent.

Dilute 5 ml of solution S to 20 ml with *distilled water R*. 15 ml of the solution complies with the limit test for sulphates.

Loss on drying (*2.2.32*): 5.0 per cent to 7.5 per cent, determined on 0.500 g by drying in an oven at 100-105 °C.

ASSAY

Dissolve 0.350 g in a mixture of 10 ml of *anhydrous acetic acid R* and 20 ml of *dioxan R*. Titrate with *0.1 M perchloric acid* using 0.05 ml of *crystal violet solution R* as indicator.

1 ml of *0.1 M perchloric acid* is equivalent to 39.74 mg of $C_{18}H_{24}NO_7P$.

STORAGE

Protected from light.

IMPURITIES

Specified impurities (see note for information p. xli): A, B, C, D, E.

Other detectable impurities: F, G.

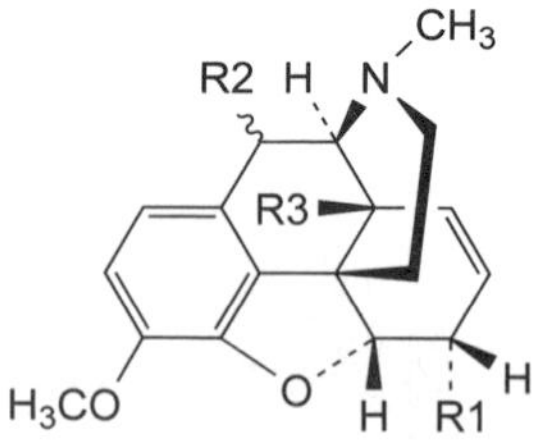

A. R1 = OCH_3, R2 = R3 = H: 7,8-didehydro-4,5α-epoxy-3,6α-dimethoxy-17-methylmorphinan (methylcodeine),

E. R1 = R2 = OH, R3 = H: 7,8-didehydro-4,5α-epoxy-3-methoxy-17-methylmorphinan-6α,10-diol,

F. R1 = R3 = OH, R2 = H: 7,8-didehydro-4,5α-epoxy-3-methoxy-17-methylmorphinan-6α,14-diol,

B. morphine,

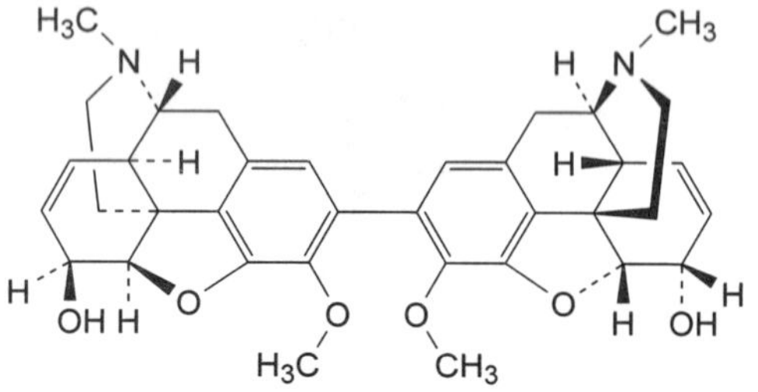

C. 7,7′,8,8′-tetradehydro-4,5α:4′,5′α-diepoxy-3,3′-dimethoxy-17,17′-dimethyl-2,2′-bimorphinanyl-6α,6′α-diol (codeine dimer),

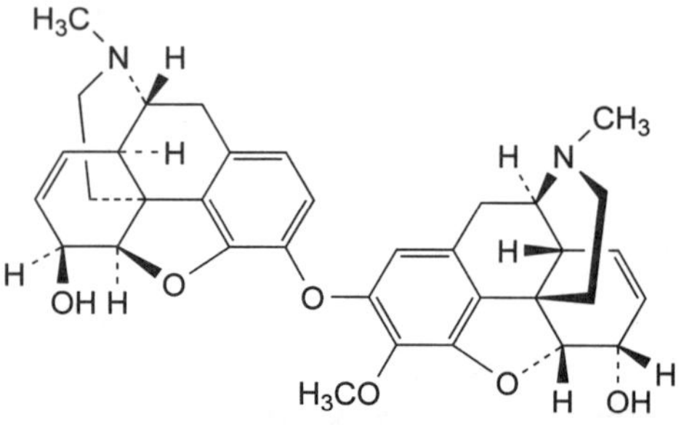

D. 7,8-didehydro-2-[(7,8-didehydro-4,5α-epoxy-6α-hydroxy-17-methylmorphinan-3-yl)oxy]-4,5α-epoxy-3-methoxy-17-methylmorphinan-6α-ol (3-*O*-(codein-2-yl)morphine),

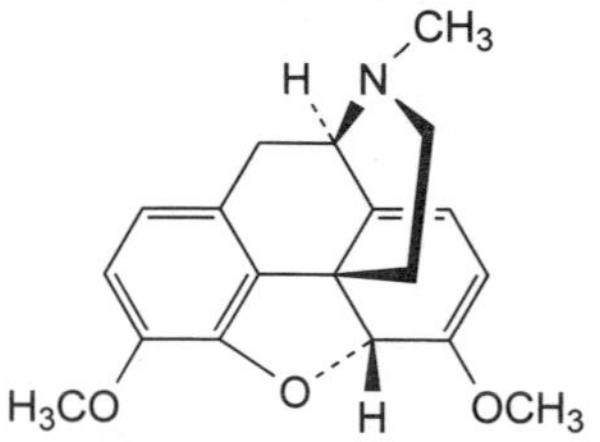

G. 6,7,8,14-tetradehydro-4,5α-epoxy-3,6-dimethoxy-17-methylmorphinan (thebaine).

D

07/2004:0232

DISODIUM EDETATE

Dinatrii edetas

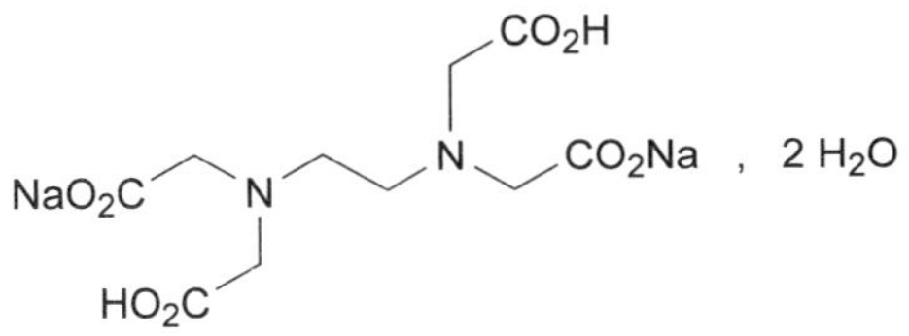

$C_{10}H_{14}N_2Na_2O_8,2H_2O$ M_r 372.2

DEFINITION

Disodium dihydrogen (ethylenedinitrilo)tetraacetate dihydrate.

Content: 98.5 per cent to 101.0 per cent.

CHARACTERS

Appearance: white, crystalline powder.

Solubility: soluble in water, practically insoluble in alcohol.

IDENTIFICATION

First identification: A, B, D.

Second identification: B, C, D.

A. Infrared absorption spectrophotometry (*2.2.24*).

Preparation: discs.

Comparison: *disodium edetate CRS.*

B. Dissolve 2 g in 25 ml of *water R*, add 6 ml of *lead nitrate solution R*, shake and add 3 ml of *potassium iodide solution R*. No yellow precipitate is formed. Make alkaline to *red litmus paper R* by the addition of *dilute ammonia R2.* Add 3 ml of *ammonium oxalate solution R*. No precipitate is formed.

C. Dissolve 0.5 g in 10 ml of *water R* and add 0.5 ml of *calcium chloride solution R*. Make alkaline to *red litmus paper R* by the addition of *dilute ammonia R2* and add 3 ml of *ammonium oxalate solution R*. No precipitate is formed.

D. It gives the reactions of sodium (*2.3.1*).

TESTS

Solution S. Dissolve 5.0 g in *carbon dioxide-free water R* and dilute to 100 ml with the same solvent.

Appearance of solution. Solution S is clear (*2.2.1*) and colourless (*2.2.2, Method II*).

pH (*2.2.3*): 4.0 to 5.5 for solution S.

Impurity A. Liquid chromatography (*2.2.29*). *Carry out the test protected from light.*

Solvent mixture. Dissolve 10.0 g of *ferric sulphate pentahydrate R* in 20 ml of *0.5 M sulphuric acid* and add 780 ml of *water R*. Adjust to pH 2.0 with *1 M sodium hydroxide* and dilute to 1000 ml with *water R*.

Test solution. Dissolve 0.100 g of the substance to be examined in the solvent mixture and dilute to 25.0 ml with the solvent mixture.

Reference solution. Dissolve 40.0 mg of *nitrilotriacetic acid R* in the solvent mixture and dilute to 100.0 ml with the solvent mixture. To 1.0 ml of the solution add 0.1 ml of the test solution and dilute to 100.0 ml with the solvent mixture.

Column:

– *size*: *l* = 0.10 m, Ø = 4.6 mm,

– *stationary phase*: spherical *graphitised carbon for chromatography R1* (5 µm) with a specific surface area of 120 m^2/g and a pore size of 25 nm.

Mobile phase: dissolve 50.0 mg of *ferric sulphate pentahydrate R* in 50 ml of *0.5 M sulphuric acid* and add 750 ml of *water R*. Adjust to pH 1.5 with *0.5 M sulphuric acid* or *1 M sodium hydroxide*, add 20 ml of *ethylene glycol R* and dilute to 1000 ml with *water R*.

Flow rate: 1 ml/min.

Detection: spectrophotometer at 273 nm.

Injection: 20 µl; filter the solutions and inject immediately.

Run time: 4 times the retention time of the iron complex of impurity A.

Retention times: iron complex of impurity A = about 5 min; iron complex of edetic acid = about 10 min.

System suitability: reference solution:

– *resolution*: minimum 7 between the peaks due to the iron complex of impurity A and the iron complex of edetic acid,

– *signal-to-noise ratio*: minimum 50 for the peak due to impurity A.

Limits:

– *impurity A*: not more than the area of the corresponding peak in the chromatogram obtained with the reference solution (0.1 per cent).

Iron (*2.4.9*): maximum 80 ppm.

Dilute 2.5 ml of solution S to 10 ml with *water R*. Add 0.25 g of *calcium chloride R* to the test solution and the standard before the addition of the *thioglycollic acid R*.

Heavy metals (*2.4.8*): maximum 20 ppm.

1.0 g complies with limit test D. Prepare the standard using 2 ml of *lead standard solution (10 ppm Pb) R*.

ASSAY

Dissolve 0.300 g in *water R* and dilute to 300 ml with the same solvent. Add 2 g of *hexamethylenetetramine R* and 2 ml of *dilute hydrochloric acid R*. Titrate with *0.1 M lead nitrate*, using about 50 mg of *xylenol orange triturate R* as indicator.

1 ml of *0.1 M lead nitrate* is equivalent to 37.22 mg of $C_{10}H_{14}N_2Na_2O_8,2H_2O$.

STORAGE

Protected from light.

IMPURITIES

Specified impurities (see note for information p. xli): A.

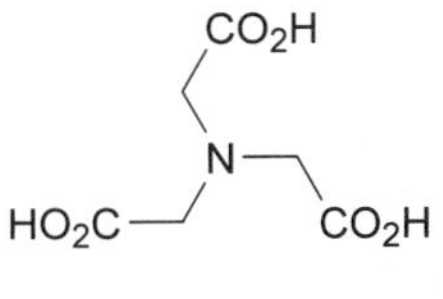

A. nitrilotriacetic acid.

07/2004:1007

DITHRANOL

Dithranolum

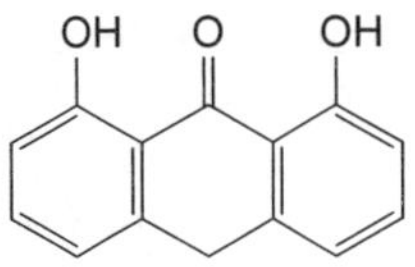

$C_{14}H_{10}O_3$ M_r 226.2

DEFINITION

Dithranol contains not less than 98.5 per cent and not more than the equivalent of 101.0 per cent of 1,8-dihydroxyanthracen-9(10*H*)-one, calculated with reference to the dried substance.

CHARACTERS

A yellow or brownish-yellow, crystalline powder, practically insoluble in water, soluble in methylene chloride, sparingly soluble in acetone, slightly soluble in alcohol. It dissolves in dilute solutions of alkali hydroxides.

Carry out all tests protected from bright light and use freshly prepared solutions.

IDENTIFICATION

First identification: A, B.

Second identification: A, C, D.

A. It melts (*2.2.14*) at 178 °C to 182 °C.

B. Examine by infrared absorption spectrophotometry (*2.2.24*), comparing with the spectrum obtained with *dithranol CRS*.

C. Examine by thin-layer chromatography (*2.2.27*), using *silica gel H R* as the coating substance.

Test solution. Dissolve 10 mg of the substance to be examined in *methylene chloride R* and dilute to 10 ml with the same solvent.

Reference solution (a). Dissolve 10 mg of *dithranol CRS* in *methylene chloride R* and dilute to 10 ml with the same solvent.

Reference solution (b). Dissolve about 5 mg of *dantron R* in 5 ml of reference solution (a).

Apply to the plate 10 µl of each solution. Develop over a path of 12 cm using a mixture of equal volumes of *hexane R* and *methylene chloride R*. Allow the plate to dry in air. Place the plate in a tank saturated with ammonia vapour until the spots appear. Examine in daylight. The principal spot in the chromatogram obtained with the test solution is similar in position, colour and size to the principal spot in the chromatogram obtained with reference solution (a). The test is not valid unless the chromatogram obtained with reference solution (b) shows 2 clearly separated spots.

D. To 5 mg add 0.1 g of *anhydrous sodium acetate R* and 1 ml of *acetic anhydride R*. Boil for 30 s. Add 20 ml of *alcohol R*. Examined in ultraviolet light at 365 nm, the solution shows a blue fluorescence.

TESTS

Related substances

A. Examine by liquid chromatography (*2.2.29*).

Test solution. Dissolve 0.200 g of the substance to be examined in 20 ml of *methylene chloride R*, add 1.0 ml of *glacial acetic acid R* and dilute to 100.0 ml with *hexane R*.

Reference solution. Dissolve 5.0 mg each of *anthrone R*, *dantron R*, *dithranol impurity C CRS* and *dithranol CRS* in *methylene chloride R* and dilute to 5.0 ml with the same solvent. To 1.0 ml of the solution, add 19.0 ml of *methylene chloride R* and 1.0 ml of *glacial acetic acid R*, and dilute to 50.0 ml with *hexane R*.

The chromatographic procedure may be carried out using:

- a stainless steel column 0.25 m long and 4.6 mm in internal diameter packed with *silica gel for chromatography R* (5 µm),
- as mobile phase at a flow rate of 2 ml/min a mixture of 1 volume of *glacial acetic acid R*, 5 volumes of *methylene chloride R* and 82 volumes of *hexane R*,
- as detector a spectrophotometer set at 260 nm.

Inject 20 µl of each solution. Continue the chromatography for 1.5 times the retention time of dithranol impurity C. Adjust the sensitivity of the system so that the height of the principal peak in the chromatogram obtained with the reference solution is about 70 per cent of the full scale of the recorder. When the chromatograms are recorded in the prescribed conditions, the substances are eluted in the following sequence: dithranol, dantron, anthrone, dithranol impurity C. The test is not valid unless, in the chromatogram obtained with the reference solution, the resolution between the peaks due to dithranol and dantron is greater than 2.0. In the chromatogram obtained with the test solution: the area of any peak corresponding to anthrone, dantron or dithranol impurity C is not greater than that of the corresponding peak in the chromatogram obtained with the reference solution (1 per cent); the area of any peak apart from the principal peak and any peaks due to anthrone, dantron and dithranol impurity C is not greater than that of the peak due to dithranol in the chromatogram obtained with the reference solution (1 per cent).

B. Examine by liquid chromatography (*2.2.29*).

Test solution. Dissolve 25.0 mg of the substance to be examined in 5 ml of *tetrahydrofuran R* and dilute to 25.0 ml with the mobile phase.

Reference solution. Dissolve 5.0 mg of *dithranol impurity D CRS* and 5.0 mg of *dithranol CRS* in 5 ml of *tetrahydrofuran R* and dilute to 10.0 ml with the mobile phase. Dilute 1.0 ml of the solution to 20.0 ml with the mobile phase.

The chromatographic procedure may be carried out using:

- a stainless steel column 0.20 m long and 4.6 mm in internal diameter packed with *octadecylsilyl silica gel for chromatography R* (5 µm),
- as mobile phase at a flow rate of 0.9 ml/min a mixture of 2.5 volumes of *glacial acetic acid R*, 40 volumes of *tetrahydrofuran R* and 60 volumes of *water R*,
- as detector a spectrophotometer set at 254 nm.

Inject 20 µl of each solution. Continue the chromatography for 3 times the retention time of the peak due to dithranol. Adjust the sensitivity of the system so that the height of the principal peak in the chromatogram obtained with the reference solution is about 50 per cent of the full scale of the recorder. The test is not valid unless, in the chromatogram obtained with the reference solution, the resolution between the peaks due to dithranol impurity D and dithranol is greater than 2.5. In the chromatogram obtained with the test solution, the area of any peak corresponding to dithranol impurity Dis not greater than that of the corresponding peak in the chromatogram obtained with the reference solution (2.5 per cent).

The total content of related substances as determined in tests A and B is not more than 3.0 per cent.

Chlorides (*2.4.4*). Shake 1.0 g with 20 ml of *water R* for 1 min and filter. Dilute 10 ml of the filtrate to 15 ml with *water R*. The solution complies with the limit test for chlorides (100 ppm).

Loss on drying (*2.2.32*). Not more than 0.5 per cent, determined on 1.000 g by drying in an oven at 100-105 °C

Sulphated ash (*2.4.14*). Not more than 0.1 per cent, determined on 1.0 g.

ASSAY

Dissolve 0.200 g in 50 ml of *anhydrous pyridine R*. Titrate with *0.1 M tetrabutylammonium hydroxide* under *nitrogen R*. Determine the end-point potentiometrically

(*2.2.20*), using a glass indicator electrode and a calomel reference electrode containing, as the electrolyte, a saturated solution of *potassium chloride R* in *methanol R*.

1 ml of *0.1 M tetrabutylammonium hydroxide* is equivalent to 22.62 mg of $C_{14}H_{10}O_3$.

STORAGE

Store protected from light.

IMPURITIES

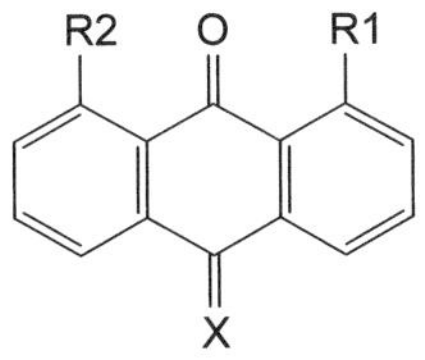

A. R1 = R2 = H, X = H_2: anthracen-9(10*H*)-one (anthrone),

B. R1 = R2 = OH, X = O: 1,8-dihydroxyanthracene-9,10-dione (danthron),

D. R1 = OH, R2 = H, X = H_2: 1-hydroxyanthracen-9(10*H*)-one,

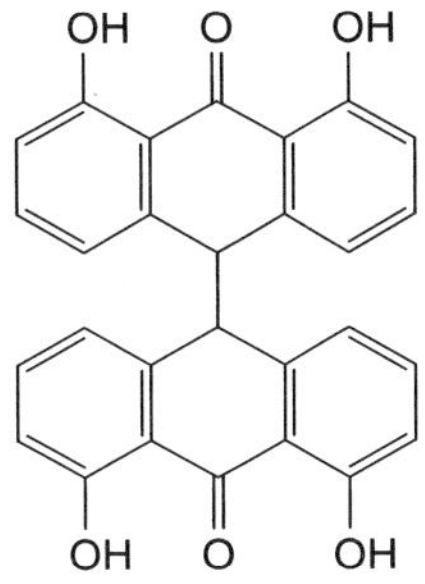

C. C. 4,4′,5,5′-tetrahydroxy-9,9′-bianthracenyl-10,10′(9*H*,9′*H*)-dione.

E

07/2004:1612

EDETIC ACID

Acidum edeticum

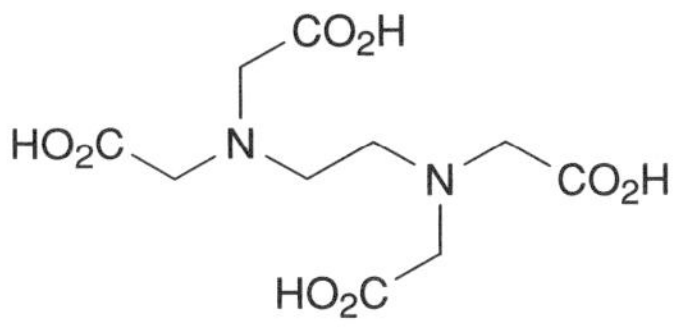

$C_{10}H_{16}N_2O_8$ M_r 292.2

DEFINITION

(Ethylenedinitrilo)tetraacetic acid.

Content: 98.0 per cent to 101.0 per cent.

CHARACTERS

Appearance: white, crystalline powder or colourless crystals.

Solubility: practically insoluble in water and in alcohol. It dissolves in dilute solutions of alkali hydroxides.

IDENTIFICATION

First identification: A.

Second identification: B, C.

A. Infrared absorption spectrophotometry (*2.2.24*).

Preparation: discs, after drying the substance to be examined in an oven at 100-105 °C for 2 h.

Comparison: *sodium edetate R*, treated as follows: dissolve 0.25 g of *sodium edetate R* in 5 ml of *water R*, add 1.0 ml of *dilute hydrochloric acid R*. Filter, wash the residue with 2 quantities, each of 5 ml, of *water R* and dry the residue in an oven at 100-105 °C for 2 h.

B. To 5 ml of *water R* add 0.1 ml of *ammonium thiocyanate solution R* and 0.1 ml of *ferric chloride solution R1* and mix. The solution is red. Add 0.5 ml of solution S (see Tests). The solution becomes yellowish.

C. To 10 ml of solution S add 0.5 ml of *calcium chloride solution R*. Make alkaline to *red litmus paper R* by the addition of *dilute ammonia R2* and add 3 ml of *ammonium oxalate solution R*. No precipitate is formed.

TESTS

Solution S. Dissolve 5.0 g in 20 ml of *dilute sodium hydroxide solution R* and dilute to 100 ml with *water R*.

Appearance of solution. Solution S is clear (*2.2.1*) and colourless (*2.2.2, Method II*).

Impurity A. Liquid chromatography (*2.2.29*). *Carry out the test protected from light.*

Solvent mixture. Dissolve 10.0 g of *ferric sulphate pentahydrate R* in 20 ml of *0.5 M sulphuric acid* and add 780 ml of *water R*. Adjust to pH 2.0 with *1 M sodium hydroxide* and dilute to 1000 ml with *water R*.

Test solution. Dissolve 0.100 g of the substance to be examined in 1.0 ml of *1 M sodium hydroxide* and dilute to 25.0 ml with the solvent mixture.

Reference solution. Dissolve 40.0 mg of *nitrilotriacetic acid R* in the solvent mixture and dilute to 100.0 ml with the solvent mixture. To 1.0 ml of the solution add 0.1 ml of the test solution and dilute to 100.0 ml with the solvent mixture.

Column:

- *size*: l = 0.10 m, Ø = 4.6 mm,
- *stationary phase*: spherical *graphitised carbon for chromatography R1* (5 µm) with a specific surface area of 120 m^2/g and a pore size of 25 nm.

Mobile phase: dissolve 50.0 mg of *ferric sulphate pentahydrate R* in 50 ml of *0.5 M sulphuric acid* and add 750 ml of *water R*. Adjust to pH 1.5 with *0.5 M sulphuric acid* or *1 M sodium hydroxide*, add 20 ml of *ethylene glycol R* and dilute to 1000 ml with *water R*.

Flow rate: 1 ml/min.

Detection: spectrophotometer at 273 nm.

Injection: 20 µl; filter the solutions and inject immediately.

Run time: 4 times the retention time of the iron complex of impurity A.

Retention time: iron complex of impurity A = about 5 min; iron complex of edetic acid = about 10 min.

System suitability: reference solution:

- *resolution*: minimum 7 between the peaks due to the iron complex of impurity A and the iron complex of edetic acid,
- *signal-to-noise ratio*: minimum 50 for the peak due to impurity A.

Limits:

- *impurity A*: not more than the area of the corresponding peak in the chromatogram obtained with the reference solution (0.1 per cent).

Chlorides (*2.4.4*): maximum 200 ppm.

To 10 ml of solution S add 8 ml of *nitric acid R* and stir for 10 min. A precipitate is formed. Filter and wash the filter with *water R*. Collect the filtrate and the washings and dilute to 20 ml with *water R*. Dilute 10 ml of this solution to 15 ml with *water R*.

Iron (*2.4.9*): maximum 80 ppm.

Dilute 2.5 ml of solution S to 10 ml with *water R* and add 0.25 g of *calcium chloride R* before adding the *thioglycollic acid R*. Allow to stand for 5 min. Also add 0.25 g of *calcium chloride R* to the standard.

Heavy metals (*2.4.8*): maximum 20 ppm.

1.0 g complies with limit test D. Use a fused-silica crucible. If necessary moisten the residue on ignition with *nitric acid R* and ignite until a white residue is obtained. Prepare the standard using 2 ml of *lead standard solution (10 ppm Pb) R*.

Sulphated ash (*2.4.14*): maximum 0.2 per cent, determined on 1.0 g.

ASSAY

Dissolve 0.250 g in 2.0 ml of *dilute sodium hydroxide solution R* and dilute to 300 ml with *water R*. Add 2 g of *hexamethylenetetramine R* and 2 ml of *dilute hydrochloric acid R*. Titrate with *0.1 M zinc sulphate* using about 50 mg of *xylenol orange triturate R* as indicator.

1 ml of *0.1 M zinc sulphate* corresponds to 29.22 mg of $C_{10}H_{16}N_2O_8$.

STORAGE

Protected from light.

IMPURITIES

Specified impurities (see note for information p. xli): A.

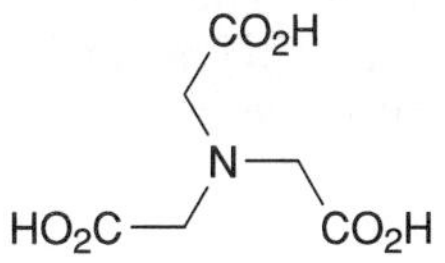

A. nitrilotriacetic acid.

Monographs D - K

07/2004:0821

ESTRADIOL HEMIHYDRATE

Estradiolum hemihydricum

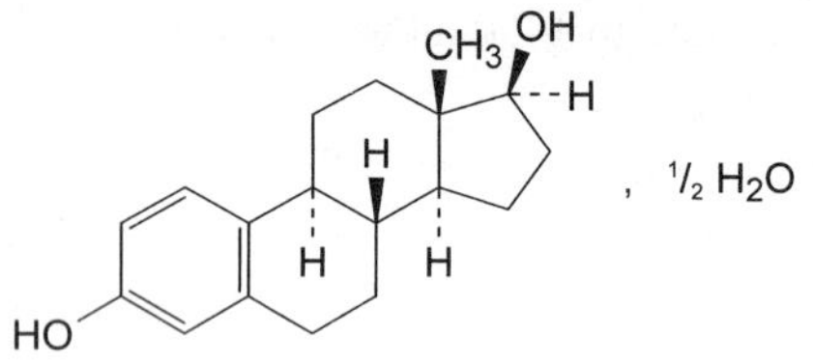

$C_{18}H_{24}O_2, ^1/_2\ H_2O$ M_r 281.4

DEFINITION

Estra-1,3,5(10)-triene-3,17β-diol hemihydrate.

Content: 97.0 per cent to 103.0 per cent (anhydrous substance).

CHARACTERS

Appearance: white or almost white, crystalline powder or colourless crystals.

Solubility: practically insoluble in water, soluble in acetone, sparingly soluble in alcohol, slightly soluble in methylene chloride.

IDENTIFICATION

First identification: B.

Second identification: A, C, D, E.

A. Melting point (*2.2.14*): 175 °C to 180 °C.

B. Infrared absorption spectrophotometry (*2.2.24*).

Comparison: *estradiol hemihydrate CRS.*

C. Thin-layer chromatography (*2.2.27*).

Test solution. Dissolve 50 mg of the substance to be examined in *methanol R* and dilute to 50 ml with the same solvent.

Reference solution (a). Dissolve 50 mg of *estradiol hemihydrate CRS* in *methanol R* and dilute to 50 ml with the same solvent.

Reference solution (b). Dissolve 25 mg of *ethinylestradiol CRS* in reference solution (a) and dilute to 25 ml with reference solution (a).

Plate: *TLC silica gel plate R.*

Mobile phase: *alcohol R, toluene R* (20:80 *V/V*).

Application: 5 μl.

Development: over 3/4 of the plate.

Drying: in air until the solvent has evaporated.

Detection: heat at 110 °C for 10 min. Spray the hot plate with *alcoholic solution of sulphuric acid R.* Heat again at 110 °C for 10 min. Allow to cool. Examine in daylight and in ultraviolet light at 365 nm.

System suitability: the chromatogram obtained with reference solution (b) shows 2 spots which may however not be completely separated.

Results: the principal spot in the chromatogram obtained with the test solution is similar in position, colour in daylight, fluorescence in ultraviolet light at 365 nm and size to the principal spot in the chromatogram obtained with reference solution (a).

D. To about 1 mg add 0.5 ml of freshly prepared *sulphomolybdic reagent R2.* A blue colour develops which in ultraviolet light at 365 nm has an intense green fluorescence. Add 1 ml of *sulphuric acid R* and 9 ml of *water R*. The colour becomes pink with a yellowish fluorescence.

E. It complies with the test for water (see Tests).

TESTS

Specific optical rotation (*2.2.7*): + 76.0 to + 83.0 (anhydrous substance).

Dissolve 0.250 g in *alcohol R* and dilute to 25.0 ml with the same solvent.

Related substances. Liquid chromatography (*2.2.29*).

Test solution. Dissolve 25.0 mg of the substance to be examined in 10 ml of *acetonitrile R* and dilute to 25.0 ml with *methanol R2.*

Reference solution (a). Dilute 1.0 ml of the test solution to 100.0 ml with the mobile phase. Dilute 2.0 ml of the solution to 10.0 ml with the mobile phase.

Reference solution (b). Dissolve 2 mg of *17α-estradiol R* in 5.0 ml of *acetonitrile R.* Mix 2.0 ml of this solution with 1.0 ml of the test solution and dilute to 5.0 ml with the mobile phase.

Reference solution (c). Mix equal volumes of a 1 mg/ml solution of the substance to be examined in *methanol R2* and of a 1 mg/ml solution of *2,3-dichloro-5,6-dicyanobenzoquinone R* in *methanol R2.* Allow to stand for 30 min before injection.

Reference solution (d). Dissolve 5 mg of *estradiol for peak identification CRS* (estradiol hemihydrate spiked with impurities A, B and C at about 0.5 per cent) in 2 ml of *acetonitrile R* and dilute to 5 ml with *methanol R2.*

Column:

- size: l = 0.25 m, Ø = 4.6 mm,
- *stationary phase*: *end-capped octadecylsilyl silica gel for chromatography R* (5 μm).

Mobile phase: to 400 ml of *acetonitrile R* add 50 ml of *methanol R2* and 400 ml of *water R*; allow to stand for 10 min, dilute to 1000 ml with *water R* and mix again.

Flow rate: 1 ml/min.

Detection: spectrophotometer at 280 nm.

Equilibration: about 60 min.

Injection: 20 μl.

Run time: twice the retention time of the principal peak.

Relative retention with reference to estradiol (retention time = about 13 min): impurity D = about 0.9; impurity B = about 1.1; impurity A = about 1.4; impurity C = about 1.9.

System suitability: reference solution (b):

- *resolution*: minimum 2.5 between the peaks due to estradiol and impurity B.

Limits:

- *correction factor*: for the calculation of content, multiply the peak area of impurity D by 0.4 (use the chromatogram obtained with reference solution (c) to identify this peak),
- *impurities A, B, C, D*: for each impurity, not more than 1.5 times the area of the principal peak obtained with reference solution (a) (0.3 per cent),
- *any other impurity*: for each impurity, not more than 0.5 times the area of the principal peak obtained with reference solution (a) (0.1 per cent),
- *total*: not more than 2.5 times the area of the principal peak in the chromatogram obtained with reference solution (a) (0.5 per cent),

– *disregard limit*: 0.25 times the area of the principal peak in the chromatogram obtained with reference solution (a) (0.05 per cent).

Water (*2.5.12*): 2.9 per cent to 3.5 per cent, determined on 0.500 g.

ASSAY

Dissolve 20.0 mg in *alcohol R* and dilute to 100.0 ml with the same solvent. Dilute 5.0 ml of the solution to 50.0 ml with *0.1 M sodium hydroxide*. Allow to cool to room temperature. Measure the absorbance (*2.2.25*) of the solution at the maximum at 238 nm.

Calculate the content of $C_{18}H_{24}O_2$ taking the specific absorbance to be 335.

IMPURITIES

Specified impurities (see note for information p. xli): A, B, C, D.

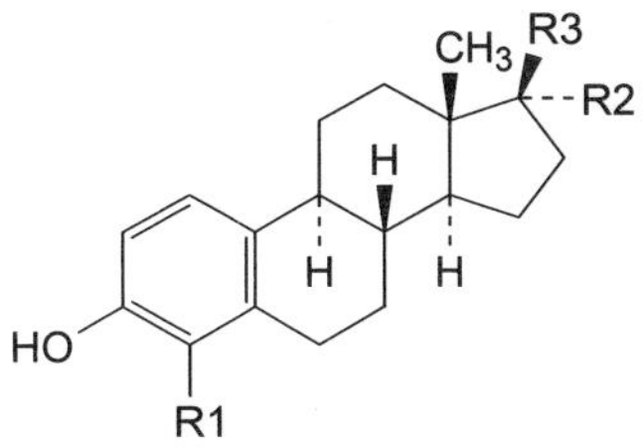

A. R1 = H, R2 + R3 = O: 3-hydroxyestra-1,3,5(10)-trien-17-one (estrone),

B. R1 = R3 = H, R2 = OH: estra-1,3,5(10)-triene-3,17α-diol (17α-estradiol),

C. R1 = CH_3, R2 = H, R3 = OH: 4-methylestra-1,3,5(10)-triene-3,17β-diol,

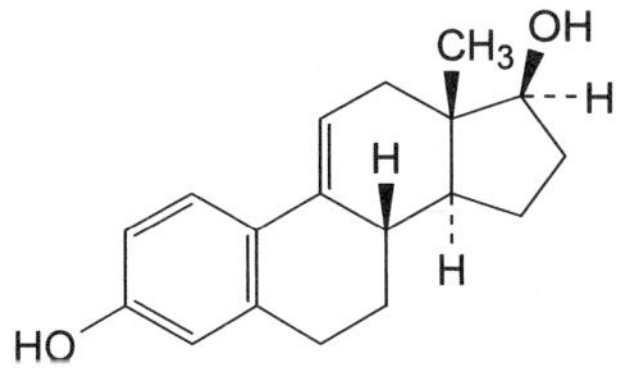

D. estra-1,3,5(10),9(11)-tetraene-3,17β-diol.

F

07/2004:1326

FLUMAZENIL

Flumazenilum

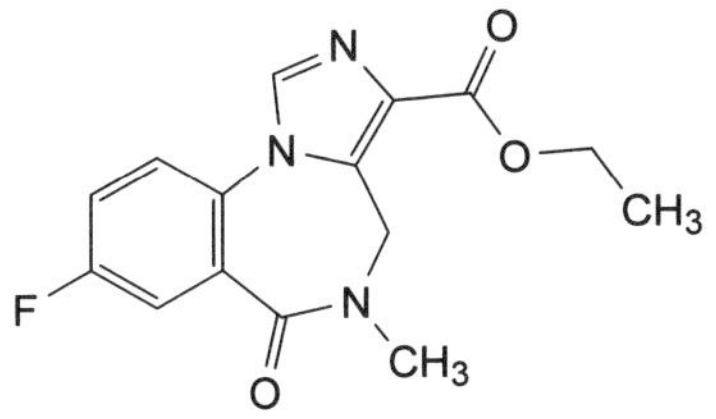

$C_{15}H_{14}FN_3O_3$ M_r 303.3

DEFINITION

Ethyl 8-fluoro-5-methyl-6-oxo-5,6-dihydro-4*H*-imidazo[1,5-*a*][1,4]benzodiazepine-3-carboxylate.

Content: 99.0 per cent to 101.0 per cent (dried substance).

CHARACTERS

Appearance: white or almost white, crystalline powder.

Solubility: very slightly soluble in water, freely soluble in methylene chloride, sparingly soluble in methanol.

mp: 198 °C to 202 °C.

IDENTIFICATION

Infrared absorption spectrophotometry (*2.2.24*).

Comparison: *Ph. Eur. reference spectrum of flumazenil.*

TESTS

Appearance of solution. The solution is clear (*2.2.1*) and is not more intensely coloured than reference solution BY_7 (*2.2.2, Method II*).

Dissolve 0.10 g in *methanol R* and dilute to 10 ml with the same solvent.

Impurity C: maximum 1 per cent.

Dissolve 0.10 g in 0.5 ml of *methylene chloride R* and dilute to 10 ml with *butanol R*. To 5.0 ml of this solution add 2.0 ml of *ninhydrin solution R* and heat in a water-bath at 95 °C for 15 min. Any blue-purple colour in the solution is not more intense than that in a standard prepared at the same time and in the same manner using 5.0 ml of a 0.1 g/l solution of *dimethylformamide diethylacetal R* in *butanol R*.

Related substances. Liquid chromatography (*2.2.29*).

Test solution. Dissolve 50.0 mg of the substance to be examined in 5 ml of *methanol R* and dilute to 25.0 ml with the mobile phase.

Reference solution (a). Dissolve 2.0 mg of *flumazenil impurity B CRS* and 2.0 mg of the substance to be examined in the mobile phase and dilute to 25.0 ml with the mobile phase. Dilute 2.0 ml of this solution to 25.0 ml with the mobile phase.

Reference solution (b). Dilute 10.0 ml of the test solution to 100.0 ml with the mobile phase. Dilute 1.0 ml of this solution to 100.0 ml with the mobile phase.

Column:

- *size*: l = 0.25 m, Ø = 4.6 mm,
- *stationary phase*: *end-capped octadecylsilyl silica gel for chromatography R* (5 μm).

Mobile phase: to 800 ml of *water R* adjusted to pH 2.0 with *phosphoric acid R*, add 130 ml of *methanol R* and 70 ml of *tetrahydrofuran R* and mix.

Flow rate: 1 ml/min.

Detection: spectrophotometer at 230 nm.

Injection: 20 μl.

Run time: 3 times the retention time of flumazenil.

Relative retention with reference to flumazenil (retention time = about 14 min): impurity A = about 0.4; impurity D = about 0.5; impurity E = about 0.6; impurity B = about 0.7; impurity F = about 2.4.

System suitability: reference solution (a):

- *resolution*: minimum 3.0 between the peaks due to impurity B and flumazenil.

Limits:

- *impurity B*: not more than twice the area of the principal peak in the chromatogram obtained with reference solution (b) (0.2 per cent),
- *any other impurity*: for each impurity, not more than the area of the principal peak in the chromatogram obtained with reference solution (b) (0.1 per cent),
- *total*: not more than twice the area of the principal peak in the chromatogram obtained with reference solution (b) (0.2 per cent),
- *disregard limit*: 0.5 times the area of the principal peak in the chromatogram obtained with reference solution (b) (0.05 per cent).

Loss on drying (*2.2.32*): maximum 0.5 per cent, determined on 1.000 g by drying in an oven at 100-105 °C.

Sulphated ash (*2.4.14*): maximum 0.1 per cent, determined on 1.0 g in a platinum crucible.

ASSAY

Dissolve 0.250 g in 50 ml of a mixture of 2 volumes of *acetic anhydride R* and 3 volumes of *anhydrous acetic acid R*. Titrate with *0.1 M perchloric acid*, determining the end-point potentiometrically (*2.2.20*).

1 ml of *0.1 M perchloric acid* is equivalent to 30.33 mg of $C_{15}H_{14}FN_3O_3$.

IMPURITIES

Specified impurities (see note for information p. xli): B, C.

Other detectable impurities: A, D, E, F.

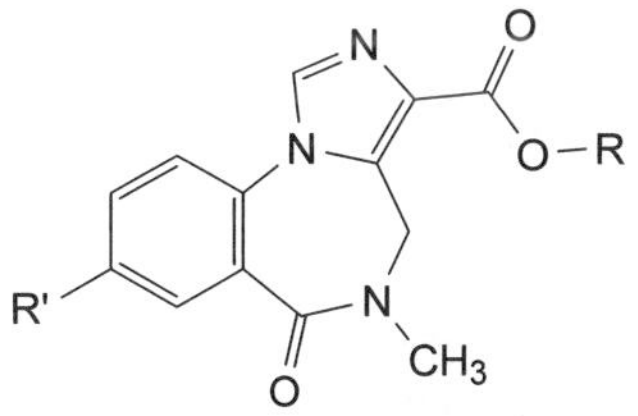

A. R = H, R′ = F: 8-fluoro-5-methyl-6-oxo-5,6-dihydro-4*H*-imidazo[1,5-*a*][1,4]benzodiazepine-3-carboxylic acid,

B. R = C_2-H_5, R′ = OH: ethyl 8-hydroxy-5-methyl-6-oxo-5,6-dihydro-4*H*-imidazo[1,5-*a*][1,4]benzodiazepine-3-carboxylate,

E. R = C_2H_5, R′ = H: ethyl 5-methyl-6-oxo-5,6-dihydro-4*H*-imidazo[1,5-*a*][1,4]benzodiazepine-3-carboxylate,

F. R = C_2H_5, R′ = Cl: ethyl 8-chloro-5-methyl-6-oxo-5,6-dihydro-4*H*-imidazo[1,5-*a*][1,4]benzodiazepine-3-carboxylate,

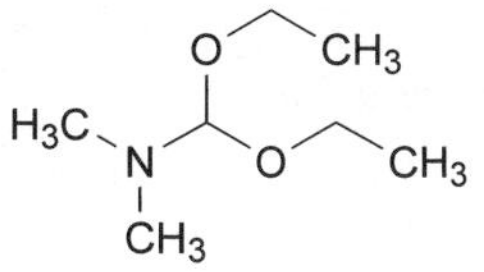

C. diethoxy-*N*,*N*-dimethylmethanamine,

Monographs D - K

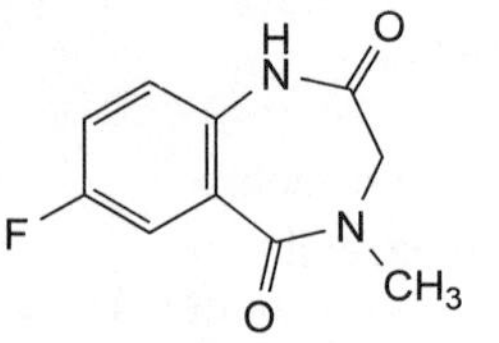

D. 7-fluoro-4-methyl-3,4-dihydro-1*H*-1,4-benzodiazepine-2,5-dione.

01/2003:0717
corrected

FLUNITRAZEPAM

Flunitrazepamum

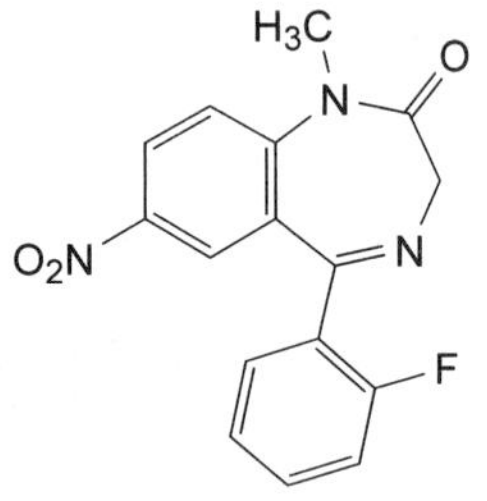

$C_{16}H_{12}FN_3O_3$ M_r 313.3

DEFINITION

5-(2-Fluorophenyl)-1-methyl-7-nitro-1,3-dihydro-2*H*-1,4-benzodiazepin-2-one.

Content: 99.0 per cent to 101.0 per cent (dried substance).

CHARACTERS

Appearance: white or yellowish, crystalline powder.

Solubility: practically insoluble in water, soluble in acetone, slightly soluble in alcohol.

IDENTIFICATION

Infrared absorption spectrophotometry (*2.2.24*).

Comparison: *Ph. Eur. reference spectrum of flunitrazepam.*

TESTS

Related substances. Liquid chromatography (*2.2.29*). *Prepare the solutions immediately before use.*

Test solution. Dissolve 100.0 mg of the substance to be examined in 10 ml of *acetonitrile R* and dilute to 50.0 ml with the mobile phase.

Reference solution (a). Dilute 1.0 ml of the test solution to 100.0 ml with the mobile phase. Dilute 5.0 ml of this solution to 50.0 ml with the mobile phase.

Reference solution (b). Dissolve 4 mg of the substance to be examined and 4 mg of *nitrazepam R* in 5 ml of *acetonitrile R* and dilute to 20.0 ml with the mobile phase. Dilute 1.0 ml of the solution to 20.0 ml with the mobile phase.

Column:

- *size*: *l* = 0.15 m, Ø = 4.6 mm,
- *stationary phase*: *octadecylsilyl silica gel for chromatography R* (5 µm).

Mobile phase: *methanol R, acetonitrile R, water R* (50:305:645 *V/V/V*).

Flow rate: 1.0 ml/min.

Detection: spectrophotometer at 254 nm.

Injection: 20 µl.

Run time: 6 times the retention time of flunitrazepam.

Relative retention with reference to flunitrazepam (retention time = about 11 min): impurity A = about 0.2; impurity B = about 0.6; impurity C = about 2.3; impurity D = about 4.0.

System suitability: reference solution (b):

- *resolution*: minimum 4.0 between the peaks due to nitrazepam and flunitrazepam.

Limits:

- *correction factor*: for the calculation of content, multiply the peak area of impurity C by 2.44,
- *any impurity*: not more than the area of the principal peak in the chromatogram obtained with reference solution (a) (0.1 per cent),
- *total*: not more than 3 times the area of the principal peak in the chromatogram obtained with reference solution (a) (0.3 per cent),
- *disregard limit*: 0.5 times the area of the principal peak in the chromatogram obtained with reference solution (a) (0.05 per cent).

Loss on drying (*2.2.32*): maximum 0.5 per cent, determined on 1.000 g by drying in an oven at 100-105 °C.

Sulphated ash (*2.4.14*): maximum 0.1 per cent, determined on 1.0 g.

ASSAY

Dissolve 0.250 g in 20 ml of *anhydrous acetic acid R* and add 50 ml of *acetic anhydride R*. Titrate with *0.1 M perchloric acid*, determining the end-point potentiometrically (*2.2.20*).

1 ml of *0.1 M perchloric acid* is equivalent to 31.33 mg of $C_{16}H_{12}FN_3O_3$.

STORAGE

Protected from light.

IMPURITIES

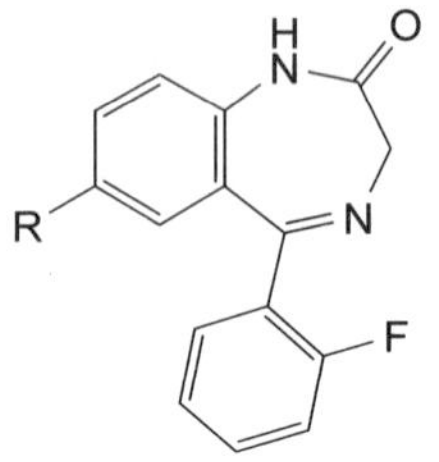

A. R = NH_2: 7-amino-5-(2-fluorophenyl)-1,3-dihydro-2*H*-1,4-benzodiazepin-2-one (7-aminodemethylflunitrazepam),

B. R = NO_2: 5-(2-fluorophenyl)-7-nitro-1,3-dihydro-2*H*-1,4-benzodiazepin-2-one (demethylflunitrazepam),

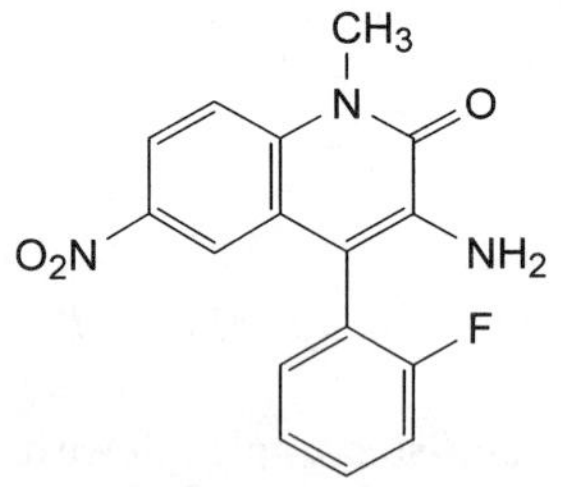

C. 3-amino-4-(2-fluorophenyl)-1-methyl-6-nitroquinolin-2(1*H*)-one,

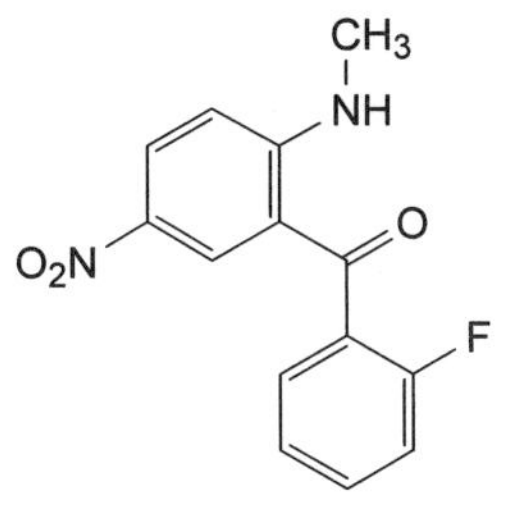

D. (2-fluorophenyl)[2-(methylamino)-5-nitrophenyl]methanone.

G

07/2004:0331

GENTAMICIN SULPHATE

Gentamicini sulfas

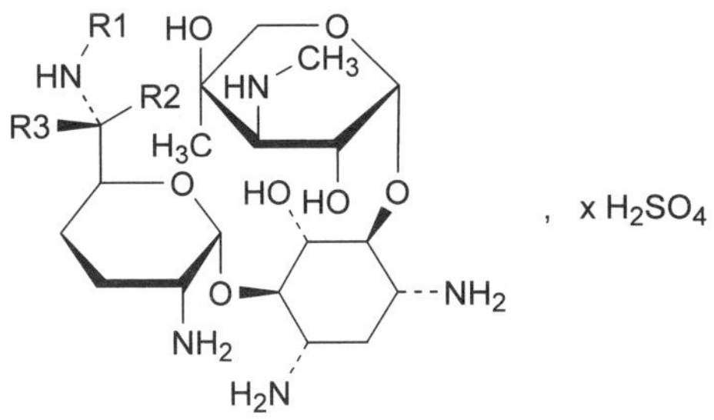

Gentamicin	Mol. Formula	R1	R2	R3
C1	$C_{21}H_{43}N_5O_7$	CH_3	CH_3	H
C1a	$C_{19}H_{39}N_5O_7$	H	H	H
C2	$C_{20}H_{41}N_5O_7$	H	CH_3	H
C2a	$C_{20}H_{41}N_5O_7$	H	H	CH_3
C2b	$C_{20}H_{41}N_5O_7$	CH_3	H	H

DEFINITION

Mixture of the sulphates of antimicrobial substances produced by *Micromonospora purpurea*, the main components being gentamicins C1, C1a, C2, C2a and C2b.

Content: minimum 590 IU/mg (anhydrous substance).

CHARACTERS

Appearance: white or almost white, hygroscopic powder.

Solubility: freely soluble in water, practically insoluble in alcohol.

IDENTIFICATION

First identification: C, D.

Second identification: A, B, D.

A. Dissolve about 10 mg in 1 ml of *water R* and add 5 ml of a 400 g/l solution of *sulphuric acid R*. Heat on a water-bath for 100 min, cool and dilute to 25 ml with *water R*. Examined between 240 nm and 330 nm (*2.2.25*), the solution shows no absorption maximum.

B. Thin-layer chromatography (*2.2.27*).

Test solution. Dissolve 25 mg of the substance to be examined in *water R* and dilute to 5 ml with the same solvent.

Reference solution. Dissolve 25 mg of *gentamicin sulphate CRS* in *water R* and dilute to 5 ml with the same solvent.

Plate: *TLC silica gel plate R*.

Mobile phase: the lower layer of a mixture of equal volumes of *concentrated ammonia R*, *methanol R* and *methylene chloride R*.

Application: 10 µl.

Development: over 2/3 of the plate.

Drying: in air.

Detection: spray with *ninhydrin solution R1* and heat at 110 °C for 5 min.

Results: the 3 principal spots in the chromatogram obtained with the test solution are similar in position, colour and size to the 3 principal spots in the chromatogram obtained with the reference solution.

C. Examine the chromatograms obtained in the test for composition.

Results: the chromatogram obtained with the test solution shows 5 principal peaks having the same retention times as the 5 principal peaks in the chromatogram obtained with reference solution (a).

D. It gives reaction (a) of sulphates (*2.3.1*).

TESTS

Solution S. Dissolve 0.8 g in *carbon dioxide-free water R* and dilute to 20 ml with the same solvent.

Appearance of solution. Solution S is clear (*2.2.1*) and not more intensely coloured than intensity 6 of the range of reference solutions of the most appropriate colour (*2.2.2, Method II*).

pH (*2.2.3*): 3.5 to 5.5 for solution S.

Specific optical rotation (*2.2.7*): + 107 to + 121 (anhydrous substance).

Dissolve 2.5 g in *water R* and dilute to 25.0 ml with the same solvent.

Composition. Liquid chromatography (*2.2.29*): use the normalisation procedure.

Test solution. Dissolve 50 mg of the substance to be examined in the mobile phase and dilute to 100.0 ml with the mobile phase.

Reference solution (a). Dissolve 50 mg of *gentamicin sulphate CRS* in the mobile phase and dilute to 100.0 ml with the mobile phase.

Reference solution (b). Dilute 5.0 ml of reference solution (a) to 100.0 ml with the mobile phase.

Column:

- *size*: l = 0.25 m, Ø = 4.6 mm,
- *stationary phase*: *styrene-divinylbenzene copolymer R* (8 µm) with a pore size of 100 nm,
- *temperature*: 55 °C.

Mobile phase: a mixture prepared with *carbon dioxide-free water R* containing 60 g/l of *anhydrous sodium sulphate R*, 1.75 g/l of *sodium octanesulphonate R*, 8 ml/l of *tetrahydrofuran R*, 50 ml/l of *0.2 M potassium dihydrogen phosphate R* previously adjusted to pH 3.0 with *dilute phosphoric acid R* and degassed.

Flow rate: 1.0 ml/min.

Post-column solution: a *carbonate-free sodium hydroxide solution R* diluted 1 to 25, previously degassed, which is added pulse-less to the column effluent using a 375 µl polymeric mixing coil.

Flow rate: 0.3 ml/min.

Detection: pulsed amperometric detector or equivalent with a gold indicator electrode, a silver-silver chloride reference electrode, and a stainless steel auxiliary electrode which is the cell body, held at respectively + 0.05 V detection, + 0.75 V oxidation and − 0.15 V reduction potentials, with pulse durations according to the instrument used.

Injection: 20 µl.

Run time: 1.2 times the retention time of gentamicin C1.

System suitability: reference solution (a):

- *peak-to-valley ratio*: minimum 2.0 where H_p = height above the baseline of the peak due to gentamicin C2a, and H_v = height above the baseline of the lowest point of the curve separating this peak from the peak due to gentamicin C2.

Limits:

- *gentamicin C1*: 20.0 per cent to 40.0 per cent,
- *gentamicin C1a*: 10.0 per cent to 30.0 per cent,

– *sum of gentamicins C2, C2a, and C2b*: 40.0 per cent to 60.0 per cent,

– *disregard limit*: the area of the peak due to gentamicin C1a in the chromatogram obtained with reference solution (b).

Related substances. Liquid chromatography (*2.2.29*) as described in the test for composition.

Limits (for related substances eluting before gentamicin C1a):

– *any impurity*: maximum 3.0 per cent,

– *total*: maximum 10.0 per cent.

Methanol (*2.4.24, System B*): maximum 1.0 per cent.

Sulphate: 32.0 per cent to 35.0 per cent (anhydrous substance).

Dissolve 0.250 g in 100 ml of *distilled water R* and adjust the solution to pH 11 using *concentrated ammonia R.* Add 10.0 ml of *0.1 M barium chloride* and about 0.5 mg of *phthalein purple R.* Titrate with *0.1 M sodium edetate,* adding 50 ml of *alcohol R* when the colour of the solution begins to change and continue the titration until the violet-blue colour disappears.

1 ml of *0.1 M barium chloride* is equivalent to 9.606 mg of SO_4.

Water (*2.5.12*): maximum 15.0 per cent, determined on 0.300 g.

Sulphated ash (*2.4.14*): maximum 1.0 per cent, determined on 0.50 g.

Sterility (*2.6.1*). If intended for use in the manufacture of parenteral or ophthalmic dosage forms without a further appropriate sterilisation procedure, it complies with the test for sterility.

Bacterial endotoxins (*2.6.14*): less than 0.71 IU/mg, if intended for use in the manufacture of parenteral dosage forms without a further appropriate procedure for the removal of bacterial endotoxins.

ASSAY

Carry out the microbiological assay of antibiotics (*2.7.2*).

STORAGE

In an airtight container. If the substance is sterile, store in a sterile, airtight, tamper-proof container.

LABELLING

The label states:

– where applicable, that the substance is sterile,

– where applicable, that the substance is free from bacterial endotoxins.

IMPURITIES

Specified impurities (see note for information p. xli): A, B, C.

Other detectable impurities: D, E.

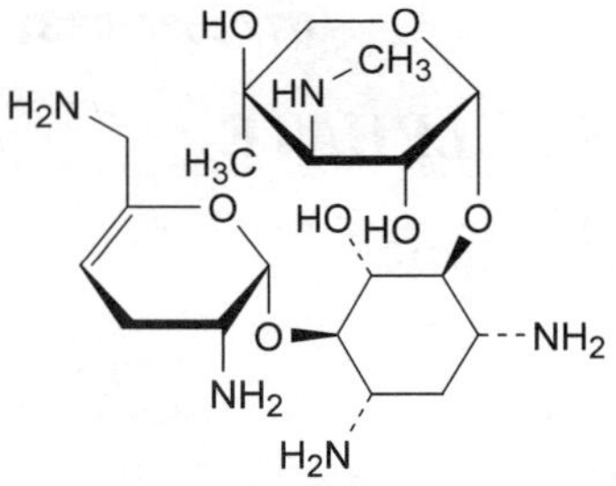

A. 2-deoxy-4-*O*-[3-deoxy-4-*C*-methyl-3-(methylamino)-β-L-arabinopyranosyl]-6-*O*-(2,6-diamino-2,3,4,6-tetradeoxy-α-D-*glycero*-hex-4-enopyranosyl)-L-streptamine (sisomicin),

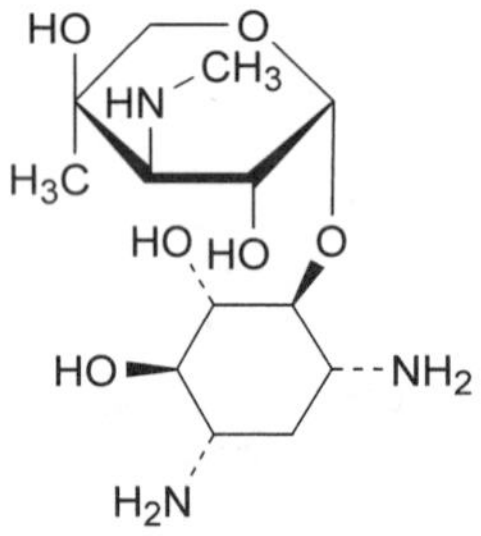

B. 2-deoxy-4-*O*-[3-deoxy-4-*C*-methyl-3-(methylamino)-β-L-arabinopyranosyl]-L-streptamine (garamine),

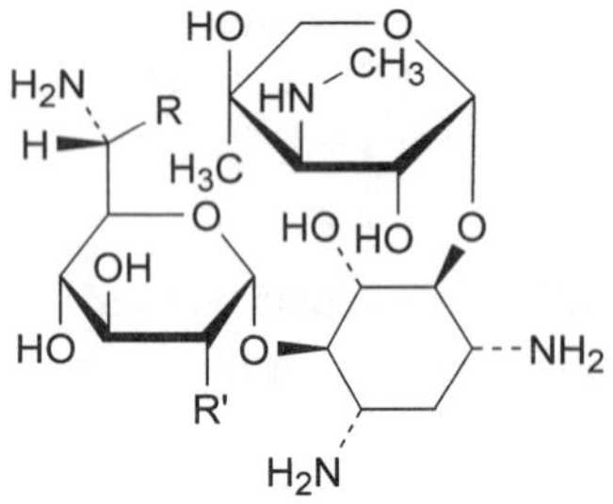

C. R = CH_3, R′ = OH: 4-*O*-(6-amino-6,7-dideoxy-D-*glycero*-α-D-*gluco*-heptopyranosyl)-2-deoxy-6-*O*-[3-deoxy-4-*C*-methyl-3-(methylamino)-β-L-arabinopyranosyl]-D-streptamine (gentamicin B_1),

D. R = H, R′ = NH_2: 2-deoxy-4-*O*-[3-deoxy-4-*C*-methyl-3-(methylamino)-β-L-arabinopyranosyl]-6-*O*-(2,6-diamino-2,6-dideoxy-α-D-*gluco*-hexopyranosyl)-L-streptamine,

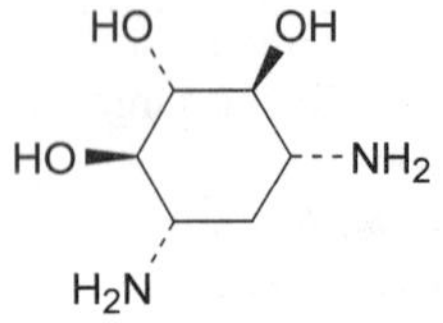

E. 2-deoxystreptamine.

07/2004:1330

GLUCOSE, LIQUID

Glucosum liquidum

DEFINITION

Liquid glucose is an aqueous solution containing a mixture of glucose, oligosaccharides and polysaccharides obtained by hydrolysis of starch. It contains not less than 70.0 per cent of dry matter. The degree of hydrolysis expressed as dextrose equivalent (DE) is not less than 20 (nominal value).

CHARACTERS

A clear, colourless or brown, viscous liquid, miscible with water. The substance may partly or totally solidify at room temperature and liquefies again when heated to 50 °C.

IDENTIFICATION

A. Dissolve 0.1 g in 2.5 ml of *water R* and heat with 2.5 ml of *cupri-tartaric solution R*. A red precipitate is formed.

B. Dip, for 1 s, a suitable stick with a reactive pad containing glucose-oxidase, peroxidase and a hydrogen-donating substance, such as tetramethylbenzidine, in a 5 g/l solution of the substance to be examined. Observe the colour of the reactive pad; within 60 s the colour changes from yellow to green or blue.

C. It is a clear, colourless or brown, viscous liquid, miscible with water. The substance may partly or totally solidify at room temperature and liquefies again when heated to 50 °C.

D. It complies with the test for dextrose equivalent (see Tests).

TESTS

Solution S. Dissolve 25.0 g in *carbon dioxide-free water R* and dilute to 50.0 ml with the same solvent.

pH (*2.2.3*). The pH of a mixture of 1 ml of a 223.6 g/l solution of *potassium chloride R* and 30 ml of solution S is 4.0 to 6.0.

Sulphur dioxide (*2.5.29*). Not more than 20 ppm. Not more than 400 ppm if intended for the production of lozenges or pastilles obtained by high boiling techniques, provided that the final product does not contain more than 50 ppm of sulphur dioxide.

Heavy metals (*2.4.8*). Dilute 2 ml of solution S to 30 ml with *water R*. The solution complies with limit test E for heavy metals (10 ppm). Prepare the standard using 10 ml of *lead standard solution (1 ppm Pb) R*.

Loss on drying (*2.2.32*). Not more than 30.0 per cent, determined on 1.000 g. Triturate the sample with 3.000 g of *kieselguhr G R*, previously dried at 80 °C under reduced pressure for 2 h, and dry at 80 °C under reduced pressure for 2 h.

Sulphated ash (*2.4.14*). Not more than 0.5 per cent, determined on 1.0 g.

Dextrose equivalent. Weigh an amount of the substance to be examined equivalent to 2.85-3.15 g of reducing carbohydrates, calculated as dextrose equivalent, into a 500 ml volumetric flask. Dissolve in *water R* and dilute to 500.0 ml with the same solvent. Transfer the solution to a 50 ml burette.

Pipette 25.0 ml of *cupri-tartaric solution R* into a 250 ml flask and add 18.5 ml of the test solution from the burette, mix and add boiling chips. Place the flask on a hot plate, previously adjusted so that the solution begins to boil after 2 min ± 15 s. Leave to boil for exactly 120 s, add 1 ml of a 1 g/l solution of *methylene blue R* and titrate with the test solution (V_1) until the blue colour disappears. Maintain the solution at boiling throughout the titration.

Standardise the cupri-tartaric solution using a 6.00 g/l solution of *glucose R* (V_0).

Calculate the dextrose equivalent (DE) from the equation:

$$\mathrm{DE} = \frac{300 \times V_0 \times 100}{V_1 \times M \times D}$$

V_0 = total volume of glucose standard solution, in millilitres,

V_1 = total volume of test solution, in millilitres,

M = mass of the sample, in grams,

D = percentage content of dry matter in the substance.

The dextrose equivalent (DE) is within 10 per cent of the nominal value.

LABELLING

The label states the dextrose equivalent (DE) (= nominal value).

07/2004:1525

GLUCOSE, LIQUID, SPRAY-DRIED

Glucosum liquidum dispersione desiccatum

DEFINITION

Spray-dried liquid glucose is a mixture of glucose, oligosaccharides and polysaccharides, obtained by the partial hydrolysis of starch. The degree of hydrolysis, expressed as dextrose equivalent (DE), is not less than 20 (nominal value).

CHARACTERS

A white or almost white, slightly hygroscopic powder or granules, freely soluble in water.

IDENTIFICATION

A. Dissolve 0.1 g in 2.5 ml of *water R* and heat with 2.5 ml of *cupri-tartaric solution R*. A red precipitate is formed.

B. Dip, for 1 s, a suitable stick with a reactive pad containing glucose-oxidase, peroxidase and a hydrogen-donating substance, such as tetramethylbenzidine, in a 5 g/l solution of the substance to be examined. Observe the colour of the reactive pad; within 60 s the colour changes from yellow to green or blue.

C. It is a powder or granules.

D. It complies with the test for dextrose equivalent (see Tests).

TESTS

Solution S. Dissolve 12.5 g in *carbon dioxide-free water R* and dilute to 50.0 ml with the same solvent.

pH (*2.2.3*). The pH of a mixture of 1 ml of a 223.6 g/l solution of *potassium chloride R* and 30 ml of solution S is 4.0 to 7.0.

Sulphur dioxide (*2.5.29*). Not more than 20 ppm.

Heavy metals (*2.4.8*). Dilute 4 ml of solution S to 30 ml with *water R*. The solution complies with limit test E (10 ppm). Prepare the standard using 10 ml of *lead standard solution (1 ppm Pb) R*.

Loss on drying (*2.2.32*). Not more than 6.0 per cent, determined on 10.00 g by drying in an oven at 100-105 °C.

Sulphated ash (*2.4.14*). Not more than 0.5 per cent, determined on 1.0 g.

Dextrose equivalent. Weigh an amount of the substance to be examined equivalent to 2.85-3.15 g of reducing carbohydrates, calculated as dextrose equivalent, into a

500 ml volumetric flask. Dissolve in *water R* and dilute to 500.0 ml with the same solvent. Transfer the solution to a 50 ml burette.

Pipette 25.0 ml of *cupri-tartaric solution R* into a 250 ml flask and add 18.5 ml of the test solution from the burette, mix and add boiling chips. Place the flask on a hot plate, previously adjusted so that the solution begins to boil after 2 min ± 15 s. Allow to boil for exactly 120 s, add 1 ml of a 1 g/l solution of *methylene blue R* and titrate with the test solution (V_1) until the blue colour disappears. Maintain the solution at boiling throughout the titration.

Standardise the cupri-tartaric solution using a 6.00 g/l solution of *glucose R* (V_0).

Calculate the dextrose equivalent (DE) from the equation:

$$DE = \frac{300 \times V_0 \times 100}{V_1 \times M \times D}$$

V_0 = total volume of glucose standard solution, in millilitres,

V_1 = total volume of test solution, in millilitres,

M = mass of the sample, in grams,

D = percentage content of dry matter in the substance.

The dextrose equivalent (DE) is within 10 per cent of the nominal value.

Microbial contamination. Total viable aerobic count (*2.6.12*) not more than 10^3 bacteria and 10^2 fungi per gram, determined by plate count. It complies with the tests for *Escherichia coli* and *Salmonella* (*2.6.13*).

LABELLING

The label states the dextrose equivalent (DE) (= nominal value).

Monographs D - K

07/2004:1831

GOLDENSEAL RHIZOME

Hydrastis rhizoma

DEFINITION

Whole or cut, dried rhizome and root of *Hydrastis canadensis* L.

Content:

– hydrastine ($C_{21}H_{21}NO_6$; M_r 383.4): minimum 2.5 per cent (dried drug),

– berberine ($C_{20}H_{19}NO_5$; M_r 353.4): minimum 3.0 per cent (dried drug).

CHARACTERS

Macroscopic and microscopic characters described under identification tests A and B.

IDENTIFICATION

A. The rhizome is tortuous and knotty, about 5 cm long and 5 mm to 10 mm thick. The surface is yellowish to brownish-grey and irregularly wrinkled, and bears the remains of numerous slender, wiry roots; stem bases and scale leaves occur on the upper surface. The fracture is short and resinous. The transversely-cut surface is yellowish-brown and shows a fairly wide bark, a ring of from about 12 to 20 widely separated xylem bundles and a large, central pith.

B. Reduce to a powder (180). The powder is greenish-yellow. Examine under a microscope using *chloral hydrate solution R*. The powder shows the following diagnostic characters: abundant thin-walled parenchyma; occasional fragments of yellowish-brown cork from the rhizome and roots; groups of small vessels with conspicuous perforations in the oblique end walls and with simple or bordered, slit-shaped pits; infrequent groups of thin-walled, pitted fibres, usually found associated with the vessels; numerous ovoid or spherical, orange-brown granular masses. Examine under a microscope using a 50 per cent *V/V* solution of *glycerol R*. The powder shows abundant starch granules, mostly simple but sometimes compound with up to 4 components; the granules are small, spherical to ovoid, up to about 10 µm in diameter, occasionally with a small, rounded or slit-shaped hilum.

C. Thin-layer chromatography (*2.2.27*).

Test solution. Sonicate for 10 min 250 mg of powdered drug (180) in 4 ml of a mixture of 20 ml of *water R* and 80 ml of *methanol R* and filter. Wash the residue twice with 2 ml of *methanol R*. Combine the solutions and dilute to 20 ml with *methanol R*.

Reference solution. Dissolve 5 mg of *hydrastine hydrochloride R* and 5 mg of *berberine chloride R* in 20 ml of *methanol R*.

Plate: *TLC silica gel plate R*.

Mobile phase: *anhydrous formic acid R, water R, ethyl acetate R* (10:10:80 *V/V/V*).

Application: 20 µl as bands.

Development: over a path of 15 cm.

Drying: in air.

Detection: examine in ultraviolet light at 365 nm.

Results: see below the sequence of the zones present in the chromatograms obtained with the reference solution and the test solution. Furthermore other fluorescent zones may be present in the chromatogram obtained with the test solution.

Top of the plate	
———	———
Berberine: a bright yellow fluorescent zone	A bright yellow fluorescent zone (berberine)
Hydrastine: a deep blue fluorescent zone	A deep blue fluorescent zone (hydrastine)
———	———
	A bright light blue fluorescent zone (hydrastinine)
	A deep blue fluorescent zone
Reference solution	**Test solution**

TESTS

Foreign matter (*2.8.2*): maximum 2 per cent *m/m*.

Loss on drying (*2.2.32*): maximum 10.0 per cent, determined on 1.000 g of the powdered drug (180) by drying in an oven at 100-105 °C for 2 h.

Total ash (*2.4.16*): maximum 8.0 per cent.

Ash insoluble in hydrochloric acid (*2.8.1*): maximum 4.0 per cent.

ASSAY

Liquid chromatography (*2.2.29*).

Test solution. To 1.000 g of the powdered drug (355) in a 100 ml round-bottomed flask, add 50 ml of a 10 ml/l solution of *concentrated ammonia R* in *alcohol R* and boil the mixture under a reflux condenser for 30 min. Allow to cool to room temperature and filter the liquid through a plug of absorbent cotton into a flask. Add the absorbent cotton to the residue in the round-bottomed flask and repeat the extraction with a further 2 quantities, each of 30 ml of a 10 ml/l solution of *concentrated ammonia R* in *alcohol R*, each time boiling under a reflux condenser for 10 min and filtering through a plug of absorbent cotton in the same flask as previously. Filter the combined filtrates through a filter-paper into a 250 ml round-bottomed flask, and rinse flask and filter with 20 ml of a 10 ml/l solution of *concentrated ammonia R* in *alcohol R*. Evaporate the filtrate to dryness *in vacuo* in a water-bath at 55 °C. Dissolve the residue in 50.0 ml of the mobile phase. Dilute 10.0 ml of this solution to 250.0 ml with the mobile phase.

Reference solution. Dissolve 10 mg of *hydrastine hydrochloride R* and 10 mg of *berberine chloride R* in *methanol R* and dilute to 100.0 ml with the same solvent.

Column:

- *size*: l = 0.125 m, Ø = 4 mm,
- *stationary phase*: *end-capped octadecylsilyl silica gel for chromatography R* (5 μm).

Mobile phase: dissolve 9.93 g of *potassium dihydrogen phosphate R* in 730 ml of *water R*, add 270 ml of *acetonitrile R* and mix.

Flow rate: 1.2 ml/min.

Detection: spectrophotometer at 235 nm.

Injection: 10 μl.

System suitability: reference solution:

- *elution order*: when the chromatograms are recorded in the prescribed conditions, the components elute in the order indicated in the composition of the reference solution; record the retention times of these substances;
- *resolution*: minimum 1.5 between the peaks due to hydrastine and berberine.

Using the retention times determined from the chromatogram obtained with the reference solution, locate the components of the reference solution on the chromatogram obtained with the test solution.

Calculate the percentage content of each alkaloid (hydrastine and berberine) from the following expression:

$$\frac{A_1 \times m_2 \times p}{A_2 \times m_1} \times 12.5$$

A_1 = area of the peak due to hydrastine or berberine in the chromatogram obtained with the test solution,

A_2 = area of the peak due to hydrastine or berberine in the chromatogram obtained with the reference solution,

m_1 = mass of the drug to be examined, in grams,

m_2 = mass of hydrastine hydrochloride or berberine chloride in the reference solution, in grams,

p = percentage content of hydrastine in *hydrastine hydrochloride R* or berberine in *berberine chloride R*.

07/2004:1861

GREATER CELANDINE

Chelidonii herba

DEFINITION

Dried, whole or cut aerial parts of *Chelidonium majus* L. collected during flowering.

Content: minimum 0.6 per cent of total alkaloids, expressed as chelidonine ($C_{20}H_{19}NO_5$; M_r 353.4) (dried drug).

CHARACTERS

Macroscopic and microscopic characters described under identification tests A and B.

IDENTIFICATION

A. The stems are rounded, ribbed, yellowish to greenish-brown, somewhat pubescent, about 3 mm to 7 mm in diameter, hollow and mostly collapsed. The leaves are thin, irregularly pinnate, the leaflets ovate to oblong with coarsely dentate margins, the terminal leaflet often three-lobed; the adaxial surface is bluish-green and glabrous, the abaxial surface paler and pubescent, especially on the veins. The flowers have 2 deeply concavo-convex sepals, readily removed, and 4 yellow, broadly ovate, spreading petals about 8 mm to 10 mm long; the stamens are numerous, yellow, and a short style arises from a superior ovary; long, capsular, immature fruits are rarely present.

B. Reduce to a powder (355). The powder is dark greyish-green to brownish-green. Examine under a microscope using *chloral hydrate solution R*. The powder shows the following diagnostic characters: numerous fragments of leaves in surface view, the epidermal cells with sinuous walls; anomocytic stomata (*2.8.3*) occur on the abaxial surface only; covering trichomes long, uniseriate, with thin walls and usually fragmented; vascular tissue from the leaves and stems with groups of fibres, pitted and spirally thickened vessels and associated latex tubes with yellowish-brown contents; occasional fragments of the corolla with thin-walled, partly papillose cells containing numerous pale yellow droplets of oil; spherical pollen grains about 30 μm to 40 μm in diameter with 3 pores and a finely pitted exine.

C. Thin-layer chromatography (*2.2.27*).

Test solution. To 0.4 g of the powdered drug (710) add 50 ml of *dilute acetic acid R*. Boil the mixture under a reflux condenser in a water-bath for 30 min. Cool and filter. To the filtrate add *concentrated ammonia R* until a strong alkaline reaction is produced. Shake with 30 ml of *methylene chloride R*. Dry the organic layer over *anhydrous sodium sulphate R*, filter and evaporate *in vacuo* to dryness. Dissolve the residue in 1.0 ml of *methanol R*.

Reference solution. Dissolve 2 mg of *papaverine hydrochloride R* and 2 mg of *methyl red R* in 10 ml of *alcohol R*.

Plate: *TLC silica gel plate R*.

Mobile phase: *anhydrous formic acid R*, *water R*, *propanol R* (1:9:90 *V/V/V*).

Application: 10 μl as bands.

Development: over a path of 10 cm.

Drying: in air.

Monographs D - K

Detection: spray with *potassium iodobismuthate solution R* and dry the plate in air; spray with *sodium nitrite solution R* and allow the plate to dry in air; examine in daylight.

Results: see below the sequence of the zones present in the chromatograms obtained with the reference solution and the test solution. Furthermore, other weaker zones may be present in the chromatogram obtained with the test solution.

Top of the plate	
———	———
Methyl red: a red zone	A brown zone
	A brown zone
Papaverine: a greyish-brown zone	A greyish-brown zone
———	———
	A brown zone
	A brown zone
Reference solution	**Test solution**

TESTS

Foreign matter (*2.8.2*): maximum 10 per cent.

Loss on drying (*2.2.32*): maximum 10.0 per cent, determined on 1.000 g of the powdered drug (355) by drying in an oven at 100-105 °C for 2 h.

Total ash (*2.4.16*): maximum 13.0 per cent.

ASSAY

Test solution. To 0.750 g of the powdered drug (710), add 200 ml of *dilute acetic acid R* and heat on a water-bath for 30 min, shaking frequently. Cool and dilute to 250.0 ml with *dilute acetic acid R*. Filter. Discard the first 20 ml of the filtrate. To 30.0 ml of the filtrate add 6.0 ml of *concentrated ammonia R* and 100.0 ml of *methylene chloride R*. Shake for 30 min. Separate the organic layer, place 50.0 ml in a 100 ml round-bottomed flask and evaporate to dryness *in vacuo* at a temperature not exceeding 40 °C. Dissolve the residue in about 2-3 ml of *alcohol R*, warming slightly. Transfer the solution to a 25 ml volumetric flask by rinsing the round-bottomed flask with *dilute sulphuric acid R* and dilute to 25.0 ml with the same solvent. To 5.0 ml of the solution, add 5.0 ml of a 10 g/l solution of *chromotropic acid, sodium salt R* in *sulphuric acid R* in a 25 ml volumetric flask, stopper the flask and mix carefully. Dilute to 25.0 ml with *sulphuric acid R* and stopper the flask.

Compensation solution. At the same time and in the same manner, place in a 25 ml volumetric flask 5.0 ml of *dilute sulphuric acid R* and 5.0 ml of a 10 g/l solution of *chromotropic acid, sodium salt R* in *sulphuric acid R*, stopper the flask and mix carefully. Dilute to 25.0 ml with *sulphuric acid R* and stopper the flask.

Place both solutions on a water-bath for 10 min. Cool to about 20 °C and dilute if necessary to 25.0 ml with *sulphuric acid R*. Measure the absorbance (*2.2.25*) of the test solution at 570 nm.

Calculate the percentage content of total alkaloids, expressed as chelidonine, from the expression:

$$\frac{A \times 2.23}{m}$$

i.e. taking the specific absorbance of chelidonine to be 933.

A = absorbance at 570 nm,

m = mass of the substance to be examined, in grams.

H

07/2004:0911

HISTIDINE

Histidinum

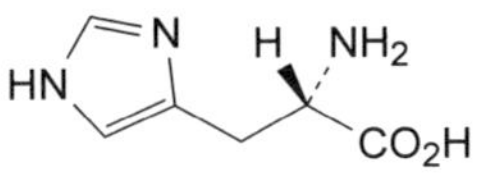

$C_6H_9N_3O_2$ M_r 155.2

DEFINITION

(*S*)-2-Amino-3-(imidazol-4-yl)propanoic acid.

Content: 98.5 per cent to 101.0 per cent (dried substance).

CHARACTERS

Appearance: white, crystalline powder or colourless crystals.

Solubility: soluble in water, very slightly soluble in alcohol.

IDENTIFICATION

First identification: A, B.

Second identification: A, C, D.

A. It complies with the test for specific optical rotation (see Tests).

B. Infrared absorption spectrophotometry (*2.2.24*).

Preparation: discs.

Comparison: *histidine CRS.*

If the spectra obtained show differences, dissolve the substance to be examined and the reference substance separately in the minimum volume of *water R*, evaporate to dryness at 60 °C and record new spectra using the residues.

C. Examine the chromatograms obtained in the test for ninhydrin-positive substances. The principal spot in the chromatogram obtained with test solution (b) is similar in position, colour and size to the principal spot in the chromatogram obtained with reference solution (a).

D. Dissolve 0.1 g in 7 ml of *water R* and add 3 ml of a 200 g/l solution of *sodium hydroxide R*. Dissolve 50 mg of *sulphanilic acid R* in a mixture of 0.1 ml of *hydrochloric acid R* and 10 ml of *water R* and add 0.1 ml of *sodium nitrite solution R*. Add the second solution to the first and mix. An orange-red colour develops.

TESTS

Solution S. Dissolve 2.5 g in *distilled water R*, heating in a water-bath and dilute to 50 ml with the same solvent.

Appearance of solution. Solution S is clear (*2.2.1*) and not more intensely coloured than reference solution BY_7 (*2.2.2, Method II*).

Specific optical rotation (*2.2.7*): + 11.4 to + 12.4 (dried substance).

Dissolve 2.75 g in 12.0 ml of *hydrochloric acid R1* and dilute to 25.0 ml with *water R*.

Ninhydrin-positive substances. Thin-layer chromatography (*2.2.27*).

Test solution (a). Dissolve 0.10 g of the substance to be examined in *water R* and dilute to 10 ml with the same solvent.

Test solution (b). Dilute 1 ml of test solution (a) to 50 ml with *water R.*

Reference solution (a). Dissolve 10 mg of *histidine CRS* in *water R* and dilute to 50 ml with the same solvent.

Reference solution (b). Dilute 5 ml of test solution (b) to 20 ml with *water R.*

Reference solution (c). Dissolve 10 mg of *histidine CRS* and 10 mg of *proline CRS* in *water R* and dilute to 25 ml with the same solvent.

Plate: *TLC silica gel plate R.*

Mobile phase: *glacial acetic acid R, water R, butanol R* (20:20:60 *V/V/V*).

Application: 5 µl.

Development: over 2/3 of the plate.

Drying: in air.

Detection: spray with *ninhydrin solution R* and heat at 100-105 °C for 15 min.

System suitability: the chromatogram obtained with reference solution (c) shows 2 clearly separated spots.

Limits:

– *any impurity*: any spots in the chromatogram obtained with test solution (a), apart from the principal spot, are not more intense than the spot in the chromatogram obtained with reference solution (b) (0.5 per cent).

Chlorides (*2.4.4*): maximum 200 ppm.

Dilute 5 ml of solution S to 15 ml with *water R.*

Sulphates (*2.4.13*): maximum 300 ppm.

Dilute 10 ml of solution S to 15 ml with *distilled water R.*

Ammonium (*2.4.1*): maximum 200 ppm, determined on 50 mg.

Prepare the standard using 0.1 ml of *ammonium standard solution (100 ppm NH_4) R.*

Iron (*2.4.9*): maximum 10 ppm.

In a separating funnel, dissolve 1.0 g in 10 ml of *dilute hydrochloric acid R.* Shake with 3 quantities, each of 10 ml, of *methyl isobutyl ketone R1,* shaking for 3 min each time. To the combined organic layers add 10 ml of *water R* and shake for 3 min. The aqueous layer complies with the limit test for iron.

Heavy metals (*2.4.8*): maximum 10 ppm.

Dissolve 2.0 g in a mixture of 3 ml of *dilute hydrochloric acid R* and 15 ml of *water R,* with gentle warming if necessary, and dilute to 20 ml with *water R.* 12 ml of the solution complies with limit test A. Prepare the standard using *lead standard solution (1 ppm Pb) R.*

Loss on drying (*2.2.32*): maximum 0.5 per cent, determined on 1.000 g by drying in an oven at 100-105 °C.

Sulphated ash (*2.4.14*): maximum 0.1 per cent, determined on 1.0 g.

ASSAY

Dissolve 0.130 g in 50 ml of *water R.* Titrate with *0.1 M hydrochloric acid,* determining the end-point potentiometrically (*2.2.20*).

1 ml of *0.1 M hydrochloric acid* is equivalent to 15.52 mg of $C_6H_9N_3O_2$.

STORAGE

Protected from light.

Monographs D - K

04/2004:0500
corrected

HOMATROPINE HYDROBROMIDE

Homatropini hydrobromidum

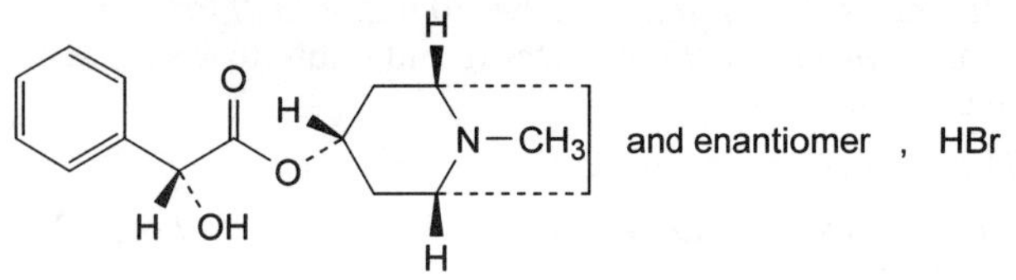

$C_{16}H_{22}BrNO_3$ M_r 356.3

DEFINITION

(1*R*,3*r*,5*S*)-8-Methyl-8-azabicyclo[3.2.1]oct-3-yl (2*RS*)-2-hydroxy-2-phenylacetate hydrobromide.

Content: 99.0 per cent to 101.0 per cent (dried substance).

CHARACTERS

Appearance: white, crystalline powder or colourless crystals.

Solubility: freely soluble in water, sparingly soluble in alcohol.

mp: about 215 °C, with decomposition.

IDENTIFICATION

First identification: A, C.

Second identification: B, C.

A. Infrared absorption spectrophotometry (*2.2.24*).
Comparison: *homatropine hydrobromide CRS*.

B. Dissolve 50 mg in 1 ml of *water R* and add 2 ml of *dilute acetic acid R*. Heat and add 4 ml of *picric acid solution R*. Allow to cool, shaking occasionally. Collect the crystals, wash with 2 quantities, each of 3 ml, of iced *water R* and dry at 100-105 °C. The crystals melt (*2.2.14*) at 182 °C to 186 °C.

C. It gives reaction (a) of bromides (*2.3.1*).

TESTS

Solution S. Dissolve 1.25 g in *carbon dioxide-free water R* and dilute to 25 ml with the same solvent.

Appearance of solution. Solution S is clear (*2.2.1*) and colourless (*2.2.2, Method II*).

pH (*2.2.3*): 5.0 to 6.5 for solution S.

Related substances. Liquid chromatography (*2.2.29*).

Test solution. Dissolve 50.0 mg of the substance to be examined in the mobile phase and dilute to 25.0 ml with the mobile phase.

Reference solution (a). Dilute 5.0 ml of the test solution to 100.0 ml with the mobile phase. Dilute 5.0 ml of this solution to 50.0 ml with the mobile phase.

Reference solution (b). Dilute 5.0 ml of reference solution (a) to 25.0 ml with the mobile phase.

Reference solution (c). Dissolve 5.0 mg of *hyoscine hydrobromide CRS* in the mobile phase and dilute to 50.0 ml with the mobile phase. To 10.0 ml of this solution add 0.5 ml of the test solution and dilute to 100.0 ml with the mobile phase.

Column:

– *size*: l = 0.1 m, Ø = 4.6 mm,
– *stationary phase*: *octadecylsilyl silica gel for chromatography R* (3 µm),
– *temperature*: 40 °C.

Mobile phase: mix 33 volumes of *methanol R2* and 67 volumes of a solution prepared as follows: dissolve 6.8 g of *potassium dihydrogen phosphate R* and 7.0 g of *sodium heptanesulphonate monohydrate R* in 1000 ml of *water R* and adjust to pH 2.7 with a 330 g/l solution of *phosphoric acid R*.

Flow rate: 1.5 ml/min.

Detection: spectrophotometer at 210 nm.

Injection: 10 µl.

Run time: 3 times the retention time of homatropine.

Relative retention with reference to homatropine (retention time = about 6.8 min): impurity C = about 0.2; impurity A = about 0.9; impurity B = about 1.1; impurity D = about 1.9.

System suitability: reference solution (c):

– *resolution*: minimum 1.5 between the peaks due to homatropine and impurity B,
– *symmetry factor*: maximum 2.5 for the peak due to homatropine.

Limits:

– *impurity A*: not more than the area of the principal peak in the chromatogram obtained with reference solution (a) (0.5 per cent),
– *impurities B, C, D*: for each impurity, not more than the area of the principal peak in the chromatogram obtained with reference solution (b) (0.1 per cent),
– *any other impurity*: for each impurity, not more than the area of the principal peak in the chromatogram obtained with reference solution (b) (0.1 per cent),
– *total*: not more than twice the area of the principal peak in the chromatogram obtained with reference solution (a) (1.0 per cent); disregard the peak due to the bromide ion which appears close to the peak due to the solvent,
– *disregard limit*: 0.5 times the area of the principal peak in the chromatogram obtained with reference solution (b) (0.05 per cent).

Loss on drying (*2.2.32*): maximum 0.5 per cent, determined on 1.000 g by drying in an oven at 100-105 °C.

Sulphated ash (*2.4.14*): maximum 0.1 per cent, determined on 1.0 g.

ASSAY

Dissolve 0.300 g in a mixture of 5.0 ml of *0.01 M hydrochloric acid* and 50 ml of *alcohol R*. Carry out a potentiometric titration (*2.2.20*), using *0.1 M sodium hydroxide*. Read the volume added between the 2 points of inflexion.

1 ml of *0.1 M sodium hydroxide* is equivalent to 35.63 mg of $C_{16}H_{22}BrNO_3$.

STORAGE

Protected from light.

IMPURITIES

Specified impurities (see note for information p. xli): A, B, C, D.

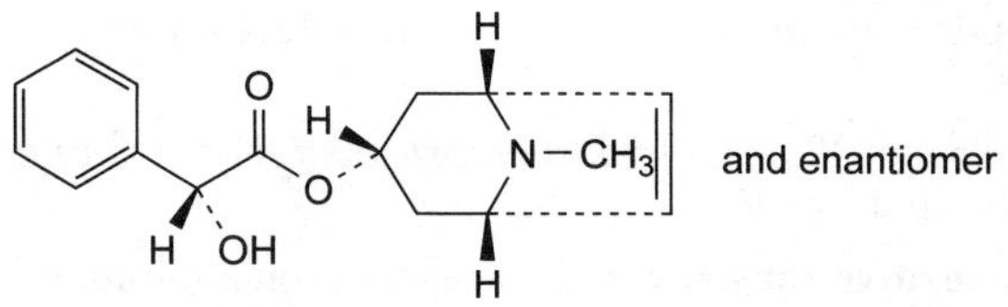

A. (1*R*,3*s*,5*S*)-8-methyl-8-azabicyclo[3.2.1]oct-6-en-3-yl (2*RS*)-2-hydroxy-2-phenylacetate (dehydrohomatropine),

B. hyoscine,

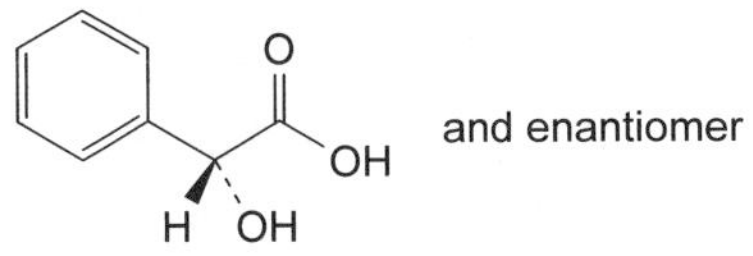

C. (2*RS*)-2-hydroxy-2-phenylacetic acid (mandelic acid),

D. atropine.

04/2004:0720
corrected

HOMATROPINE METHYLBROMIDE

Homatropini methylbromidum

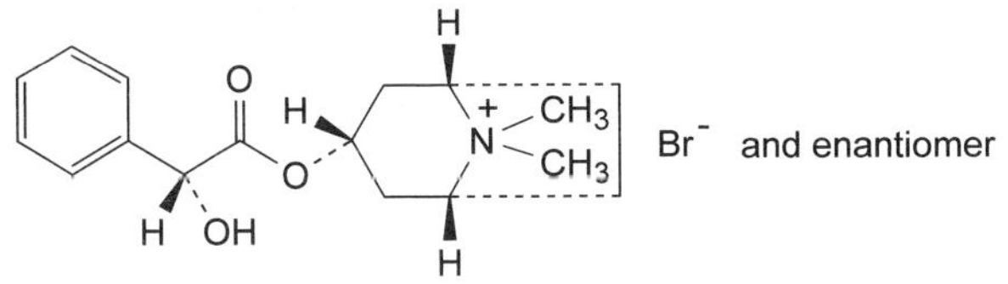

$C_{17}H_{24}BrNO_3$ M_r 370.3

DEFINITION

(1*R*,3*r*,5*S*)-3-[[(2*RS*)-2-hydroxy-2-phenylacetyl]oxy]-8,8-dimethyl-8-azoniabicyclo[3.2.1]octane bromide.

Content: 98.5 per cent to 101.0 per cent (dried substance).

CHARACTERS

Appearance: white, crystalline powder or colourless crystals.

Solubility: freely soluble in water, soluble in alcohol.

mp: about 190 °C.

IDENTIFICATION

First identification: A, C.

Second identification: B, C.

A. Infrared absorption spectrophotometry (*2.2.24*),
Comparison: *homatropine methylbromide CRS*.

B. Dissolve 50 mg in 1 ml of *water R* and add 2 ml of *dilute acetic acid R*. Heat and add 4 ml of *picric acid solution R*. Allow to cool, shaking occasionally. The crystals, washed with 2 quantities, each of 3 ml, of iced *water R* and dried at 100-105 °C melt (*2.2.14*) at 132 °C to 138 °C.

C. It gives reaction (a) of bromides (*2.3.1*).

TESTS

Solution S. Dissolve 1.25 g in *carbon dioxide-free water R* and dilute to 25 ml with the same solvent.

Appearance of solution. Solution S is clear (*2.2.1*) and colourless (*2.2.2, Method II*).

pH (*2.2.3*): 4.5 to 6.5 for solution S.

Related substances. Liquid chromatography (*2.2.29*).

Solvent mixture: *acetonitrile R*, mobile phase A (9:41 *V/V*).

Test solution. Dissolve 50.0 mg of the substance to be examined in the solvent mixture and dilute to 25.0 ml with the solvent mixture.

Reference solution (a). Dilute 5.0 ml of the test solution to 100.0 ml with the solvent mixture. Dilute 5.0 ml of the solution to 50.0 ml with the solvent mixture.

Reference solution (b). Dilute 5.0 ml of reference solution (a) to 25.0 ml with the solvent mixture.

Reference solution (c). Dissolve 5.0 mg of *homatropine hydrobromide CRS* in the solvent mixture and dilute to 50.0 ml with the solvent mixture. To 10.0 ml of the solution add 0.5 ml of the test solution and dilute to 100.0 ml with the solvent mixture.

Column:

- *size*: l = 0.15 m, Ø = 4.6 mm,
- *stationary phase*: *octadecylsilyl silica gel for chromatography R* (3 µm),
- *temperature*: 25 °C.

Mobile phase:

- *mobile phase A*: dissolve 3.4 g of *potassium dihydrogen phosphate R* and 5.0 g of *sodium heptanesulphonate monohydrate R* in 1000 ml of *water R*, and adjust to pH 3.0 with a 330 g/l solution of *phosphoric acid R*,
- *mobile phase B*: mix 400 ml of mobile phase A and 600 ml of *acetonitrile R*,

Time (min)	Mobile phase A (per cent *V/V*)	Mobile phase B (per cent *V/V*)
0 - 2	70	30
2 - 15	70 → 30	30 → 70
15 - 20	30 → 70	70 → 30

Flow rate: 1.4 ml/min.

Detection: spectrophotometer at 210 nm.

Injection: 10 µl.

Relative retention with reference to homatropine methylbromide (retention time = about 4.8 min): impurity C = about 0.7; impurity A = about 0.9; impurity B = about 1.2; impurity D = about 1.3; impurity E = about 1.4; impurity F = about 1.7.

System suitability: reference solution (c):

- *resolution*: minimum 2.5 between the peaks due to homatropine methylbromide and impurity B,
- *symmetry factor*: maximum 2.5 for the peak due to homatropine methylbromide.

Limits:

- *impurities A, B*: for each impurity, not more than the area of the principal peak in the chromatogram obtained with reference solution (a) (0.5 per cent),
- *impurities C, D, E, F*: for each impurity, not more than the area of the principal peak in the chromatogram obtained with reference solution (b) (0.1 per cent),
- *any other impurity*: for each impurity, not more than the area of the principal peak in the chromatogram obtained with reference solution (b) (0.1 per cent),
- *total*: not more than twice the area of the principal peak in the chromatogram obtained with reference solution (a) (1.0 per cent); disregard the peak due to the bromide ion which appears close to the peak due to the solvent,
- *disregard limit*: 0.5 times the area of the principal peak in the chromatogram obtained with reference solution (b) (0.05 per cent).

Loss on drying (*2.2.32*): maximum 0.5 per cent, determined on 1.000 g by drying in an oven at 100-105 °C.

Sulphated ash (*2.4.14*): maximum 0.1 per cent, determined on 1.0 g.

ASSAY

Dissolve 0.300 g in 10 ml of *water R*. Titrate with *0.1 M silver nitrate*. Determine the end-point potentiometrically (*2.2.20*), using a silver indicator electrode and a silver-silver chloride reference electrode.

1 ml of *0.1 M silver nitrate* is equivalent to 37.03 mg of $C_{17}H_{24}BrNO_3$.

STORAGE

Protected from light.

IMPURITIES

Specified impurities (see note for information p. xli): A, B, C, D, E, F.

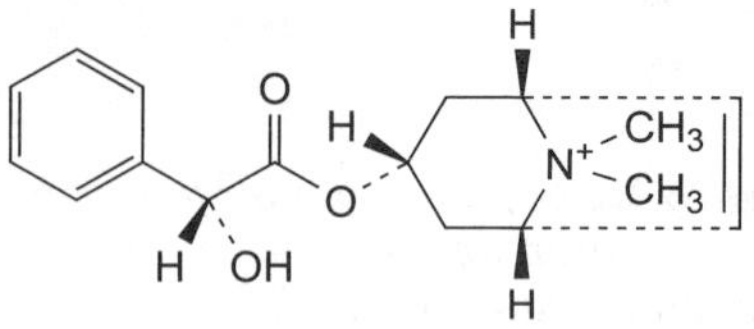

A. (1*R*,3*s*,5*S*)-3-[[(2*RS*)-2-hydroxy-2-phenylacetyl]oxy]-8,8-dimethyl-8-azoniabicyclo[3.2.1]oct-6-ene (methyldehydrohomatropine),

B. homatropine,

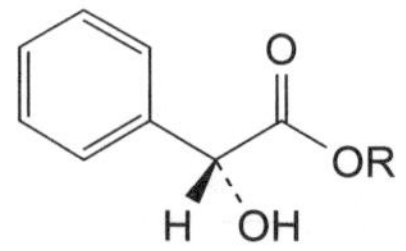

C. R = H: (2*RS*)-2-hydroxy-2-phenylacetic acid (mandelic acid),

F. R = CH_3: methyl (2*RS*)-2-hydroxy-2-phenylacetate (methyl mandelate),

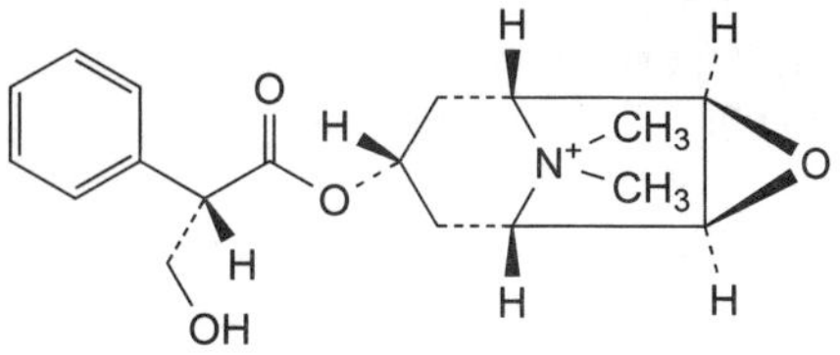

D. (1*R*,2*R*,4*S*,5*S*,7*s*)-7-[[(2*S*)-3-hydroxy-2-phenylpropanoyl]oxy]-9,9-dimethyl-3-oxa-9-azoniatricyclo[3.3.1.0^{2,4}]nonane (methylhyoscine),

E. methylatropine.

07/2004:1646

HUMAN PLASMA (POOLED AND TREATED FOR VIRUS INACTIVATION)

Plasma humanum collectum deinde conditum ad viros exstinguendos

DEFINITION

Human plasma pooled and treated for virus inactivation is a frozen or freeze-dried, sterile, non-pyrogenic preparation obtained from human plasma derived from donors belonging to the same ABO blood group. The preparation is thawed or reconstituted before use to give a solution for infusion.

The human plasma used complies with the monograph on *Human plasma for fractionation (0853).*

PRODUCTION

The units of plasma to be used are cooled to −30 °C or lower within 6 h of separation of cells and in any case within 24 h of collection.

The pool is prepared by mixing units of plasma belonging to the same ABO blood group.

The pool of plasma is tested for hepatitis B surface antigen (HBsAg), for hepatitis C virus antibodies and for HIV antibodies using test methods of suitable sensitivity and specificity; the pool must give negative results in these tests.

The plasma pool is also tested for hepatitis C virus RNA using a validated nucleic acid amplification technique (*2.6.21*). A positive control with 100 IU of hepatitis C virus RNA per millilitre and, to test for inhibitors, an internal control prepared by addition of a suitable marker to a sample of the plasma pool are included in the test. The test is invalid if the positive control is non-reactive or if the result obtained with the internal control indicates the presence of inhibitors. The pool complies with the test if it is found non-reactive for hepatitis C virus RNA.

To limit the potential burden of B19 virus in plasma pools, the plasma pool is also tested for B19 virus using a validated nucleic acid amplification technique (*2.6.21*).

A positive control with 10^4 IU of B19 virus DNA per millilitre and, to test for inhibitors, an internal control prepared by addition of a suitable marker to a sample of the plasma pool are included in the test. The test is invalid if the positive control is non-reactive or if the result obtained with the internal control indicates the presence of inhibitors. The plasma pool contains not more than 10^4 IU of B19 virus DNA per millilitre.

The method of preparation is designed to minimise activation of any coagulation factor (to minimise potential thrombogenicity) and includes a step, or steps that have been shown to inactivate known agents of infection; if substances are used for the inactivation of viruses during production, the subsequent purification procedure must be validated to demonstrate that the concentration of these substances is reduced to a suitable level and that any residues are such as not to compromise the safety of the preparation for patients.

A typical method to inactivate enveloped viruses is the solvent-detergent process which uses treatment with a combination of tributyl phosphate and octoxinol 10; these reagents are subsequently removed by oil extraction or by solid phase extraction so that the amount in the final product is less than 2 µg/ml for tributyl phosphate and less than 5 µg/ml for octoxinol 10.

No antimicrobial preservative is added.

The solution is passed through a bacteria-retentive filter, distributed aseptically into the final containers and immediately frozen; it may subsequently be freeze-dried.

Plastic containers comply with the requirements for sterile plastic containers for human blood and blood components (*3.2.3*).

Glass containers comply with the requirements for glass containers for pharmaceutical use (*3.2.1*).

CHARACTERS

The frozen preparation, after thawing, is a clear or slightly opalescent liquid free from solid and gelatinous particles. The freeze-dried preparation is an almost white or slightly yellow powder or friable solid.

Thaw or reconstitute the preparation to be examined as stated on the label immediately before carrying out the identification, tests and assay.

IDENTIFICATION

A. Examine by electrophoresis (*2.2.31*) comparing with normal human plasma. The electropherograms show the same bands.

B. Using a suitable range of species-specific antisera, carry out precipitation tests on the preparation to be examined. It is recommended that the test be carried out using antisera specific to the plasma proteins of each species of domestic animal commonly used in the preparation of materials of biological origin in the country concerned. The preparation is shown to contain proteins of human origin and gives negative results with all antisera specific to plasma proteins of other species.

C. It complies with the test for anti-A and anti-B haemagglutinins (see Tests).

TESTS

pH (*2.2.3*): 6.5 to 7.6.

Osmolality (*2.2.35*): minimum 240 mosmol/kg.

Total protein: minimum 45 g/l.

Dilute with a 9 g/l solution of *sodium chloride R* to obtain a solution containing about 15 mg of protein in 2 ml. To 2.0 ml of this solution in a round-bottomed centrifuge tube add 2 ml of a 75 g/l solution of *sodium molybdate R* and 2 ml of a mixture of 1 volume of *nitrogen-free sulphuric acid R* and 30 volumes of *water R*. Shake, centrifuge for 5 min, decant the supernatant liquid and allow the inverted tube to drain on filter paper. Determine the nitrogen in the residue by the method of sulphuric acid digestion (*2.5.9*) and calculate the quantity of protein by multiplying the result by 6.25.

Activated coagulation factors (*2.6.22*). It complies with the test for activated coagulation factors. Carry out the test with 0.1 ml of the preparation to be examined instead of 1 to 10 and 1 to 100 dilutions. The coagulation time for the tube containing the preparation to be examined is not less than 150 s.

Anti-A and anti-B haemagglutinins (*2.6.20*). The presence of haemagglutinin (anti-A or anti-B) corresponds to the blood group stated on the label.

Hepatitis A virus antibodies: minimum 2 IU/ml, determined by a suitable immunochemical method (*2.7.1*).

Irregular erythrocyte antibodies. The preparation to be examined does not show the presence of irregular erythrocyte antibodies when examined without dilution by an indirect antiglobulin test.

Citrate. Liquid chromatography (*2.2.29*).

Test solution. Dilute the preparation to be examined with an equal volume of a 9 g/l solution of *sodium chloride R*. Filter the solution using a filter with 0.45 μm pores.

Reference solution. Dissolve 0.300 g of *sodium citrate R* in *water R* and dilute to 100.0 ml with the same solvent.

Column:

– *size*: l = 0.3 m, Ø = 7.8 mm,

– *stationary phase*: *cation exchange resin R* (9 μm).

Mobile phase: 0.51 g/l solution of *sulphuric acid R*.

Flow rate: 0.5 ml/min.

Detection: spectrophotometer at 215 nm.

Equilibration: 15 min.

Injection: 10 μl.

Retention time: citrate = about 10 min.

Limit:

– *citrate*: maximum 25 mmol/l.

Calcium: maximum 5.0 mmol/l.

Atomic absorption spectrometry (*2.2.23, Method I*).

Source: calcium hollow-cathode lamp using a transmission band preferably of 0.5 nm.

Wavelength: 622 nm.

Atomisation device: air-acetylene or acetylene-propane flame.

Potassium: maximum 5.0 mmol/l.

Atomic emission spectrometry (*2.2.22, Method I*).

Wavelength: 766.5 nm.

Sodium: maximum 200 mmol/l.

Atomic emission spectrometry (*2.2.22, Method I*).

Wavelength: 589 nm.

Water: for the freeze-dried product: determined by a suitable method, such as the semi-micro determination of water (*2.5.12*), loss on drying (*2.2.32*) or near-infrared spectrometry (*2.2.40*), the water content is within the limits approved by the competent authority.

Sterility (*2.6.1*). It complies with the test for sterility.

Pyrogens (*2.6.8*). It complies with the test for pyrogens. Inject 3 ml per kilogram of the rabbit's mass.

ASSAY

Factor VIII. Carry out the assay of coagulation factor VIII (*2.7.4*) using a reference plasma calibrated against the International Standard for blood coagulation factor VIII in plasma.

The estimated potency is not less than 0.5 IU/ml. The confidence interval (P = 0.95) of the estimated potency is not greater than 80 per cent to 120 per cent.

Factor V. Using *imidazole buffer solution pH 7.3 R*, prepare 3 twofold dilutions of the preparation to be examined, preferably in duplicate, from 1 in 10 to 1 in 40. Test each dilution as follows: mix 0.1 ml of *plasma substrate deficient in factor V R*, 0.1 ml of the dilution to be examined, 0.1 ml of *thromboplastin R* and 0.1 ml of a 3.5 g/l solution of *calcium chloride R*; measure the coagulation times, i.e. the interval between the moment at which the calcium chloride solution is added and the first indication of the formation of fibrin, which may be observed visually or by means of a suitable apparatus.

In the same manner, determine the coagulation time of 4 twofold dilutions (1 in 10 to 1 in 80) of human normal plasma in *imidazole buffer solution pH 7.3 R*. 1 unit of factor V is equal to the activity of 1 ml of human normal plasma. Human normal plasma is prepared by pooling plasma units from not fewer than 30 donors and stored at −30 °C or lower.

Check the validity of the assay and calculate the potency of the test preparation by the usual statistical methods for a parallel-line assay (for example, *5.3*).

The estimated potency is not less than 0.5 units/ml. The confidence interval (P = 0.95) of the estimated potency is not greater than 80 per cent to 120 per cent.

Factor XI. Carry out the assay of human coagulation factor XI (*2.7.22*) using as reference human normal plasma (see above under Factor V).

The estimated potency is not less than 0.5 units/ml. The confidence interval (P = 0.95) of the estimated potency is not greater than 80 per cent to 125 per cent.

LABELLING

The label states:

– the ABO blood group,

– the method used for virus inactivation.

K

Monographs
D - K

07/2004:1746

KETOBEMIDONE HYDROCHLORIDE

Cetobemidoni hydrochloridum

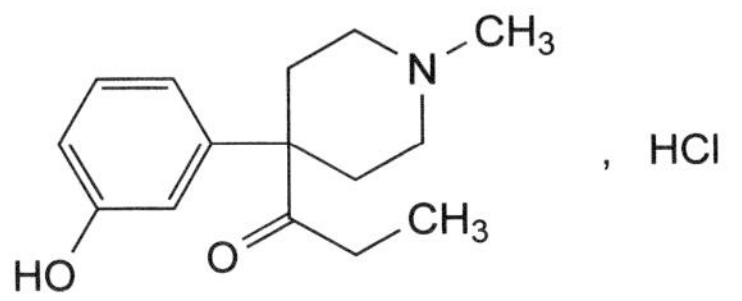

$C_{15}H_{22}ClNO_2$ M_r 283.8

DEFINITION

1-[4-(3-Hydroxyphenyl)-1-methylpiperidin-4-yl]propan-1-one hydrochloride.

Content: 99.0 per cent to 101.0 per cent (anhydrous substance).

CHARACTERS

Appearance: white or almost white, crystalline powder.

Solubility: freely soluble in water, soluble in alcohol, very slightly soluble in methylene chloride.

IDENTIFICATION

A. Infrared absorption spectrophotometry (*2.2.24*).

Comparison: *Ph. Eur. reference spectrum of ketobemidone hydrochloride.*

B. Solution S (see Tests) gives reaction (a) of chlorides (*2.3.1*).

TESTS

Solution S. Dissolve 0.250 g in *carbon dioxide-free water R* and dilute to 25.0 ml with the same solvent.

Appearance of solution. Solution S is clear (*2.2.1*) and not more intensely coloured than reference solution B_8 (*2.2.2, Method II*).

pH (*2.2.3*): 4.5 to 5.5 for solution S.

Related substances. Liquid chromatography (*2.2.29*).

Solution A: 1.54 g/l solution of *ammonium acetate R* adjusted to pH 8.0 with *dilute ammonia R1*.

Test solution. Dissolve 50.0 mg of the substance to be examined in solution A and dilute to 25.0 ml with the same solution.

Reference solution (a). Dissolve 1 mg of *ketobemidone impurity B CRS* and 1 mg of *ketobemidone impurity C CRS* in solution A and dilute to 25 ml with the same solution.

Reference solution (b). Dilute 1.0 ml of the test solution to 100.0 ml with solution A. Dilute 20.0 ml of this solution to 100.0 ml with solution A.

Column:

- *size*: l = 0.25 m, Ø = 4.6 mm,
- *stationary phase*: *phenylhexylsilyl silica gel for chromatography R* (5 μm),
- *temperature*: 40 °C.

Mobile phase: *acetonitrile R*, solution A (20:80 *V/V*).

Flow rate: 1.5 ml/min.

Detection: spectrophotometer at 278 nm.

Injection: 20 μl.

Run time: 4.5 times the retention time of ketobemidone.

Relative retention with reference to ketobemidone (retention time = about 10 min): impurity A = about 0.4; impurity B = about 0.6; impurity C = about 0.7; impurity D = about 3.5; impurity E = about 4.2.

System suitability: reference solution (a):

- *resolution*: minimum 4.0 between the peaks due to impurity B and impurity C.

Limits:

- *impurities A, B, C, D*: for each impurity, not more than the area of the principal peak in the chromatogram obtained with reference solution (b) (0.2 per cent),
- *any other impurity*: for each impurity, not more than 0.5 times the area of the principal peak in the chromatogram obtained with reference solution (b) (0.1 per cent),
- *total*: not more than 3.5 times the area of the principal peak in the chromatogram obtained with reference solution (b) (0.7 per cent),
- *disregard limit*: 0.25 times the area of the principal peak in the chromatogram obtained with reference solution (b) (0.05 per cent).

Water (*2.5.12*): maximum 1.0 per cent, determined on 0.50 g.

Sulphated ash (*2.4.14*): maximum 0.1 per cent, determined on 1.0 g.

ASSAY

Dissolve 0.200 g in a mixture of 5.0 ml of *0.01 M hydrochloric acid* and 50 ml of *alcohol R*. Carry out a potentiometric titration (*2.2.20*) using *0.1 M sodium hydroxide*. Read the volume added between the 2 points of inflexion.

1 ml of *0.1 M sodium hydroxide* is equivalent to 28.38 mg of $C_{15}H_{22}ClNO_2$.

IMPURITIES

Specified impurities (see note for information p. xli): A, B, C, D.

Other detectable impurities: E.

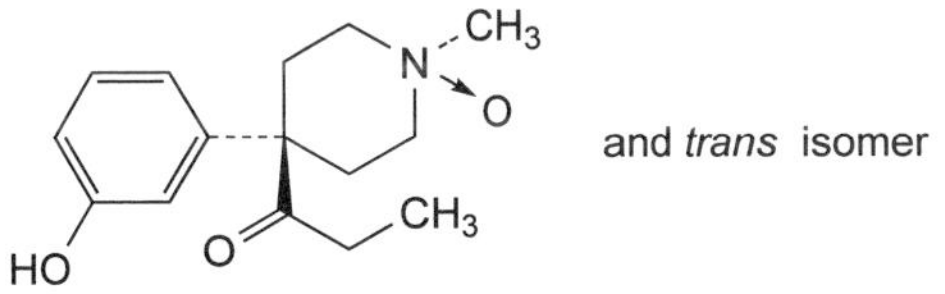

A. 1-[4-(3-hydroxyphenyl)-1-methyl-1-oxidopiperidin-4-yl]propan-1-one (*cis* and *trans* isomers),

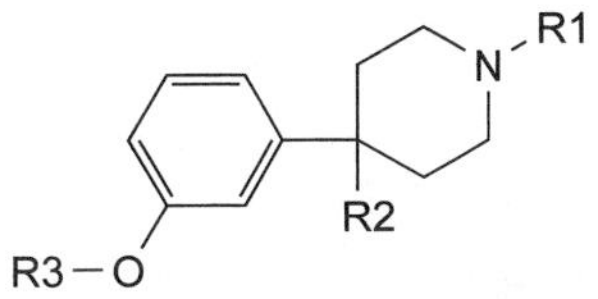

B. R1 = CH_3, R2 = CO-CH_3, R3 = H: 1-[4-(3-hydroxyphenyl)-1-methylpiperidin-4-yl]ethanone,

C. R1 = R3 = H, R2 = CO-CH_2-CH_3: 1-[4-(3-hydroxyphenyl)piperidin-4-yl]propan-1-one,

D. R1 = R3 = CH_3, R2 = CO-CH_2-CH_3: 1-[4-(3-methoxyphenyl)-1-methylpiperidin-4-yl]propan-1-one,

E. R1 = CH_3, R2 = CN, R3 = H: 4-(3-hydroxyphenyl)-1-methylpiperidin-4-carbonitrile.

L

07/2004:1442

LEUPRORELIN

Leuprorelinum

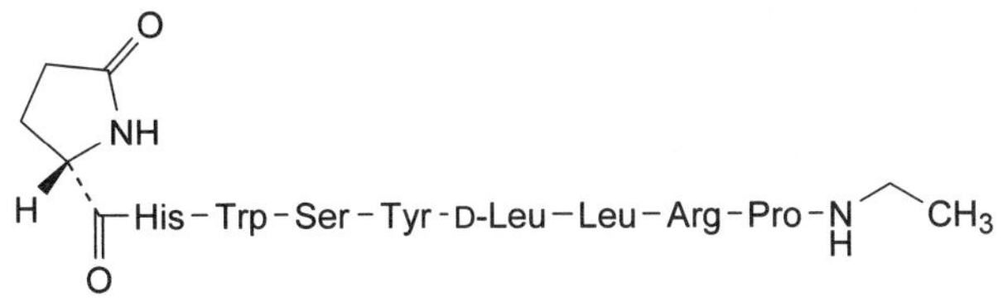

$C_{59}H_{84}N_{16}O_{12}$ M_r 1209

DEFINITION

5-Oxo-L-prolyl-L-histidyl-L-tryptophyl-L-seryl-L-tyrosyl-D-leucyl-L-leucyl-L-arginyl-*N*-ethyl-L-prolinamide.

Synthetic nonapeptide analogue of the hypothalamic peptide, gonadorelin. It is obtained by chemical synthesis and is available as an acetate.

Content: 97.0 per cent to 103.0 per cent (anhydrous and acetic acid-free substance).

CHARACTERS

Appearance: hygroscopic, white or almost white powder.

IDENTIFICATION

A. Infrared absorption spectrophotometry (*2.2.24*).

Preparation: discs of *potassium bromide R*.

Comparison: *Ph. Eur. reference spectrum of leuprorelin.*

B. Examine the chromatograms obtained in the assay.

Results: the principal peak in the chromatogram obtained with test solution (b) is similar in retention time and size to the principal peak in the chromatogram obtained with reference solution (b).

C. Amino acid analysis (*2.2.56*). For hydrolysis use Method 1 and for analysis use Method 1.

Express the content of each amino acid in moles. Calculate the relative proportions of the amino acids taking one seventh of the sum of the number of moles of histidine, glutamic acid, leucine, proline, tyrosine and arginine as equal to 1. The values fall within the following limits: serine present; glutamic acid = 0.85 to 1.1; proline = 0.85 to 1.1; leucine = 1.8 to 2.2; tyrosine = 0.85 to 1.1; histidine = 0.85 to 1.1 and arginine = 0.85 to 1.1. Not more than traces of other amino acids are present, with the exception of tryptophan.

TESTS

Specific optical rotation (*2.2.7*): − 38.0 to − 42.0 (anhydrous and acetic acid-free substance).

Dissolve the substance to be examined in a 1 per cent *V/V* solution of *glacial acetic acid R* to obtain a concentration of 10.0 mg/ml.

Related substances. Liquid chromatography (*2.2.29*): use the normalisation procedure.

Test solution (a). Dissolve the substance to be examined in the mobile phase to obtain a concentration of 1.0 mg/ml.

Test solution (b). Dilute 1.0 ml of test solution (a) to 20.0 ml with the mobile phase.

Reference solution (a). Dissolve *leuprorelin CRS* in the mobile phase to obtain a concentration of 1.0 mg/ml.

Reference solution (b). Dilute 1.0 ml of reference solution (a) to 20.0 ml with the mobile phase.

Resolution solution. Dilute 5.0 ml of reference solution (a) to 50.0 ml with *water R*. To 5 ml of the solution add 100 µl of *1 M sodium hydroxide* and shake vigorously. Heat in an oven at 100 °C for 60 min, cool immediately and add 50 µl of *dilute phosphoric acid R*. Shake vigorously.

Column:

– *size*: *l* = 0.10 m, Ø = 4.6 mm,
– *stationary phase*: *octadecylsilyl silica gel for chromatography R* (3 µm).

Mobile phase: dissolve about 15.2 g of *triethylamine R* in 800 ml of *water R*, adjust to pH 3.0 with *phosphoric acid R* and dilute to 1000 ml with *water R*. Add 850 ml of this solution to 150 ml of a mixture of 2 volumes of *propanol R* and 3 volumes of *acetonitrile R*.

Flow rate: 1.0-1.5 ml/min.

Detection: spectrophotometer at 220 nm.

Injection: 20 µl of test solution (a) and the resolution solution.

Run time: 90 min.

Relative retention with reference to leuprorelin (retention time = 41-49 min): impurity E = about 0.7; impurity F = about 0.7; impurity H = about 0.78; impurity A = about 0.8; impurity B = about 0.9; impurity I = about 0.94; impurity J = about 1.09; impurity C = about 1.2; impurity G = about 1.3; impurity K = about 1.31; impurity D = about 1.5.

System suitability: resolution solution:

– *resolution*: minimum 1.5 between the peaks due to impurity B and leuprorelin.

Limits:

– *impurity D*: maximum 1.0 per cent,
– *impurities A, B, C*: for each impurity, maximum 0.5 per cent,
– *any other impurity*: for each impurity, maximum 0.5 per cent,
– *total*: maximum 2.5 per cent,
– *disregard limit*: 0.1 per cent.

Acetic acid (*2.5.34*): 4.7 per cent to 9.0 per cent.

Test solution. Dissolve 10.0 mg of the substance to be examined in a mixture of 5 volumes of mobile phase B and 95 volumes of mobile phase A and dilute to 10.0 ml with the same mixture of mobile phases.

Water (*2.5.32*): maximum 5.0 per cent.

Sulphated ash (*2.4.14*): maximum 0.3 per cent.

Bacterial endotoxins (*2.6.14, Method D*): less than 16.7 IU/mg, if intended for use in the manufacture of parenteral dosage forms without a further appropriate procedure for removal of bacterial endotoxins.

ASSAY

Liquid chromatography (*2.2.29*) as described in the test for related substances with the following modifications.

Run time: 60 min.

Injection: 20 µl of test solution (b) and reference solution (b).

Calculate the content of leuprorelin ($C_{59}H_{84}N_{16}O_{12}$) using the areas of the peaks and the declared content of $C_{59}H_{84}N_{16}O_{12}$ in *leuprorelin CRS*.

STORAGE

In an airtight container, protected from light, at a temperature not exceeding 30 °C.

If the substance is sterile, store in a sterile, airtight, tamper-proof container.

LABELLING

The label states:

– the mass of peptide in the container,

– where applicable, that the substance is free from bacterial endotoxins.

IMPURITIES

Specified impurities (see note for information p. xli): A, B, C, D.

Other detectable impurities: E, F, G, H, I, J, K.

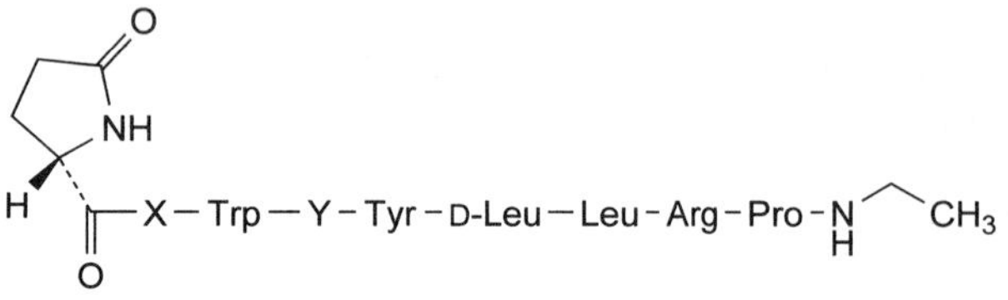

A. X = L-His, Y = D-Ser: [4-D-serine]leuprorelin,

B. X = D-His, Y = L-Ser: [2-D-histidine]leuprorelin,

F. X = D-His, Y = D-Ser: [2-D-histidine,4-D-serine]leuprorelin,

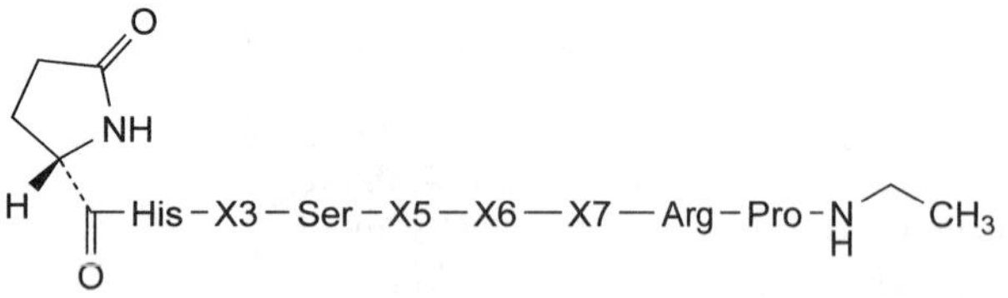

C. X3 = L-Trp, X5 = L-Tyr, X6 = X7 = L-Leu: [6-L-leucine]leuprorelin,

E. X3 = D-Trp, X5 = L-Tyr, X6 = D-Leu, X7 = L-Leu: [3-D-tryptophane]leuprorelin,

G. X3 = L-Trp, X5 = D-Tyr, X6 = D-Leu, X7 = L-Leu: [5-D-tyrosine]leuprorelin,

H. X3 = L-Trp, X5 = L-Tyr, X6 = X7 = D-Leu: [7-D-leucine]leuprorelin,

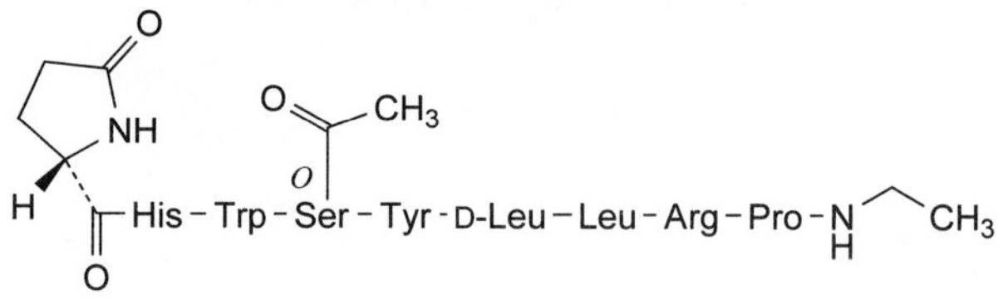

D. [4-(*O*-acetyl-L-serine)]leuprorelin,

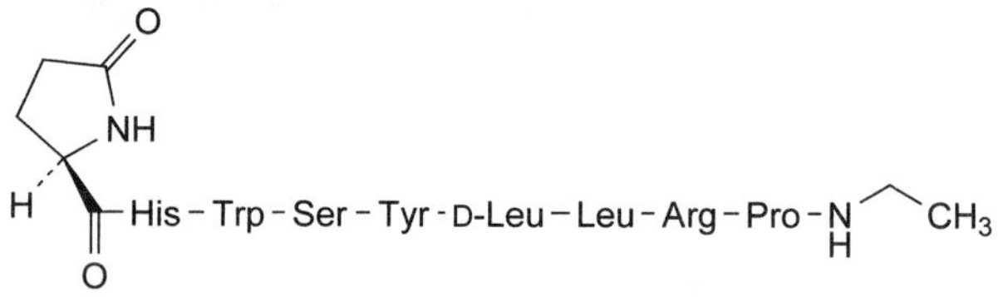

I. [1-(5-oxo-D-proline)]leuprorelin,

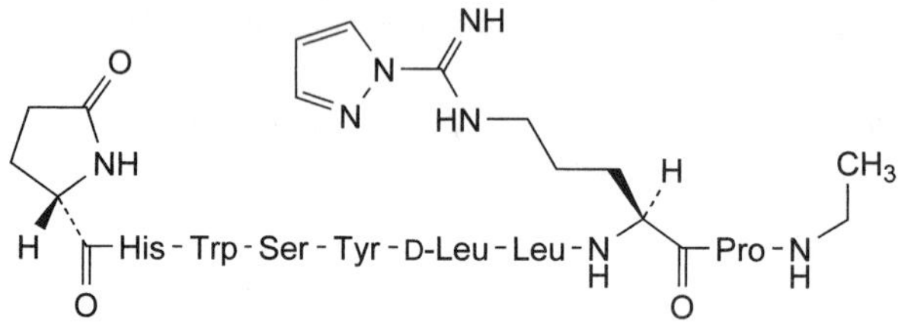

J. [8-[5-*N*-[imino(1*H*-pyrazol-1-yl)methyl]-L-ornithine]]leuprorelin,

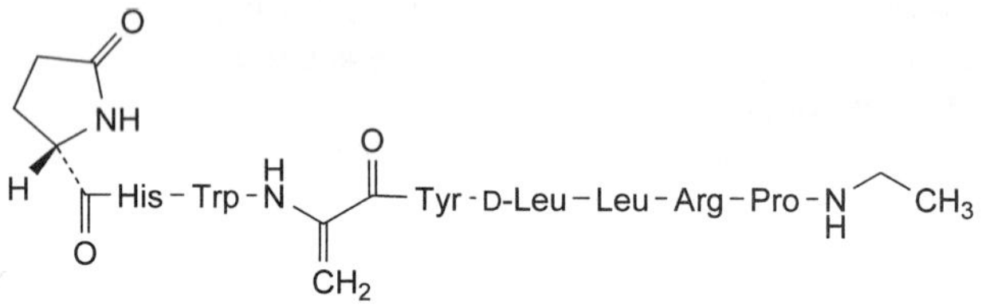

K. [4-dehydroalanine]leuprorelin.

M

07/2004:1542

MALTODEXTRIN

Maltodextrinum

DEFINITION

Maltodextrin is a mixture of glucose, disaccharides and polysaccharides, obtained by the partial hydrolysis of starch. The degree of hydrolysis, expressed as dextrose equivalent (DE), is not more than 20 (nominal value).

CHARACTERS

A white or almost white, slightly hygroscopic powder or granules, freely soluble in water.

IDENTIFICATION

A. Dissolve 0.1 g in 2.5 ml of *water R* and heat with 2.5 ml of *cupri-tartaric solution R*. A red precipitate is formed.

B. Dip, for 1 s, a suitable stick with a reactive pad containing glucose-oxidase, peroxidase and a hydrogen-donating substance, such as tetramethylbenzidine, in a 100 g/l solution of the substance to be examined. Observe the colour of the reactive pad; within 60 s the colour changes from yellow to green or blue.

C. It is a powder or granules.

D. It complies with the test for dextrose equivalent (see Tests).

TESTS

Solution S. Dissolve 12.5 g in *carbon dioxide-free water R* and dilute to 50.0 ml with the same solvent.

pH (*2.2.3*). The pH of a mixture of 30 ml of solution S and 1 ml of a 223.6 g/l solution of *potassium chloride R* is 4.0 to 7.0.

Sulphur dioxide (*2.5.29*). Not more than 20 ppm.

Heavy metals (*2.4.8*). Dilute 4 ml of solution S to 30 ml with *water R*. The solution complies with limit test E for heavy metals (10 ppm). Prepare the standard using 10 ml of *lead standard solution (1 ppm Pb) R*.

Loss on drying (*2.2.32*). Not more than 6.0 per cent, determined on 10.00 g by drying in an oven at 100-105 °C.

Sulphated ash (*2.4.14*). Not more than 0.5 per cent, determined on 1.0 g.

Dextrose equivalent. Weigh an amount of the sample to be examined equivalent to 2.85-3.15 g of reducing carbohydrates, calculated as dextrose equivalent, into a 500 ml volumetric flask. Dissolve in *water R* and dilute to 500.0 ml with the same solvent. Transfer the solution to a 50 ml burette.

Pipette 25.0 ml of *cupri-tartaric solution R* into a 250 ml flask and add 18.5 ml of the sample solution from the burette, mix and add boiling chips. Place the flask on a hot plate, previously adjusted so that the solution begins to boil within 2 min ± 15 s. Allow to boil for exactly 120 s, add 1 ml of a 1 g/l solution of *methylene blue R* and titrate with the sample solution (V_1) until the blue colour disappears. Maintain the solution at boiling throughout the titration.

Standardise the cupri-tartaric solution using a 6.00 g/l solution of *glucose R* (V_0).

Calculate the dextrose equivalent (DE) from the equation:

$$DE = \frac{300 \times V_0 \times 100}{V_1 \times M \times D}$$

V_0 = total volume of glucose standard solution, in millilitres,

V_1 = total volume of sample solution, in millilitres,

M = sample weight, in grams,

D = percentage content of dry matter in the substance.

The dextrose equivalent (DE) is within 2 DE units of the nominal value.

Microbial contamination. Total viable aerobic count (*2.6.12*) not more than 10^3 bacteria and 10^2 fungi per gram, determined by plate count. It complies with the test for *Escherichia coli* and *Salmonella* (*2.6.13*).

LABELLING

The label states the dextrose equivalent (DE) (= nominal value).

07/2004:1029

MEXILETINE HYDROCHLORIDE

Mexiletini hydrochloridum

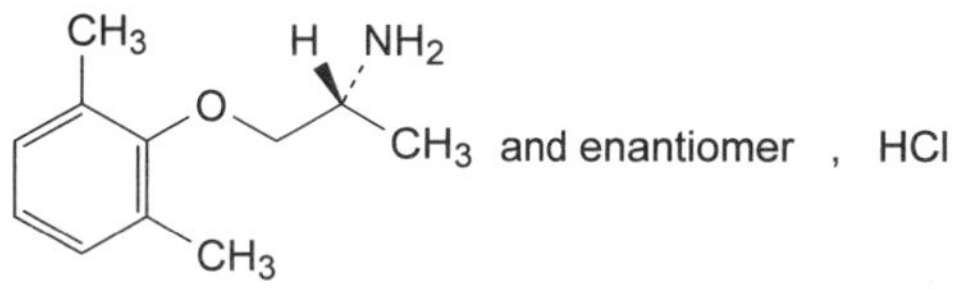

$C_{11}H_{18}ClNO$ M_r 215.7

DEFINITION

(2*RS*)-1-(2,6-Dimethylphenoxy)propan-2-amine hydrochloride.

Content: 99.0 per cent to 101.0 per cent (anhydrous substance).

CHARACTERS

Appearance: white or almost white, crystalline powder.

Solubility: freely soluble in water and in methanol, sparingly soluble in methylene chloride.

It shows polymorphism.

IDENTIFICATION

A. Infrared absorption spectrophotometry (*2.2.24*).

Comparison: *mexiletine hydrochloride CRS.*

If the spectra obtained in the solid state show differences, dissolve the substance to be examined and the reference substance separately in *methanol R*, evaporate to dryness and record new spectra using the residues.

B. Dilute 1.5 ml of solution S (see Tests) to 15 ml with *water R*. The solution gives reaction (a) of chlorides (*2.3.1*).

TESTS

Solution S. Dissolve 2.0 g in *carbon dioxide-free water R* and dilute to 20 ml with the same solvent.

Appearance of solution. The solution is clear (*2.2.1*) and colourless (*2.2.2, Method II*).

Dilute 5 ml of solution S to 10 ml with *water R*.

Monographs L - P

pH (*2.2.3*): 4.0 to 5.5 for solution S.

Impurity D. Thin-layer chromatography (*2.2.27*).

Test solution. Dissolve 0.500 g of the substance to be examined in *methanol R* and dilute to 5.0 ml with the same solvent.

Reference solution (a). Dissolve the content of a vial of *mexiletine impurity D CRS* in 4.0 ml of *methanol R.*

Reference solution (b). Dilute 1.0 ml of the test solution to 20.0 ml with *methanol R.*

Reference solution (c). Dilute 1.0 ml of reference solution (a) to 5.0 ml with *methanol R.*

Reference solution (d). Dilute 1.0 ml of reference solution (a) to 5.0 ml with reference solution (b).

Plate: *TLC silica gel plate R.*

Mobile phase: *concentrated ammonia R, alcohol R, acetone R, toluene R* (3:7:45:45 *V/V/V/V*).

Application: 5 μl of the test solution and reference solutions (c) and (d).

Development: over a path of 10 cm.

Drying: in air.

Detection: spray with *ninhydrin solution R3* and heat at 100-105 °C for 15 min or until the spots appear.

System suitability: the chromatogram obtained with reference solution (b) shows 2 clearly separated spots.

Limits:

- *impurity D*: any spot corresponding to impurity D in the chromatogram obtained with the test solution is not more intense than the spot in the chromatogram obtained with reference solution (c) (0.1 per cent).

Related substances. Liquid chromatography (*2.2.29*).

Test solution. Dissolve 0.200 g of the substance to be examined in the mobile phase and dilute to 10.0 ml with the mobile phase.

Reference solution (a). Dilute 1.0 ml of the test solution to 10.0 ml with the mobile phase.

Reference solution (b). Dissolve the content of a vial of *mexiletine impurity C CRS* in the mobile phase and transfer the solution quantitatively to a volumetric flask containing 16.0 mg of *2,6-dimethylphenol R.* Dilute to 20.0 ml with the mobile phase. Mix 1.0 ml of this solution with 2.0 ml of reference solution (a) and dilute the mixture to 100.0 ml with the mobile phase.

Column:

- *size*: l = 0.25 m, Ø = 4.6 mm,
- *stationary phase*: *end-capped octadecylsilyl silica gel for chromatography R* (5 μm).

Mobile phase: mix 65 volumes of *methanol R2* and 35 volumes of a solution prepared as follows: dissolve 11.5 g of *anhydrous sodium acetate R* in 500 ml of *water R,* add 3.2 ml of *glacial acetic acid R,* mix and allow to cool; adjust to pH 4.8 with *glacial acetic acid R* and dilute to 1000 ml with *water R.*

Flow rate: 1.0 ml/min.

Detection: spectrophotometer at 262 nm.

Injection: 20 μl.

Run time: 5.5 times the retention time of mexiletine.

Relative retention with reference to mexiletine (retention time = about 4 min): impurity C = about 0.7; impurity A = about 1.8.

System suitability: reference solution (b):

- *resolution*: minimum 5.0 between the peaks due to mexiletine and impurity C.

Limits:

- *impurity A*: not more than 2.5 times the area of the corresponding peak in the chromatogram obtained with reference solution (b) (0.1 per cent),
- *impurity C*: not more than 20 times the area of the corresponding peak in the chromatogram obtained with reference solution (b) (0.1 per cent),
- *any other impurity*: for each impurity, not more than 0.5 times the area of the peak due to mexiletine in the chromatogram obtained with reference solution (b) (0.1 per cent),
- *total*: not more than 2.5 times the area of the peak due to mexiletine in the chromatogram obtained with reference solution (b) (0.5 per cent),
- *disregard limit*: 0.25 times the area of the peak due to mexiletine in the chromatogram obtained with reference solution (b) (0.05 per cent).

Heavy metals (*2.4.8*): maximum 10 ppm.

2.0 g complies with limit test C. Prepare the standard using 2 ml of *lead standard solution (10 ppm Pb) R.*

Water (*2.5.12*): maximum 0.5 per cent, determined on 1.00 g.

Sulphated ash (*2.4.14*): maximum 0.1 per cent, determined on 1.0 g.

ASSAY

Dissolve 0.150 g in 50 ml of a mixture of equal volumes of *anhydrous acetic acid R* and *acetic anhydride R.* Titrate immediately with *0.1 M perchloric acid,* determining the end-point potentiometrically (*2.2.20*) and completing the titration within 2 min.

1 ml of *0.1 M perchloric acid* is equivalent to 21.57 mg of $C_{11}H_{18}ClNO$.

IMPURITIES

Specified impurities (see note for information p. xli): A, C, D.

Other detectable impurities: B.

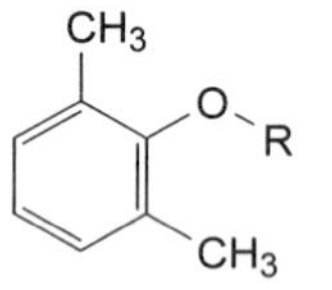

A. R = H: 2,6-dimethylphenol,

B. R = CH_2-CO-CH_3: 1-(2,6-dimethylphenoxy)propan-2-one,

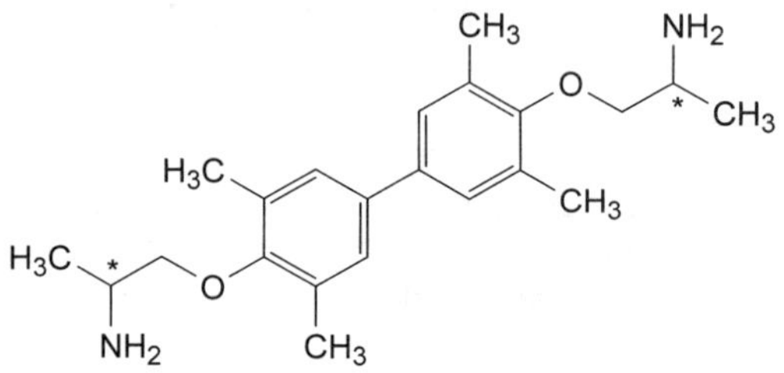

C. 1,1′-[(3,3′,5,5′-tetramethylbiphenyl-4,4′-diyl)bisoxy]dipropan-2-amine,

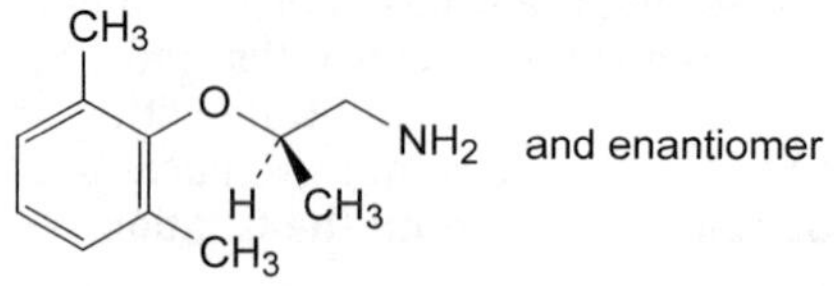

D. (2*RS*)-2-(2,6-dimethylphenoxy)propan-1-amine.

N

07/2004:1999

NIFUROXAZIDE

Nifuroxazidum

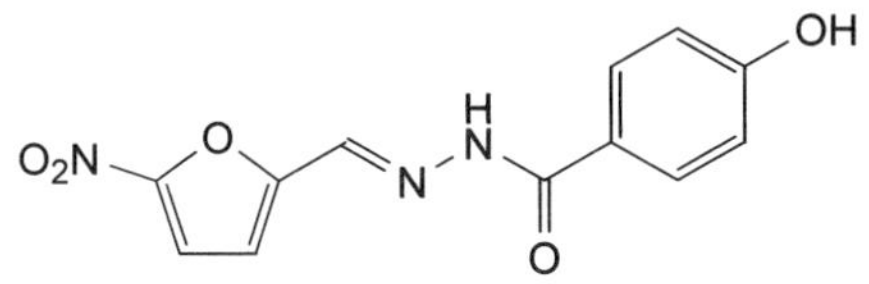

$C_{12}H_9N_3O_5$ M_r 275.2

DEFINITION

1-(4-Hydroxybenzoyl)-2-[(5-nitrofuran-2-yl)methylene]-diazane.

Content: 98.5 per cent to 101.5 per cent (dried substance).

CHARACTERS

Appearance: bright yellow, crystalline powder.

Solubility: practically insoluble in water, slightly soluble in alcohol and in methylene chloride.

IDENTIFICATION

Infrared absorption spectrophotometry (*2.2.24*).

Comparison: *Ph. Eur. reference spectrum of nifuroxazide*.

TESTS

Specific absorbance (*2.2.25*): 940 to 1000 at the absorption maximum at 367 nm.

Protected from light, dissolve 10.0 mg in 10 ml of *ethylene glycol monomethyl ether R* and dilute to 100.0 ml with *methanol R*. Dilute 5.0 ml of this solution to 100.0 ml with *methanol R*.

Impurity A: maximum 0.05 per cent.

Test solution (a). Dissolve 1.0 g of the substance to be examined in *dimethyl sulphoxide R* and dilute to 10.0 ml with the same solvent.

Test solution (b). To 5.5 ml of test solution (a) add 50.0 ml of *water R* while stirring. Allow to stand for 15 min and filter.

Reference solution. To 0.5 ml of test solution (a) add 5.0 ml of a 50 mg/l solution of *4-hydroxybenzohydrazide R* in *dimethyl sulphoxide R*. Add 50.0 ml of *water R* while stirring. Allow to stand for 15 min and filter.

Add 0.5 ml of *phosphomolybdotungstic reagent R* and 10.0 ml of *sodium carbonate solution R* separately to 10.0 ml of test solution (b) and to 10.0 ml of the reference solution. Allow to stand for 1 h. Examine the 2 solutions at 750 nm. The absorbance (*2.2.25*) of the solution obtained with test solution (b) is not greater than that obtained with the reference solution.

Related substances. Liquid chromatography (*2.2.29*). *Use freshly prepared solutions, protected from light.*

Test solution. Dissolve 0.100 g of the substance to be examined in 15.0 ml of *dimethylformamide R* and dilute to 100.0 ml with the mobile phase. If precipitation occurs, use the supernatant liquid.

Reference solution (a). Dissolve 10.0 mg of *methyl parahydroxybenzoate R* (impurity B) in 2.0 ml of *dimethylformamide R* and dilute to 20.0 ml with the mobile phase. Dilute 1.0 ml of this solution to 100.0 ml with the mobile phase.

Reference solution (b). Dissolve 5 mg of the substance to be examined and 10 mg of *methyl parahydroxybenzoate R* in 2 ml of *dimethylformamide R* and dilute to 20 ml with the mobile phase. Dilute 1 ml of this solution to 100 ml with the mobile phase.

Column:

- *size*: l = 0.25 m, Ø = 4.6 mm,
- *stationary phase*: spherical *octadecylsilyl silica gel for chromatography R* (5 µm) with a specific surface area of 340 m^2/g, a pore size of 10 nm and a carbon loading of 19 per cent.

Mobile phase: *acetonitrile R, water R* (35:65 *V/V*).

Flow rate: 1 ml/min.

Detection: spectrophotometer at 280 nm.

Injection: 20 µl.

Run time: 6 times the retention time of nifuroxazide.

Relative retention with reference to nifuroxazide (retention time = about 6.5 min): impurity A = about 0.4; impurity B = about 1.2; impurity C = about 2.8; impurity D = about 5.2.

System suitability: reference solution (b):

- *resolution*: minimum 3.0 between the peaks due to nifuroxazide and impurity B.

Limits:

- *any impurity*: not more than 0.6 times the area of the principal peak in the chromatogram obtained with reference solution (a) (0.3 per cent), and not more than 1 such peak has an area greater than 0.2 times the area of the principal peak in the chromatogram obtained with reference solution (a) (0.1 per cent),
- *total*: not more than the area of the principal peak in the chromatogram obtained with reference solution (a) (0.5 per cent),
- *disregard limit*: 0.1 times the area of the principal peak in the chromatogram obtained with reference solution (a) (0.05 per cent).

Heavy metals (*2.4.8*): maximum 20 ppm.

1.0 g complies with limit test D. Prepare the standard using 2 ml of *lead standard solution (10 ppm Pb) R.*

Loss on drying (*2.2.32*): maximum 0.5 per cent, determined on 1.000 g by drying in an oven at 100-105 °C for 3 h.

Sulphated ash (*2.4.14*): maximum 0.1 per cent, determined on 1.0 g.

ASSAY

Dissolve 0.200 g, if necessary with heating, in 30 ml of *dimethylformamide R* and add 20 ml of *water R*. Titrate with *0.1 M sodium hydroxide*, determining the end-point potentiometrically (*2.2.20*).

1 ml of *0.1 M sodium hydroxide* is equivalent to 27.52 mg of $C_{12}H_9N_3O_5$.

STORAGE

Protected from light.

Monographs L - P

IMPURITIES

Specified impurities (see note for information p. xli): A, B, C, D.

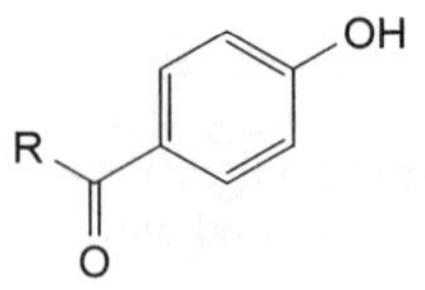

A. R = $NH\text{-}NH_2$: (4-hydroxybenzoyl)diazane (*p*-hydroxybenzohydrazide),

B. R = OCH_3: methyl 4-hydroxybenzoate,

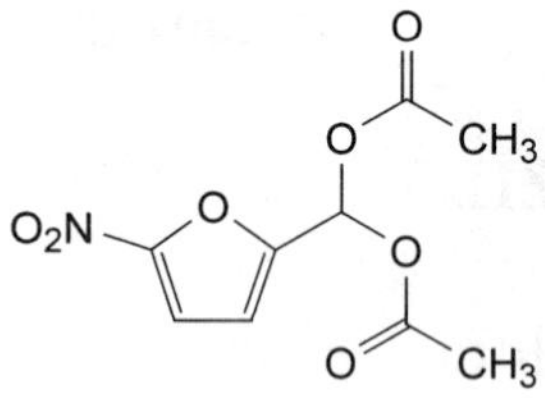

C. (5-nitrofuran-2-yl)methylene diacetate,

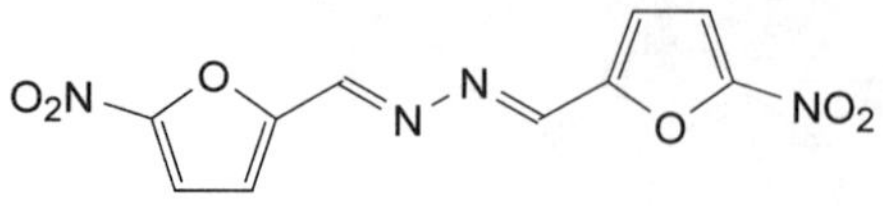

D. 1,2-bis[(5-nitrofuran-2-yl)methylene]diazane (5-nitrofurfural azine).

Monographs L - P

O

07/2004:0942

OMEPRAZOLE

Omeprazolum

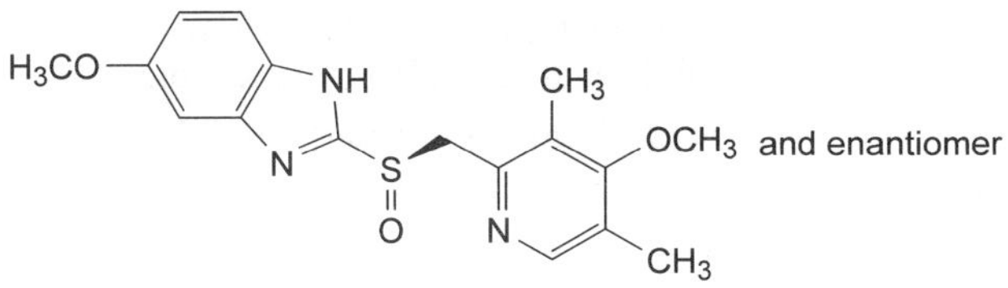

$C_{17}H_{19}N_{3}O_{3}S$ M_r 345.4

DEFINITION

Omeprazole contains not less than 99.0 per cent and not more than the equivalent of 101.0 per cent of 5-methoxy-2-[(*RS*)-[(4-methoxy-3,5-dimethylpyridin-2-yl)methyl]sulphinyl]-1*H*-benzimidazole, calculated with reference to the dried substance.

CHARACTERS

A white or almost white powder, very slightly soluble in water, soluble in methylene chloride, sparingly soluble in alcohol and in methanol. It dissolves in dilute solutions of alkali hydroxides.

It shows polymorphism.

IDENTIFICATION

First identification: B.

Second identification: A, C.

A. Dissolve 2.0 mg in *0.1 M sodium hydroxide* and dilute to 100.0 ml with the same solvent. Examined between 230 nm and 350 nm (*2.2.25*), the solution shows 2 absorption maxima at 276 nm and 305 nm. The ratio of the absorbance measured at the absorption maximum at 305 nm to that measured at the absorption maximum at 276 nm is 1.6 to 1.8.

B. Examine by infrared absorption spectrophotometry (*2.2.24*), comparing with the spectrum obtained with *omeprazole CRS*. If the spectra obtained in the solid state show differences, dissolve the substance to be examined and the reference substance separately in *methanol R*, evaporate to dryness and record new spectra using the residues.

C. Examine the chromatograms obtained in the test for impurity C. The principal spot in the chromatogram obtained with test solution (b) is similar in position and size to the principal spot in the chromatogram obtained with reference solution (a). Place the plate in a tank saturated with vapour from *acetic acid R*. The spots rapidly turn brown.

TESTS

Solution S. Dissolve 0.50 g in *methylene chloride R* and dilute to 25 ml with the same solvent.

Appearance of solution. Solution S is clear (*2.2.1*).

Absorbance (*2.2.25*). The absorbance of solution S measured at 440 nm is not more than 0.10 (this limit corresponds to 0.035 per cent of impurity F or impurity G).

Impurity C. Examine by thin-layer chromatography (*2.2.27*), using a *TLC silica gel F_{254} plate R*.

Test solution (a). Dissolve 0.10 g of the substance to be examined in 2.0 ml of a mixture of equal volumes of *methanol R* and *methylene chloride R*.

Test solution (b). Dilute 1.0 ml of test solution (a) to 10 ml with *methanol R*.

Reference solution (a). Dissolve 10 mg of *omeprazole CRS* in 2.0 ml of *methanol R*.

Reference solution (b). Dilute 1 ml of test solution (a) to 10 ml with a mixture of equal volumes of *methanol R* and *methylene chloride R*. Dilute 1 ml of this solution to 100 ml with a mixture of equal volumes of *methanol R* and *methylene chloride R*.

Apply to the plate 10 µl of each solution. Develop over a path of 15 cm using a mixture of 20 volumes of *2-propanol R*, 40 volumes of *methylene chloride R* previously shaken with *concentrated ammonia R* (shake 100 ml of *methylene chloride R* with 30 ml of *concentrated ammonia R* in a separating funnel; allow the layers to separate and use the lower layer) and 40 volumes of *methylene chloride R*. Allow the plate to dry in air. Examine in ultraviolet light at 254 nm. Any spot in the chromatogram obtained with test solution (a) with a higher R_f value than that of the spot due to omeprazole is not more intense than the spot in the chromatogram obtained with reference solution (b) (0.1 per cent).

Related substances. Examine by liquid chromatography (*2.2.29*).

Test solution. Dissolve 3.0 mg of the substance to be examined in the mobile phase and dilute to 25.0 ml with the mobile phase.

Reference solution (a). Dissolve 1.0 mg of *omeprazole CRS* and 1.0 mg of *omeprazole impurity D CRS* in the mobile phase and dilute to 10.0 ml with the mobile phase.

Reference solution (b). Dilute 1.0 ml of the test solution to 100.0 ml with the mobile phase. Dilute 1.0 ml of this solution to 10.0 ml with the mobile phase.

The chromatographic procedure may be carried out using:

– a stainless steel column 0.15 m long and 4 mm in internal diameter packed with *octylsilyl silica gel for chromatography R* (5 µm),
– as mobile phase at a flow rate of 1 ml/min a mixture of 27 volumes of *acetonitrile R* and 73 volumes of a 1.4 g/l solution of *disodium hydrogen phosphate R* previously adjusted to pH 7.6 with *phosphoric acid R*,
– as detector a spectrophotometer set at 280 nm.

When the chromatograms are recorded under the prescribed conditions, the retention time of omeprazole is about 9 min and the relative retention time of impurity D is about 0.8. Inject separately 40 µl of each solution and continue the chromatography for 3 times the retention time of omeprazole. Adjust the sensitivity of the system so that the height of the principal peak in the chromatogram obtained with reference solution (b) is at least 15 per cent of the full scale of the recorder. The test is not valid unless in the chromatogram obtained with reference solution (a), the resolution between the peaks due to impurity D and omeprazole is greater than 3. If necessary, adjust the pH of the mobile phase or the concentration of *acetonitrile R*; an increase in the pH will improve the resolution. The area of any peak, apart from the principal peak, in the chromatogram obtained with the test solution is not greater than the area of the peak in the chromatogram obtained with reference solution (b) (0.1 per cent).

Residual solvents. Examine by head-space gas chromatography (*2.2.28*), using the standard additions method. The content of chloroform is not more than 50 ppm, and the content of methylene chloride is not more than 100 ppm.

The chromatographic procedure may be carried out using:

- a fused-silica column 30 m long and 0.32 mm in internal diameter coated with a 1.8 µm film of cross-linked *poly[(cyanopropyl)(phenyl)][dimethyl]siloxane R*,
- *nitrogen for chromatography R* as the carrier gas,
- a flame-ionisation detector,
- a suitable head-space sampler.

Place 0.50 g of the substance to be examined in a 10 ml vial. Add 4.0 ml of *dimethylacetamide R* and stopper the vial. Equilibrate the vial at 80 °C for 1 h.

Loss on drying (*2.2.32*): maximum 0.2 per cent, determined on 1.000 g by drying under high vacuum at 60 °C for 4 h.

Sulphated ash (*2.4.14*): maximum 0.1 per cent, determined on 1.0 g.

ASSAY

Dissolve 1.100 g in a mixture of 10 ml of *water R* and 40 ml of *alcohol R*. Titrate with *0.5 M sodium hydroxide*, determining the end-point potentiometrically (*2.2.20*).

1 ml of *0.5 M sodium hydroxide* is equivalent to 0.1727 g of $C_{17}H_{19}N_3O_3S$.

STORAGE

In an airtight container, protected from light, at a temperature between 2 °C and 8 °C.

IMPURITIES

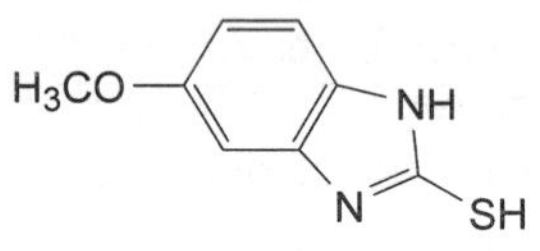

A. 5-methoxy-1*H*-benzimidazole-2-thiol,

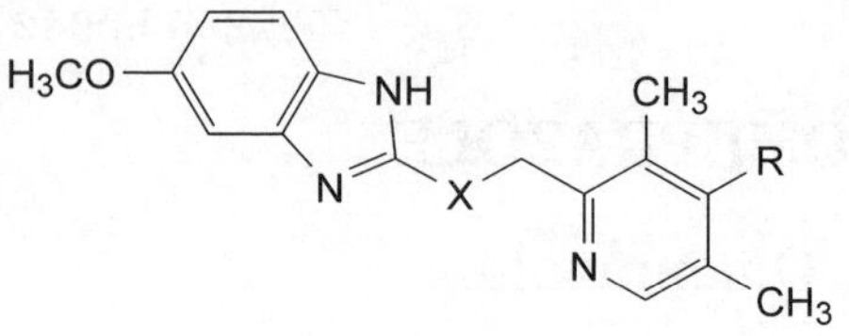

B. R = H, X = SO: 2-[(*RS*)-[(3,5-dimethylpyridin-2-yl)methyl]sulphinyl]-5-methoxy-1*H*-benzimidazole,

C. R = OCH_3, X = S: 5-methoxy-2-[[(4-methoxy-3,5-dimethylpyridin-2-yl)methyl]sulphanyl]-1*H*-benzimidazole (ufiprazole),

D. R = OCH_3, X = SO_2: 5-methoxy-2-[[(4-methoxy-3,5-dimethylpyridin-2-yl)methyl]sulphonyl]-1*H*-benzimidazole (omeprazole sulphone),

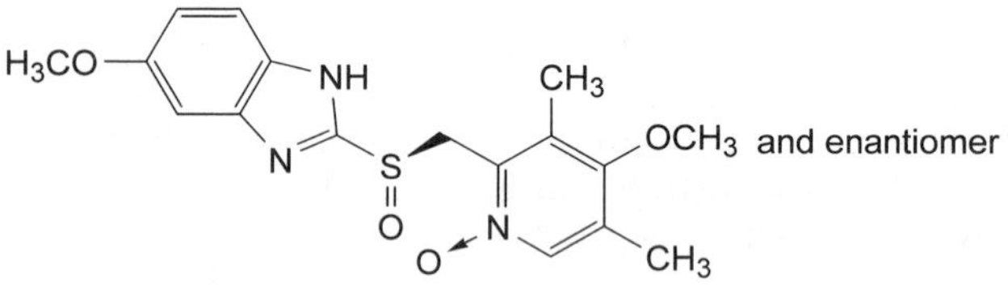

E. 4-methoxy-2-[[(*RS*)-(5-methoxy-1*H*-benzimidazol-2-yl)sulphinyl]methyl]-3,5-dimethylpyridine 1-oxide,

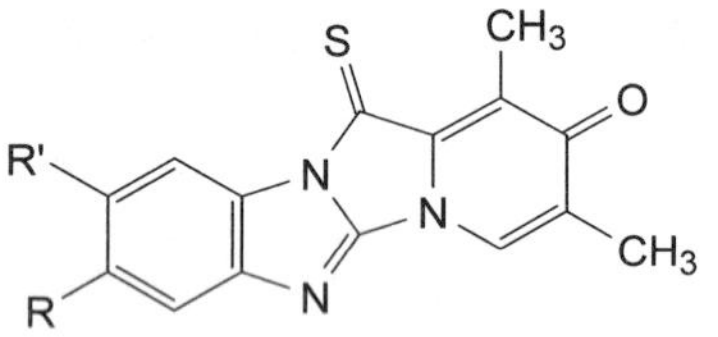

F. R = OCH_3, R′ = H: 1,3-dimethyl-8-methoxy-12-thioxopyrido[1′,2′:3,4]imidazo[1,2-*a*]benzimidazol-2(12*H*)-one,

G. R = H, R′ = OCH_3: 1,3-dimethyl-9-methoxy-12-thioxopyrido[1′,2′:3,4]imidazo[1,2-*a*]benzimidazol-2(12*H*)-one.

Monographs L - P

P

07/2003:1460
corrected

PEFLOXACIN MESILATE DIHYDRATE

Pefloxacini mesilas dihydricus

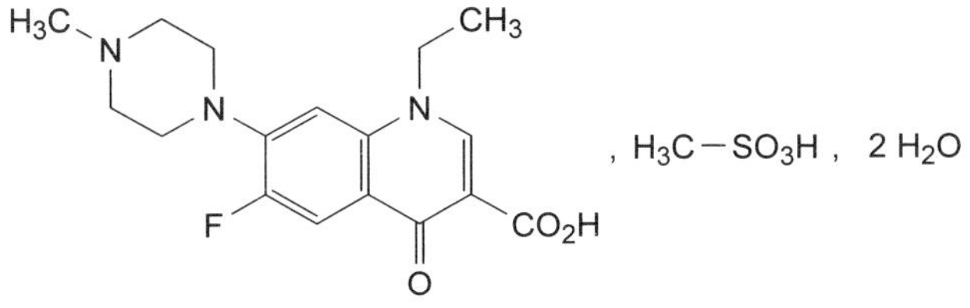

$C_{18}H_{24}FN_3O_6S,2H_2O$ M_r 465.5

DEFINITION

Pefloxacin mesilate dihydrate contains not less than 98.5 per cent and not more than the equivalent of 101.5 per cent of 1-ethyl-6-fluoro-7-(4-methylpiperazin-1-yl)-4-oxo-1,4-dihydroquinoline-3-carboxylic acid methanesulphonate, calculated with reference to the anhydrous substance.

PRODUCTION

The production method must be evaluated to determine the potential for formation of alkyl mesilates, which is particularly likely to occur if the reaction medium contains lower alcohols. Where necessary, the production method is validated to demonstrate that alkyl mesilates are not detectable in the final product.

CHARACTERS

A fine, white or almost white powder, freely soluble in water, slightly soluble in alcohol, very slightly soluble in methylene chloride.

IDENTIFICATION

A. Dissolve separately 0.1 g of the substance to be examined and 0.1 g of *pefloxacin mesilate dihydrate CRS* in 10 ml of *water R*. Add 5 ml of *1 M sodium hydroxide*. Adjust the pH of the solution to 7.4 ± 0.1 with *phosphoric acid R* and shake with 2 quantities, each of 30 ml, of *methylene chloride R*. Combine the organic layers and dry over *anhydrous sodium sulphate R*. Evaporate to dryness. Examine the residues by infrared absorption spectrophotometry (*2.2.24*), comparing the spectra obtained. Examine the residues as discs prepared using *potassium bromide R*.

B. Examine by thin-layer chromatography (*2.2.27*), using a *TLC silica gel plate R*.

Test solution. Dissolve 40 mg in *water R* and dilute to 1 ml with the same solvent.

Reference solution. Dissolve 60 mg of *methanesulphonic acid R* in *water R* and dilute to 10 ml with the same solvent.

Apply to the plate 10 µl of each solution. Develop over a path of 15 cm using a mixture of 5 volumes of *water R*, 10 volumes of *ammonia R*, 20 volumes of *butanol R* and 65 volumes of *acetone R*. Allow the plate to dry in air. Spray with a 0.4 g/l solution of *bromocresol purple R* in *alcohol (50 per cent V/V) R*, adjusted to pH 10 using *1 M sodium hydroxide*. The spot in the chromatogram obtained with the test solution is similar in position, colour and size to the spot in the chromatogram obtained with the reference solution.

TESTS

Solution S. Dissolve 1.0 g in *carbon dioxide-free water R* and dilute to 10.0 ml with the same solvent.

Appearance of solution. Examined within 1 h after its preparation, solution S is not more opalescent than reference suspension II (*2.2.1*) and not more intensely coloured than intensity 3 of the range of reference solutions of the most appropriate colour (*2.2.2, Method II*).

pH (*2.2.3*). Dilute 1 ml of solution S to 10 ml with *carbon dioxide-free water R*. The pH of the solution is 3.5 to 4.5.

Related substances. Examine by liquid chromatography (*2.2.29*).

Test solution. Dissolve 20.0 mg of the substance to be examined in the mobile phase and dilute to 100.0 ml with the mobile phase.

Reference solution (a). Dissolve 5.0 mg of *pefloxacin impurity B CRS* in the mobile phase and dilute to 50.0 ml with the mobile phase. Dilute 1.0 ml of this solution to 100.0 ml with the mobile phase. In 2.0 ml of the solution obtained, dissolve the contents of a vial of *pefloxacin impurity C CRS*.

Reference solution (b). Dissolve 10.0 mg of *norfloxacin impurity A CRS* (pefloxacin impurity F) in the mobile phase and dilute to 100.0 ml with the mobile phase. Dilute 1.0 ml of this solution to 100.0 ml with the mobile phase.

The chromatographic procedure may be carried out using:

- a stainless steel column 0.15 m long and 6 mm in internal diameter packed with *octadecylsilyl vinyl polymer for chromatography R* (5 µm),
- as mobile phase at a flow rate of 1 ml/min a mixture prepared as follows: 30 volumes of *acetonitrile R*, 70 volumes of a solution containing 2.70 g/l of *cetyltrimethylammonium bromide R* and 6.18 g/l of *boric acid R* (exactly adjusted to pH 8.30 with *1 M sodium hydroxide*), and 0.2 volumes of *thiodiethylene glycol R*,
- as detector a spectrophotometer set at 258 nm and 273 nm.

Inject 20 µl of reference solution (a). Record the chromatogram at 273 nm. The test is not valid unless the resolution between the peaks corresponding to impurity B and impurity C is at least 1.5. Inject 20 µl of the test solution and 20 µl of reference solution (b). Record the chromatograms of the test solution at 258 nm and 273 nm for 4 times the retention time of pefloxacin (about 60 min). Record the chromatogram of reference solution (b) at 258 nm. When the chromatograms are recorded in the prescribed conditions, the relative retentions are indicated in the following table.

	Approximate relative retention	Correction factor
Impurity E	0.2	-
Impurity D	0.3	-
Impurity A	0.5	-
Impurity G	0.8	1.4
Pefloxacin	1	-
Impurity C	1.7	2.4
Impurity B	1.8	-
Impurity H	2.4	1.8
Impurity F	3.5	-

From the chromatogram obtained at 258 nm with the test solution, calculate the percentage content of impurity C, F, G and H using the area of the principal peak in the chromatogram obtained at 258 nm with reference solution (b) (external standardisation) taking into account the correction factors indicated in the table.

From the chromatogram obtained at 273 nm with the test solution, calculate the percentage content of impurity A, B, D and E and of any unknown impurity from the areas of the peaks in the chromatogram obtained with the test solution by the normalisation procedure, disregarding the peaks with an area less than 0.0005 times that of the principal peak in the chromatogram obtained at 273 nm with the test solution. None of the impurities has a content of more than 0.5 per cent and not more than 3 impurities have a content between 0.2 per cent and 0.5 per cent. The sum of the contents of the impurities is not more than 1.0 per cent.

Heavy metals (*2.4.8*). 0.250 g complies with limit test E for heavy metals (10 ppm). Prepare the standard using 1.0 ml of *lead standard solution (10 ppm Pb) R*.

Water (*2.5.12*): 7.0 per cent to 8.5 per cent, determined on 50.0 mg by the semi-micro determination of water using a mixture of 10 volumes of *methanol R* and 50 volumes of *methylene chloride R*.

Sulphated ash (*2.4.14*). Not more than 0.1 per cent, determined on 1.0 g.

ASSAY

Dissolve 0.200 g in 15.0 ml of *anhydrous acetic acid R* and add 75.0 ml of *acetic anhydride R*. Titrate with *0.1 M perchloric acid*, determining the end-point potentiometrically (*2.2.20*).

1 ml of *0.1 M perchloric acid* is equivalent to 21.48 mg of $C_{18}H_{24}FN_3O_6S$.

STORAGE

Store in an airtight container, protected from light.

IMPURITIES

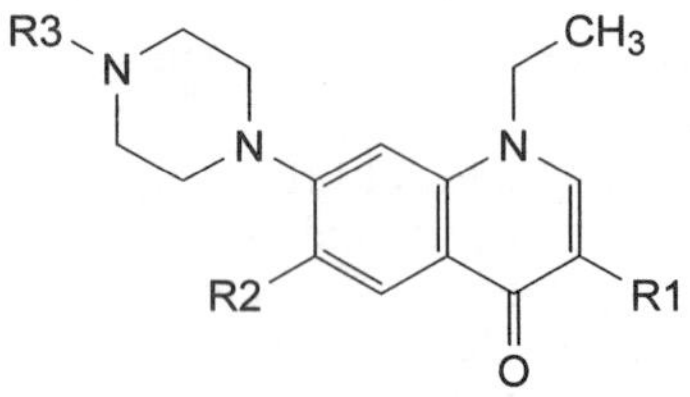

A. R1 = CO_2H, R2 = F, R3 = H: 1-ethyl-6-fluoro-4-oxo-7-(piperazin-1-yl)-1,4-dihydroquinoline-3-carboxylic acid (demethylated pefloxacin or norfloxacin),

B. R1 = CO_2H, R2 = Cl, R3 = CH_3: 6-chloro-1-ethyl-7-(4-methylpiperazin-1-yl)-4-oxo-1,4-dihydroquinoline-3-carboxylic acid (chlorinated homologue of pefloxacin),

E. R1 = H, R2 = F, R3 = CH_3: 1-ethyl-6-fluoro-7-(4-methylpiperazin-1-yl)quinoline-4(1*H*)-one (decarboxylated pefloxacin),

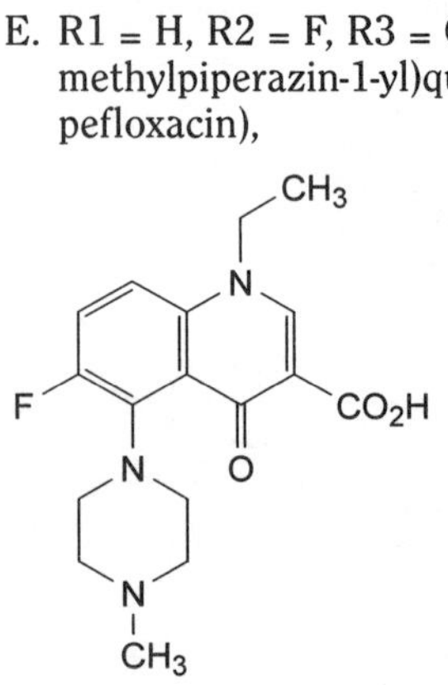

C. 1-ethyl-6-fluoro-5-(4-methylpiperazin-1-yl)-4-oxo-1,4-dihydroquinoline-3-carboxylic acid (isopefloxacin),

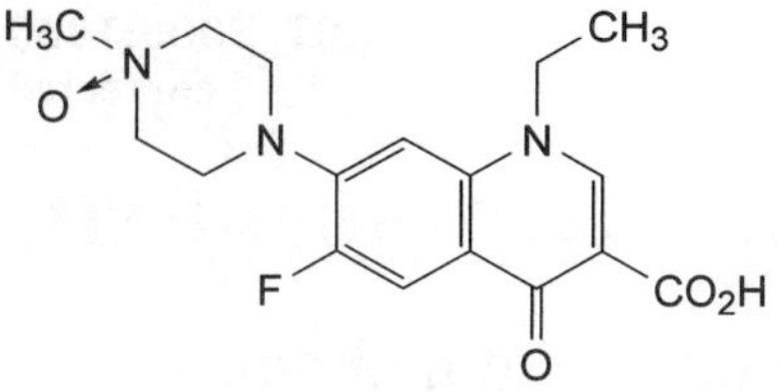

D. 4-(3-carboxy-1-ethyl-6-fluoro-4-oxo-1,4-dihydroquinolin-7-yl)-1-methylpiperazine 1-oxide (*N*-oxide of pefloxacin),

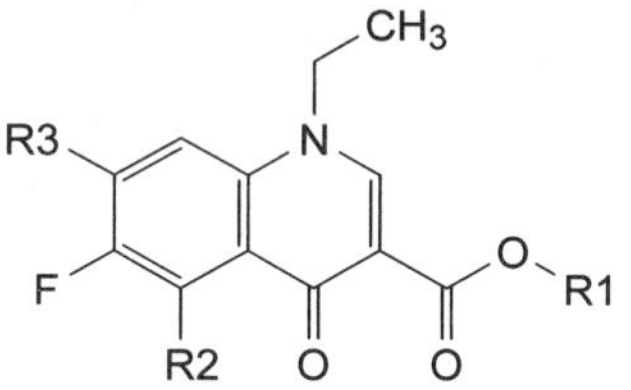

F. R1 = R2 = H, R3 = Cl: 7-chloro-1-ethyl-6-fluoro-4-oxo-1,4-dihydroquinoline-3-carboxylic acid (*N*-ethyl acid) (norfloxacin impurity A),

G. R1 = C_2H_5, R2 = H, R3 = Cl: ethyl 7-chloro-1-ethyl-6-fluoro-4-oxo-1,4-dihydroquinoline-3-carboxylate (*N*-ethyl ester),

H. R1 = R3 = H, R2 = Cl: 5-chloro-1-ethyl-6-fluoro-4-oxo-1,4-dihydroquinoline-3-carboxylic acid (iso-*N*-ethyl acid).

07/2003:0203
corrected

POLYMYXIN B SULPHATE

Polymyxini B sulfas

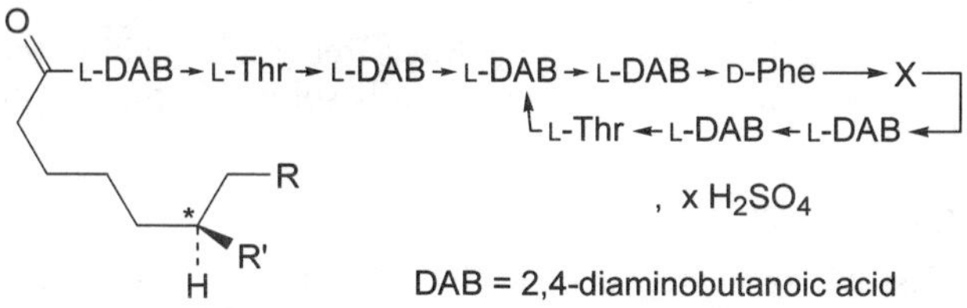

polymyxin	R	R′	X	Molecular formula	M_r
B1	CH_3	CH_3	L-Leu	$C_{56}H_{98}N_{16}O_{13}$	1204
B2	H	CH_3	L-Leu	$C_{55}H_{96}N_{16}O_{13}$	1190
B3	CH_3	H	L-Leu	$C_{55}H_{96}N_{16}O_{13}$	1190
B1-I	CH_3	CH_3	L-Ile	$C_{56}H_{98}N_{16}O_{13}$	1204

DEFINITION

Mixture of the sulphates of polypeptides produced by the growth of certain strains of *Bacillus polymyxa*, or obtained by any other means, the main component being polymyxin B1.

Content:

- sum of polymyxins B1, B2, B3 and B1-I: minimum 80.0 per cent (dried substance),
- polymyxin B3: maximum 6.0 per cent (dried substance),
- polymyxin B1-I: maximum 15.0 per cent (dried substance).

CHARACTERS

Appearance: white or almost white powder, hygroscopic.

Solubility: soluble in water, slightly soluble in alcohol.

IDENTIFICATION

First identification: B, D.

Second identification: A, C, D.

A. Thin-layer chromatography (*2.2.27*).

Test solution. Dissolve 5 mg of the substance to be examined in 1 ml of a mixture of equal volumes of *hydrochloric acid R* and *water R*. Heat at 135 °C in a sealed tube for 5 h. Evaporate to dryness on a water-bath and continue the heating until the hydrochloric acid has evaporated. Dissolve the residue in 0.5 ml of *water R*.

Reference solution (a). Dissolve 20 mg of *leucine R* in *water R* and dilute to 10 ml with the same solvent.

Reference solution (b). Dissolve 20 mg of *threonine R* in *water R* and dilute to 10 ml with the same solvent.

Reference solution (c). Dissolve 20 mg of *phenylalanine R* in *water R* and dilute to 10 ml with the same solvent.

Reference solution (d). Dissolve 20 mg of *serine R* in *water R* and dilute to 10 ml with the same solvent.

Plate: *TLC silica gel G plate R.*

Mobile phase: *water R, phenol R (25:75 V/V).*

Carry out the following procedures protected from light.

Application: 5 µl, as bands of 10 mm.

Place the plate in the chromatographic tank, so that it is not in contact with the mobile phase, and allow to become impregnated with the vapour of the solvent for at least 12 h.

Development: over a path of 12 cm using the same mobile phase.

Drying: at 100-105 °C.

Detection: spray with *ninhydrin solution R1* and heat at 110 °C for 5 min.

Results: the chromatogram obtained with the test solution shows bands corresponding to those in the chromatograms obtained with reference solutions (a), (b) and (c), but shows no band corresponding to that in the chromatogram obtained with reference solution (d). The chromatogram obtained with the test solution also shows a band with a very low R_f value (2,4-diaminobutyric acid).

B. Examine the chromatograms obtained in the assay.

Results: the peaks due to polymyxins B1, B2, B3 and B1-I in the chromatogram obtained with the test solution are similar in retention time to the corresponding peaks in the chromatogram obtained with reference solution (a).

C. Dissolve about 2 mg in 5 ml of *water R* and add 5 ml of a 100 g/l solution of *sodium hydroxide R*. Shake and add dropwise 0.25 ml of a 10 g/l solution of *copper sulphate R*, shaking after each addition. A reddish-violet colour develops.

D. It gives reaction (a) of sulphates (*2.3.1*).

TESTS

pH (*2.2.3*): 5.0 to 7.0.

Dissolve 0.2 g in *carbon dioxide-free water R* and dilute to 10 ml with the same solvent.

Specific optical rotation (*2.2.7*): − 78 to − 90 (dried substance).

Dissolve 0.50 g in *water R* and dilute to 25.0 ml with the same solvent.

Related substances. Liquid chromatography (*2.2.29*): use the normalisation procedure.

Test solution. Dissolve 50.0 mg of the substance to be examined in a mixture of 20 volumes of *acetonitrile R* and 80 volumes of *water R* and dilute to 100.0 ml with the same mixture of solvents.

Reference solution (a). Dissolve 50.0 mg of *polymyxin B sulphate CRS* in a mixture of 20 volumes of *acetonitrile R* and 80 volumes of *water R* and dilute to 100.0 ml with the same mixture of solvents.

Reference solution (b). Dilute 1.0 ml of the test solution to 100.0 ml with a mixture of 20 volumes of *acetonitrile R* and 80 volumes of *water R*.

Column:

- *size*: l = 0.25 m, Ø = 4.6 mm,
- *stationary phase*: *base-deactivated end-capped octadecylsilyl silica gel for chromatography R* (5 µm),
- *temperature*: 30 °C.

Mobile phase: mix 20 volumes of *acetonitrile R* and 80 volumes of a solution prepared as follows: dissolve 4.46 g of *anhydrous sodium sulphate R* in 900 ml of *water R*, adjust to pH 2.3 using *dilute phosphoric acid R* and dilute to 1000 ml with *water R*.

Flow rate: 1.0 ml/min.

Detection: spectrophotometer at 215 nm.

Injection: 20 µl.

Run time: 1.4 times the retention time of polymyxin B1.

Relative retention with reference to polymyxin B1 (retention time = about 35 min): polymyxin B2 = about 0.5; polymyxin B3 = about 0.6; polymyxin B1-I = about 0.8.

System suitability: reference solution (a):

- *resolution*: minimum of 3.0 between the peaks due to polymyxin B2 and polymyxin B3.

Limits:

- *any impurity*: maximum 3.0 per cent,
- *total*: maximum 17.0 per cent,
- *disregard limit*: 0.7 times the area of the principal peak in the chromatogram obtained with reference solution (b).

Sulphate: 15.5 per cent to 17.5 per cent (dried substance).

Dissolve 0.250 g in 100 ml of *water R* and adjust the solution to pH 11 using *concentrated ammonia R*. Add 10.0 ml of *0.1 M barium chloride* and about 0.5 mg of *phthalein purple R*. Titrate with *0.1 M sodium edetate*, adding 50 ml of *alcohol R* when the colour of the solution begins to change and continuing the titration until the violet-blue colour disappears.

1 ml of *0.1 M barium chloride* is equivalent to 9.606 mg of SO_4.

Loss on drying (*2.2.32*): maximum 6.0 per cent, determined on 1.000 g by drying at 60 °C over *diphosphorus pentoxide R* at a pressure not exceeding 670 Pa for 3 h.

Sulphated ash (*2.4.14*): maximum 0.75 per cent, determined on 1.0 g.

Sterility (*2.6.1*). If intended for use in the manufacture of parenteral dosage forms without a further appropriate sterilisation procedure, it complies with the test for sterility.

Pyrogens (*2.6.8*). If intended for use in the manufacture of parenteral dosage forms without a further appropriate procedure for the removal of pyrogens, it complies with the test for pyrogens. Inject, per kilogram of the rabbit's mass, 1 ml of a solution in *water for injections R* containing 1.5 mg of the substance to be examined per millilitre.

ASSAY

Liquid chromatography (*2.2.29*) as described in the test for related substances with the following modification.

Injection: test solution and reference solution (a).

Calculate the percentage content of polymyxin B3 and B1-I, and the sum of polymyxins B1, B2, B3 and B1-I.

STORAGE

In an airtight container, protected from light. If the substance is sterile, store in a sterile, airtight, tamper-proof container.

LABELLING

The label states:

– where applicable, that the substance is sterile,
– where applicable, that the substance is apyrogenic.

R

07/2004:1884

RIBWORT PLANTAIN

Plantaginis lanceolatae folium

DEFINITION

Whole or fragmented, dried leaf and scape of *Plantago lanceolata* L. s. l.

Content: minimum 1.5 per cent of total *ortho*-dihydroxycinnamic acid derivatives expressed as acteoside ($C_{29}H_{36}O_{15}$; M_r 624.6) (dried drug).

CHARACTERS

Macroscopic and microscopic characters described under identification tests A and B.

IDENTIFICATION

A. The leaf is up to 30 cm long and 4 cm wide, yellowish-green to brownish-green, with a prominent, whitish-green, almost parallel venation on the abaxial surface. It consists of a lanceolate lamina narrowing at the base into a channelled petiole. The margin is indistinctly dentate and often undulate. It has 3, 5 or 7 primary veins, nearly equal in length and running almost parallel. Hairs may be almost absent, sparsely scattered or sometimes abundant, especially on the lower surface and over the veins. The scape is brownish-green, longer than the leaves, 3 mm to 4 mm in diameter and is deeply grooved longitudinally, with 5 to 7 conspicuous ribs. The surface is usually covered with fine hairs.

B. Reduce to a powder (355). The powder is yellowish-green. Examine under a microscope using *chloral hydrate solution R*. The powder shows the following diagnostic characters: fragments of epidermis, composed of cells with irregularly sinuous anticlinal walls, the fragments from the scape with thickened outer walls and a coarsely ridged cuticle; stomata mostly of the diacytic type (*2.8.3*) and sometimes anomocytic; the multicellular, uniseriate, conical covering trichomes are highly characteristic, with a basal cell larger than the other epidermal cells followed by a short cell supporting 2 or more elongated cells with the lumen narrow and variable, occluded at intervals corresponding to slight swellings in the trichome and giving a jointed appearance; the terminal cell has an acute apex and a filiform lumen; the glandular trichomes have a unicellular cylindrical stalk and a multicellular, elongated, conical head consisting of several rows of small cells and a single terminal cell; dense groups of lignified fibro-vascular tissue with narrow, spirally and annularly thickened vessels and slender, moderately thickened fibres.

C. Examine the chromatograms obtained for *Digitalis lanata* leaves.

Results A: see below the sequence of the zones present in the chromatograms obtained with the reference solution and the test solution. Furthermore, other zones may be present in the chromatograms obtained with the test solution.

Top of the plate	
———	———
Acteoside: a yellow zone	A yellow zone (acteoside)
———	———
Aucubin: a blue zone	A blue zone (aucubin)
Reference solution	**Test solution**

TESTS

***Digitalis lanata* leaves.** Thin layer chromatography (*2.2.27*).

Test solution. Use a freshly prepared solution. To 1 g of the powdered drug (355) in a 25 ml flask, add 10 ml of a mixture of 30 volumes of *water R* and 70 volumes of *methanol R* and shake for 30 min. Filter, rinse the flask and filter with 2 quantities, each of 5 ml, with the mixture of 30 volumes of *water R* and 70 volumes of *methanol R*. Dilute to 25 ml with a mixture of 30 volumes of *water R* and 70 volumes of *methanol R*.

Reference solution. Dissolve 1 mg of *acteoside R* and 1 mg of *aucubin R* in 1 ml of a mixture of 30 volumes of *water R* and 70 volumes of *methanol R*.

Plate: *TLC silica gel F_{254} plate R*.

Mobile phase: *acetic acid R, anhydrous formic acid R, water R, ethyl acetate R* (11:11:27:100 *V/V/V/V*).

Application: 10 µl as bands.

Development: over a path of 8 cm; heat immediately after development at about 120 °C for 5-10 min.

Detection A: examine in daylight.

Detection B: examine in ultraviolet light at 365 nm.

Results B: the chromatogram obtained with the test solution shows no bright blue fluorescent zone just below the reddish-brown fluorescent zone corresponding to aucubin in the chromatogram obtained with the reference solution.

Foreign matter (*2.8.2*): maximum 5 per cent of leaves of different colour and maximum 2 per cent of other foreign matter.

Loss on drying (*2.2.32*): maximum 10.0 per cent, determined on 1.000 g of the powdered drug (355) by drying in an oven at 100-105 °C for 2 h.

Total ash (*2.4.16*): maximum 14.0 per cent.

ASSAY

Stock solution. In a flask, place 1.000 g of the powdered drug (355) and add 90 ml of *alcohol (50 per cent V/V) R*. Boil in a water-bath under a reflux condenser for 30 min. Allow to cool and filter into a 100 ml volumetric flask. Rinse the flask and the filter with 10 ml of *alcohol (50 per cent V/V) R*. Combine the filtrate and the rinsings and dilute to 100.0 ml with *alcohol (50 per cent V/V) R*.

Test solution. To a 10 ml volumetric flask add, mixing after each addition, 1.0 ml of stock solution, 2 ml of *0.5 M hydrochloric acid*, 2 ml of a solution prepared by dissolving 10 g of *sodium nitrite R* and 10 g of *sodium molybdate R* in 100 ml of *water R* and then add 2 ml of *dilute sodium hydroxide solution R*. Dilute to 10.0 ml with *water R*.

Immediately measure the absorbance (*2.2.25*) of the test solution at 525 nm using as compensation liquid a solution prepared as follows: to a 10 ml volumetric flask, add 1.0 ml of stock solution, 2 ml of *0.5 M hydrochloric acid*, 2 ml of *dilute sodium hydroxide solution R* and dilute to 10.0 ml with *water R*.

Calculate the percentage content of total *ortho*-dihydroxycinnamic acid derivatives, expressed as acteoside, from the expression:

$$\frac{A \times 1000}{185 \times m}$$

i.e. taking the specific absorbance to be 185 for acteoside at 525 nm.

A = absorbance of the test solution at 525 nm,

m = mass of the substance to be examined, in grams.

07/2004:1146

ROXITHROMYCIN

Roxithromycinum

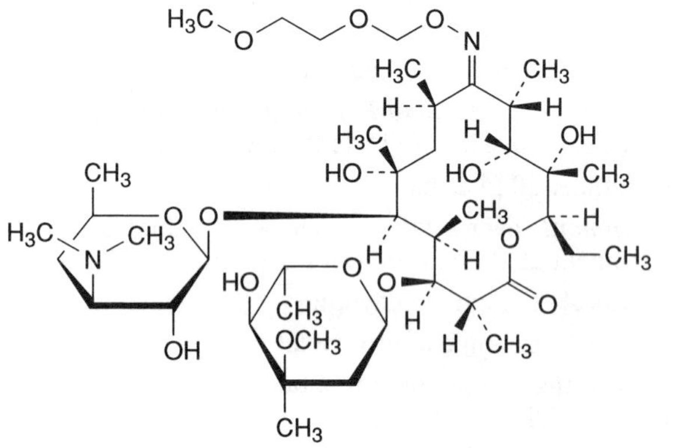

$C_{41}H_{76}N_2O_{15}$ M_r 837

DEFINITION

(3*R*,4*S*,5*S*,6*R*,7*R*,9*R*,11*S*,12*R*,13*S*,14*R*)-4-[(2,6-Dideoxy-3-*C*-methyl-3-*O*-methyl-α-L-*ribo*-hexopyranosyl)oxy]-14-ethyl-7,12,13-trihydroxy-10-[(*E*)-[(2-methoxyethoxy)methoxy]imino]-3,5,7,9,11,13-hexamethyl-6-[[3,4,6-trideoxy-3-(dimethylamino)-β-D-*xylo*-hexopyranosyl]oxy]oxacyclotetradecan-2-one (erythromycin 9-(*E*)-[*O*-[(2-methoxyethoxy)methyl]oxime]).

Content: 96.0 per cent to 102.0 per cent (anhydrous substance).

CHARACTERS

Appearance: white, crystalline powder.

Solubility: very slightly soluble in water, freely soluble in acetone, in alcohol and in methylene chloride. It is slightly soluble in dilute hydrochloric acid.

It shows polymorphism.

IDENTIFICATION

A. Infrared absorption spectrophotometry (*2.2.24*).

Comparison: *roxithromycin CRS.*

If the spectra obtained shows differences, prepare further spectra using 90 g/l solutions in *methylene chloride R*.

B. Examine the chromatograms obtained in the assay.

Results: the principal peak in the chromatogram obtained with the test solution is similar in retention time and size to the principal peak in the chromatogram obtained with reference solution (a).

TESTS

Appearance of solution. The solution is clear (*2.2.1*) and colourless (*2.2.2, Method II*).

Dissolve 0.2 g in *methanol R* and dilute to 20 ml with the same solvent.

Specific optical rotation (*2.2.7*): − 93 to − 96 (anhydrous substance).

Dissolve 0.500 g in *acetone R* and dilute to 50.0 ml with the same solvent.

Related substances. Liquid chromatography (*2.2.29*).

Solution A. Mix 30 volumes of *acetonitrile R* and 70 volumes of a 48.6 g/l solution of *ammonium dihydrogen phosphate R*, adjusted to pH 5.3 with *dilute sodium hydroxide solution R.*

Test solution. Dissolve 50.0 mg of the substance to be examined in solution A and dilute to 25.0 ml with solution A.

Reference solution (a). Dissolve 50.0 mg of *roxithromycin CRS* in solution A and dilute to 25.0 ml with solution A.

Reference solution (b). Dilute 1.0 ml of reference solution (a) to 100.0 ml with solution A.

Reference solution (c). Dissolve 2.0 mg of *roxithromycin for system suitability CRS* in solution A and dilute to 1.0 ml with solution A.

Reference solution (d). Dilute 1.0 ml of *toluene R* to 100.0 ml with *acetonitrile R.* Dilute 0.2 ml of this solution to 200.0 ml with solution A.

Column:

– *size*: l = 0.15 m, Ø = 4.6 mm,
– *stationary phase*: spherical *end-capped octadecylsilyl silica gel for chromatography R* (5 µm) with a 10 nm pore size and a carbon loading of about 19 per cent,
– *temperature*: 15 °C.

Mobile phase:

– *mobile phase A*: mix 26 volumes of *acetonitrile R* and 74 volumes of a 59.7 g/l solution of *ammonium dihydrogen phosphate R,* adjusted to pH 4.3 with *dilute sodium hydroxide solution R,*
– *mobile phase B*: *water R, acetonitrile R* (30:70 *V/V*),

Time (min)	Mobile phase A (per cent *V/V*)	Mobile phase B (per cent *V/V*)
0 - 50	100	0
50 - 51	100 → 90	0 → 10
51 - 80	90	10
80 - 81	90 → 100	10 → 0
81 - 100	100	0

Flow rate: 1.1 ml/min.

Detection: spectrophotometer at 205 nm.

Injection: 20 µl, using an injector maintained at 8 °C, of the test solution and reference solutions (b), (c) and (d).

Relative retention with reference to roxithromycin (retention time = about 22 min): impurity A = about 0.28; impurity B = about 0.31; impurity C = about 0.33; impurity D = about 0.62; impurity E = about 0.67; impurity F = about 0.83; impurity G = about 1.15; impurity K = about 1.7; impurity H = about 1.85; impurity J = about 2.65; impurity I = about 3.1.

System suitability: reference solution (c):

– *peak-to-valley ratio*: minimum 2.0, where H_p = height above the baseline of the peak due to impurity G and H_v = height above the baseline of the lowest point of the curve separating this peak from the peak due to roxithromycin.

Limits:

– *impurity G*: not more than the area of the principal peak in the chromatogram obtained with reference solution (b) (1.0 per cent),

– *impurities A, B, C, D, E, F, H, I, J*: for each impurity, not more than 0.5 times the area of the principal peak in the chromatogram obtained with reference solution (b) (0.5 per cent),

– *total*: not more than 3 times the area of the principal peak in the chromatogram obtained with reference solution (b) (3.0 per cent),

– *disregard limit*: 0.05 times the area of the principal peak in the chromatogram obtained with reference solution (b) (0.05 per cent). Disregard any peak due to toluene (use reference solution (d) to identify it).

Heavy metals (*2.4.8*): maximum 10 ppm.

Dissolve 2.0 g in a mixture of 15 volumes of *water R* and 85 volumes of *acetone R* and dilute to 20 ml with the same mixture of solvents. 12 ml of the solution complies with the limit test B. Prepare the standard using lead standard solution (1 ppm Pb) obtained by diluting *lead standard solution (100 ppm Pb) R* with a mixture of 15 volumes of *water R* and 85 volumes of *acetone R*.

Water (*2.5.12*): maximum 3.0 per cent, determined on 0.200 g.

Sulphated ash (*2.4.14*): maximum 0.1 per cent, determined on 1.0 g.

ASSAY

Liquid chromatography (*2.2.29*) as described in the test for related substances, with the following modifications.

Column:

– *size*: *l* = 0.25 m.

Mobile phase: mix 307 volumes of *acetonitrile R* and 693 volumes of a 49.1 g/l solution of *ammonium dihydrogen phosphate R* adjusted to pH 5.3 with *dilute sodium hydroxide solution R*.

Flow rate: 1.5 ml/min.

Injection: test solution and reference solutions (a) and (c).

Retention time: roxithromycin = about 12 min.

System suitability: reference solution (c):

– *peak-to-valley ratio*: minimum 1.5, where H_p = height above the baseline of the peak due to impurity G and H_v = height above the baseline of the lowest point of the curve separating this peak from the peak due to roxithromycin.

STORAGE

In an airtight container.

IMPURITIES

Specified impurities (see note for information p. xli): A, B, C, D, E, F, G, H, I, J.

Other detectable impurities: K.

A. (3*R*,4*S*,5*S*,6*R*,7*R*,9*R*,11*R*,12*R*,13*S*,14*R*)-4-[(2,6-dideoxy-3-*C*-methyl-3-*O*-methyl-α-L-*ribo*-hexopyranosyl)oxy]-14-ethyl-7,12,13-trihydroxy-3,5,7,9,11,13-hexamethyl-6-[[3,4,6-trideoxy-3-(dimethylamino)-β-D-*xylo*-hexopyranosyl]oxy]oxacyclotetradecane-2,10-dione (erythromycin A),

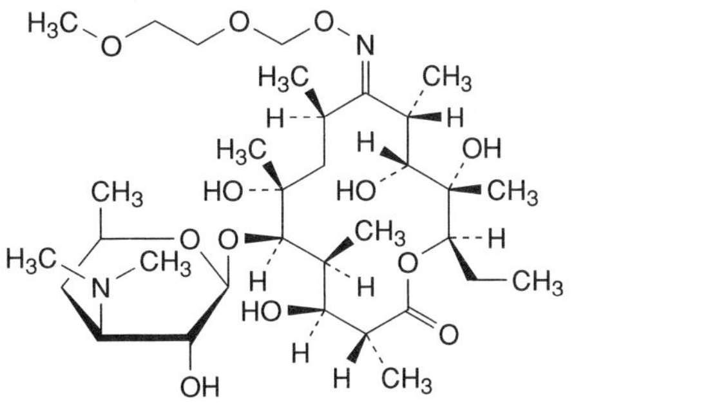

B. 3-*O*-de(2,6-dideoxy-3-*C*-methyl-3-*O*-methyl-α-L-*ribo*-hexopyranosyl)erythromycin 9-(*E*)-[*O*-[(2-methoxyethoxy)methyl]oxime],

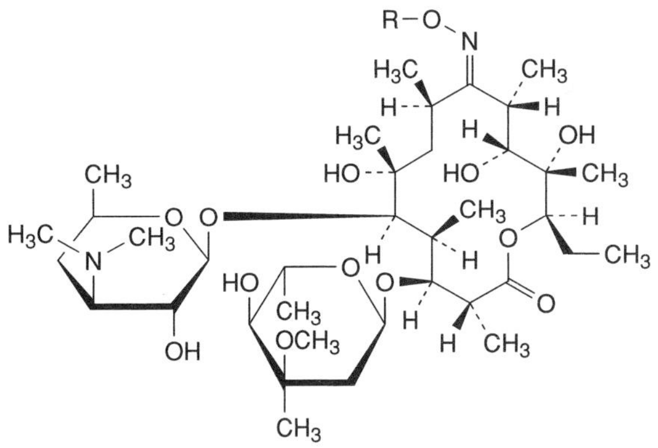

C. R = H: erythromycin 9-(*E*)-oxime,

G. R = CH_2-O-CH_2-O-CH_2-CH_2-OCH_3: erythromycin 9-(*E*)-[*O*-[[(2-methoxyethoxy)methoxy]methyl]oxime],

J. R = CH_2-O-CH_2-CH_2Cl: erythromycin 9-(*E*)-[*O*-[(2-chloroethoxy)methyl]oxime],

K. R = CH_2-O-CH_2-CH_2-O-CH_2OH: erythromycin 9-(*E*)-[*O*-[[2-(hydroxymethoxy)ethoxy]methyl]oxime],

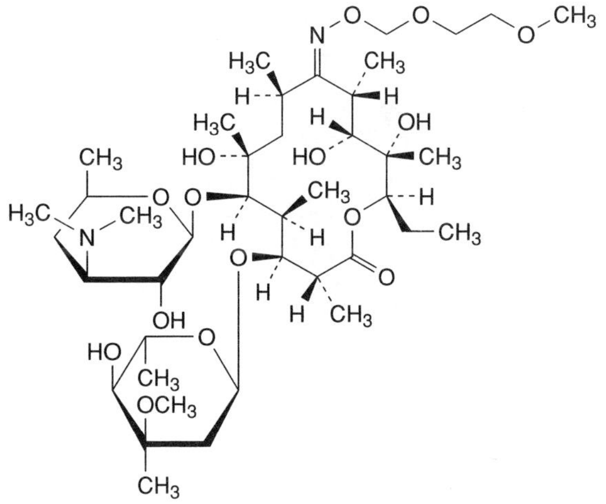

D. erythromycin 9-(*Z*)-[*O*-[(2-methoxyethoxy)methyl]oxime],

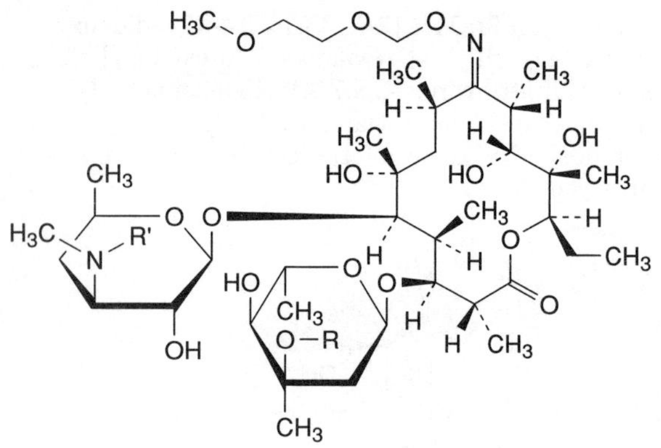

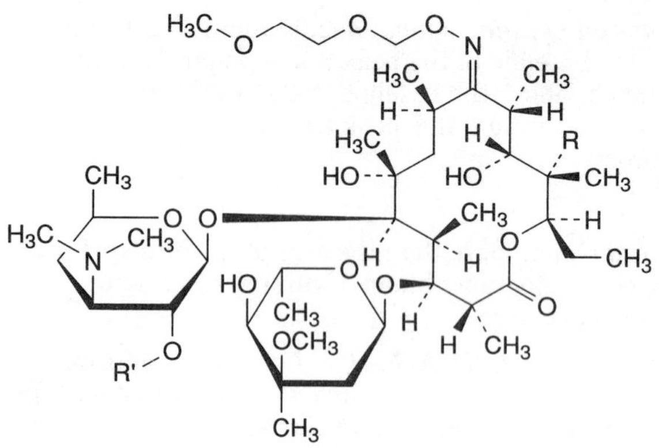

E. R = H, R′ = CH_3: 3″-*O*-demethylerythromycin 9-(*E*)-[*O*-[(2-methoxyethoxy)methyl]oxime],

F. R = CH_3, R′ = H: 3′-*N*-demethylerythromycin 9-(*E*)-[*O*-[(2-methoxyethoxy)methyl]oxime],

H. R = R′ = H: 12-deoxyerythromycin 9-(*E*)-[*O*-[(2-methoxyethoxy)methyl]oxime],

I. R = OH, R′ = CH_2-O-CH_2-CH_2-OCH_3: 2′-*O*-[(2-methoxyethoxy)methyl]erythromycin 9-(*E*)-[*O*-[(2-methoxyethoxy)methyl]oxime].

Monographs Q - Z

S

07/2004:2088

SAFFLOWER OIL, REFINED

Carthami oleum raffinatum

DEFINITION

Fatty oil obtained from seeds of *Carthamus tinctorius* L. (type I) or from seeds of hybrids of *Carthamus tinctorius* L. (type II), by expression and/or extraction followed by refining. Type II refined safflower oil is rich in oleic acid.

It may contain a suitable antioxidant.

CHARACTERS

Appearance: clear, viscous, yellow to pale yellow liquid.

Solubility: miscible with light petroleum (bp: 40-60 °C), practically insoluble in alcohol.

	Refined safflower oil (type I)	Refined safflower oil (type II)
Relative density	about 0.922	about 0.914
Refractive index	about 1.476	about 1.472

IDENTIFICATION

First identification: B.

Second identification: A.

A. Carry out the identification of fatty oils by thin-layer chromatography (*2.3.2*). The chromatogram obtained is comparable with the type chromatogram for type I or type II refined safflower oil.

B. It complies with the test for composition of fatty acids (see Tests).

TESTS

Acid value (*2.5.1*): maximum 0.5.

Peroxide value (*2.5.5*): maximum 10.0. Maximum 5.0, if intended for the manufacture of parenteral dosage forms.

Unsaponifiable matter (*2.5.7*): maximum 1.5 per cent, determined on 5.0 g.

Alkaline impurities (*2.4.19*). It complies with the test for alkaline impurities in fatty oils.

Composition of fatty acids (*2.4.22, Method A*). Use the mixture of calibrating substances in Table 2.4.22.-3.

Composition of the fatty acid fraction of type I refined safflower oil:

- *saturated fatty acids of chain length less than C14*: maximum 0.2 per cent,
- *myristic acid*: maximum 0.2 per cent,
- *palmitic acid*: 4.0 per cent to 10.0 per cent,
- *stearic acid*: 1.0 per cent to 5.0 per cent,
- *oleic acid* (equivalent chain length on polyethyleneglycol adipate 18.3): 8.0 per cent to 21.0 per cent,
- *linoleic acid* (equivalent chain length on polyethyleneglycol adipate 18.9): 68.0 per cent to 83.0 per cent,
- *linolenic acid* (equivalent chain length on polyethyleneglycol adipate 19.7): maximum 0.5 per cent,
- *arachidic acid*: maximum 0.5 per cent,
- *eicosenoic acid* (equivalent chain length on polyethyleneglycol adipate 20.3): maximum 0.5 per cent,
- *behenic acid*: maximum 1.0 per cent.

Composition of the fatty acid fraction of type II refined safflower oil:

- *saturated fatty acids of chain length less than C14*: maximum 0.2 per cent,
- *myristic acid*: maximum 0.2 per cent,
- *palmitic acid*: 3.6 per cent to 6.0 per cent,
- *stearic acid*: 1.0 per cent to 5.0 per cent,
- *oleic acid* (equivalent chain length on polyethyleneglycol adipate 18.3): 70.0 per cent to 84.0 per cent,
- *linoleic acid* (equivalent chain length on polyethyleneglycol adipate 18.9): 7.0 per cent to 23.0 per cent,
- *linolenic acid* (equivalent chain length on polyethyleneglycol adipate 19.7): maximum 0.5 per cent,
- *arachidic acid*: maximum 1.0 per cent,
- *eicosenoic acid* (equivalent chain length on polyethyleneglycol adipate 20.3): maximum 1.0 per cent,
- *behenic acid*: maximum 1.2 per cent.

Brassicasterol (*2.4.23*): maximum 0.3 per cent of brassicasterol in the sterol fraction of the oil.

Water (*2.5.32*): maximum 0.1 per cent, determined on 5.00 g, if intended for use in the manufacture of parenteral dosage forms.

STORAGE

In a well-filled, airtight container, protected from light.

LABELLING

The label states:

- where applicable, that the substance is suitable for use in the manufacture of parenteral dosage forms,
- the name and concentration of any added antioxidant,
- the type of oil (type I or type II).

07/2004:1993

SODIUM AMINOSALICYLATE DIHYDRATE

Natrii aminosalicylas dihydricus

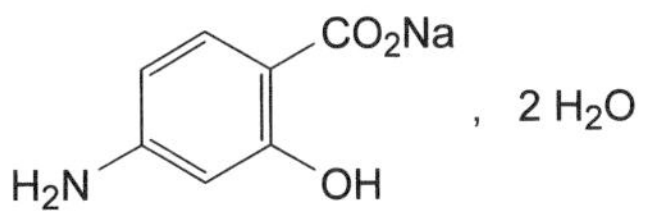

$C_7H_6NNaO_3,2H_2O$ M_r 211.2

DEFINITION

Sodium 4-amino-2-hydroxybenzoate dihydrate.

Content: 99.0 per cent to 101.0 per cent (dried substance).

CHARACTERS

Appearance: white, crystalline powder or white or almost white crystals, slightly hygroscopic.

Solubility: freely soluble in water, sparingly soluble in alcohol, practically insoluble in methylene chloride.

IDENTIFICATION

First identification: A, E.

Second identification: B, C, D, E.

A. Infrared absorption spectrophotometry (*2.2.24*).

Comparison: Ph. Eur. reference spectrum of sodium aminosalicylate dihydrate.

B. Introduce 0.3 g into a porcelain crucible. Cautiously heat on a small flame until vapour is evolved. Cover the crucible with a watch glass and collect the white sublimate. The melting point (*2.2.14*) of the sublimate is 120 °C to 124 °C.

C. To 0.1 ml of solution S (see Tests) add 5 ml of *water R* and 0.1 ml of *ferric chloride solution R1*. A reddish-brown colour develops.

D. 2 ml of solution S gives the reaction of primary aromatic amines (*2.3.1*).

E. 0.5 ml of solution S gives reaction (a) of sodium (*2.3.1*).

TESTS

Solution S. Dissolve 0.50 g in *carbon dioxide-free water R* and dilute to 25 ml with the same solvent.

Appearance of solution. The freshly prepared solution is clear (*2.2.1*) and not more intensely coloured than reference solution B_5 (*2.2.2, Method II*).

Dissolve 2.5 g in *water R* and dilute to 25 ml with the same solvent.

pH (*2.2.3*): 6.5 to 8.5 for solution S.

Related substances. Liquid chromatography (*2.2.29*). *Use freshly prepared solutions and mobile phases.*

Test solution. Dissolve 50.0 mg of the substance to be examined in *water R* and dilute to 50.0 ml with the same solvent.

Reference solution (a). Dissolve 5.0 mg of *3-aminophenol R* in *water R* and dilute to 100.0 ml with the same solvent.

Reference solution (b). Dissolve 5.0 mg of *mesalazine CRS* in *water R* and dilute to 100.0 ml with the same solvent. To 10.0 ml of this solution add 1.0 ml of reference solution (a) and dilute to 50.0 ml with *water R*.

Column:

- *size*: *l* = 0.25 m, Ø = 4.6 mm,
- *stationary phase*: spherical *base-deactivated octylsilyl silica gel for chromatography R* (5 µm).

Mobile phase:

- *mobile phase A*: dissolve 2.2 g of *perchloric acid R* and 1.0 g of *phosphoric acid R* in *water R* and dilute to 1000.0 ml with the same solvent,
- *mobile phase B*: dissolve 1.7 g of *perchloric acid R* and 1.0 g of *phosphoric acid R* in *acetonitrile R* and dilute to 1000.0 ml with the same solvent,

Time (min)	Mobile phase A (per cent *V/V*)	Mobile phase B (per cent *V/V*)
0 - 15	100	0
15 - 30	100 → 40	0 → 60
30 - 35	40 → 100	60 → 0
35 - 45	100	0

Flow rate: 1.25 ml/min.

Detection: spectrophotometer at 220 nm.

Injection: 10 µl.

Relative retention with reference to 4-aminosalicylate (retention time = about 12 min): impurity A = about 0.30; impurity B = about 0.37.

System suitability: reference solution (b):

- *resolution*: minimum 4.0 between the peaks due to impurity A and impurity B.

Limits:

- *impurity A*: not more than the area of the corresponding peak in the chromatogram obtained with reference solution (b) (0.1 per cent),
- *impurity B*: not more than the area of the corresponding peak in the chromatogram obtained with reference solution (b) (1.0 per cent),
- *any other impurity*: for each impurity, not more than 0.1 times the area of the peak due to impurity B in the chromatogram obtained with reference solution (b) (0.1 per cent),
- *total*: not more than the area of the peak due to impurity B in the chromatogram obtained with reference solution (b) (1.0 per cent),
- *disregard limit*: 0.05 times the area of the peak due to impurity B in the chromatogram obtained with reference solution (b) (0.05 per cent).

Heavy metals (*2.4.8*): maximum 10 ppm.

2.0 g complies with limit test C. Prepare the standard using 2 ml of *lead standard solution (10 ppm Pb) R*.

Loss on drying (*2.2.32*): 16.0 per cent to 17.5 per cent, determined on 1.000 g by drying in an oven at 100-105 °C.

Pyrogens (*2.6.8*). If intended for use in the manufacture of parenteral dosage forms without a further appropriate procedure for the removal of pyrogens, it complies with the test for pyrogens. Inject per kilogram of the rabbit's mass, 10 ml of a 20 mg/ml solution of the substance to be examined in *water for injections R*.

ASSAY

Dissolve 0.150 g in 20 ml of *water R*. Add 10 ml of a 500 g/l solution of *sodium bromide R* and 25 ml of *glacial acetic acid R*. Add 5 ml of *0.1 M sodium nitrite* rapidly and continue the titration with the same titrant, determining the end-point potentiometrically (*2.2.20*).

1 ml of *0.1 M sodium nitrite* is equivalent to 17.52 mg of $C_7H_6NNaO_3$.

STORAGE

In an airtight container, protected from light. If the substance is sterile, store in a sterile, airtight, tamper-proof container.

LABELLING

The label states, where applicable, that the substance is apyrogenic.

IMPURITIES

Specified impurities (see note for information p. xli): A, B.

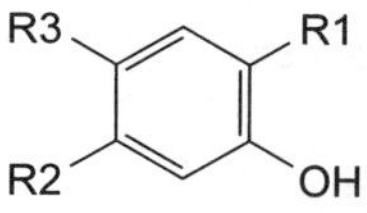

A. R1 = R3 = H, R2 = NH_2: 3-aminophenol,

B. R1 = CO_2H, R2 = H, R3 = NH_2: 5-amino-2-hydroxybenzoic acid (mesalazine).

07/2004:0231

SODIUM CALCIUM EDETATE

Natrii calcii edetas

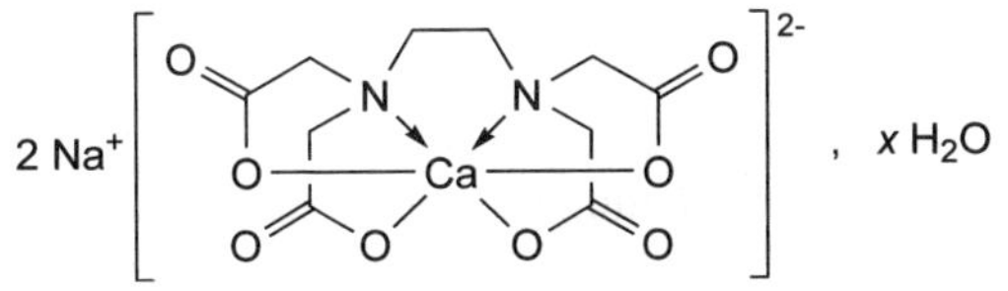

$C_{10}H_{12}CaN_2Na_2O_8,xH_2O$ M_r 374.3 (anhydrous substance)

DEFINITION

Disodium [(ethylenedinitrilo)tetraacetato]calciate(2−).

Content: 98.0 per cent to 102.0 per cent (anhydrous substance).

It contains a variable amount of water of crystallisation.

CHARACTERS

Appearance: white or almost white powder, hygroscopic.

Solubility: freely soluble in water, practically insoluble in alcohol.

IDENTIFICATION

First identification: A, C, D.

Second identification: B, C, D.

A. Infrared absorption spectrophotometry (*2.2.24*).

Preparation: discs.

Comparison: *sodium calcium edetate CRS.*

B. Dissolve 2 g in 10 ml of *water R*, add 6 ml of *lead nitrate solution R*, shake and add 3 ml of *potassium iodide solution R*. No yellow precipitate is formed. Make alkaline to *red litmus paper R* by the addition of *dilute ammonia R2* and add 3 ml of *ammonium oxalate solution R*. A white precipitate is formed.

C. Ignite. The residue gives the reactions of calcium (*2.3.1*).

D. The residue obtained in identification test C gives the reactions of sodium (*2.3.1*).

TESTS

Solution S. Dissolve 5.0 g in *water R* and dilute to 100 ml with the same solvent.

Appearance of solution. Solution S is clear (*2.2.1*) and colourless (*2.2.2, Method II*).

pH (*2.2.3*): 6.5 to 8.0.

Dissolve 5.0 g in *carbon dioxide-free water R* and dilute to 25 ml with the same solvent.

Impurity A. Liquid chromatography (*2.2.29*). *Carry out the test protected from light.*

Solvent mixture. Dissolve 10.0 g of *ferric sulphate pentahydrate R* in 20 ml of *0.5 M sulphuric acid* and add 780 ml of *water R*. Adjust to pH 2.0 with *1 M sodium hydroxide* and dilute to 1000 ml with *water R*.

Test solution. Dissolve 0.100 g of the substance to be examined in the solvent mixture and dilute to 25.0 ml with the solvent mixture.

Reference solution. Dissolve 40.0 mg of *nitrilotriacetic acid R* in the solvent mixture and dilute to 100.0 ml with the solvent mixture. To 1.0 ml of the solution add 0.1 ml of the test solution and dilute to 100.0 ml with the solvent mixture.

Column:

- *size*: l = 0.10 m, Ø = 4.6 mm,
- *stationary phase*: spherical *graphitised carbon for chromatography R1* (5 µm) with a specific surface area of 120 m^2/g and a pore size of 25 nm.

Mobile phase: dissolve 50.0 mg of *ferric sulphate pentahydrate R* in 50 ml of *0.5 M sulphuric acid* and add 750 ml of *water R*. Adjust to pH 1.5 with *0.5 M sulphuric acid* or *1 M sodium hydroxide*, add 20 ml of *ethylene glycol R* and dilute to 1000 ml with *water R*.

Flow rate: 1 ml/min.

Detection: spectrophotometer at 273 nm.

Injection: 20 µl; filter the solutions and inject immediately.

Run time: 4 times the retention time of the iron complex of impurity A.

Retention time: iron complex of impurity A = about 5 min; iron complex of edetic acid = about 10 min.

System suitability: reference solution:

- *resolution*: minimum 7 between the peaks due to the iron complex of impurity A and the iron complex of edetic acid,
- *signal-to-noise ratio*: minimum 50 for the peak due to impurity A.

Limits:

- *impurity A*: not more than the area of the corresponding peak in the chromatogram obtained with the reference solution (0.1 per cent).

Disodium edetate: maximum 1.0 per cent.

Dissolve 5.0 g in 250 ml of *water R*. Add 10 ml of *ammonium chloride buffer solution pH 10.0 R* and about 50 mg of *mordant black 11 triturate R*. Not more than 1.5 ml of *0.1 M magnesium chloride* is required to change the colour of the indicator to violet.

Chlorides (*2.4.4*): maximum 0.1 per cent.

To 20 ml of solution S add 30 ml of *dilute nitric acid R*, allow to stand for 30 min and filter. Dilute 2.5 ml of the filtrate to 15 ml with *water R*.

Iron (*2.4.9*): maximum 80 ppm.

Dilute 2.5 ml of solution S to 10 ml with *water R*. Add 0.25 g of *calcium chloride R* to the test solution and the standard before the addition of the *thioglycollic acid R*.

Heavy metals (*2.4.8*): maximum 20 ppm.

1.0 g complies with limit test D. Prepare the standard using 2 ml of *lead standard solution (10 ppm Pb) R*.

Water (*2.5.12, Method B*): 5.0 per cent to 13.0 per cent, determined on 0.100 g.

ASSAY

Dissolve 0.300 g in *water R* and dilute to 300 ml with the same solvent. Add 2 g of *hexamethylenetetramine R* and 2 ml of *dilute hydrochloric acid R*. Titrate with *0.1 M lead nitrate*, using about 50 mg of *xylenol orange triturate R* as indicator.

1 ml of *0.1 M lead nitrate* is equivalent to 37.43 mg of $C_{10}H_{12}CaN_2Na_2O_8$.

STORAGE

In an airtight container, protected from light.

IMPURITIES

Specified impurities (see note for information p. xli): A.

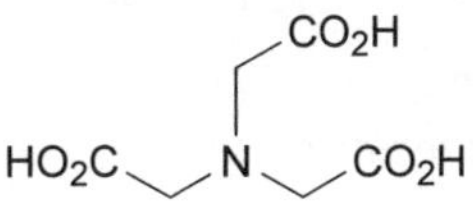

A. nitrilotriacetic acid.

07/2004:1995

SODIUM GLYCEROPHOSPHATE, HYDRATED

Natrii glycerophosphas hydricus

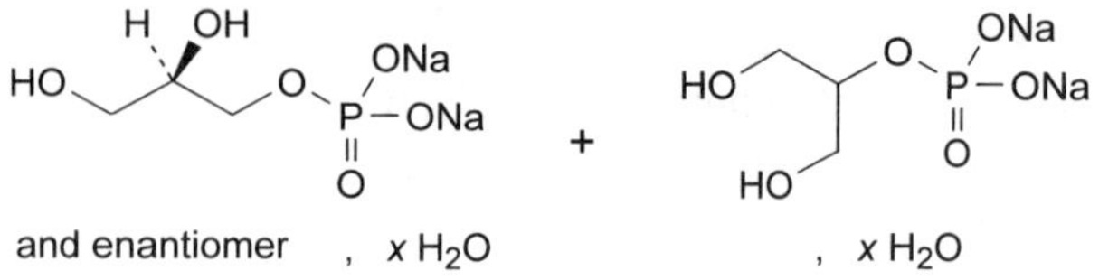

$C_3H_7Na_2O_6P, xH_2O$ M_r 216.0 (anhydrous substance)

DEFINITION

Mixture of variable proportions of sodium (2*RS*)-2,3-dihydroxypropyl phosphate and sodium 2-hydroxy-1-(hydroxymethyl)ethyl phosphate. The degree of hydration is 4 to 6.

Content: 98.0 per cent to 102.0 per cent (anhydrous substance).

CHARACTERS

Appearance: white, crystalline powder or crystals.

Solubility: freely soluble in water, practically insoluble in acetone and in alcohol.

IDENTIFICATION

A. Solution S (see Tests) gives reaction (a) of sodium (*2.3.1*).

B. To 0.1 g add 5 ml of *dilute nitric acid R*. Heat to boiling and boil for 1 min. Cool. The solution gives reaction (b) of phosphates (*2.3.1*).

C. In a test-tube fitted with a glass tube, mix 0.1 g with 5 g of *potassium hydrogen sulphate R*. Heat strongly and direct the white vapour into 5 ml of *decolorised fuchsin solution R*. A violet-red colour develops which becomes violet upon heating for 30 min on a water-bath.

TESTS

Solution S. Dissolve 10.0 g in *carbon dioxide-free water R* prepared from *distilled water R* and dilute to 100 ml with the same solvent.

Appearance of solution. Solution S is not more opalescent than reference suspension II (*2.2.1*) and not more intensely coloured than reference solution Y_6 (*2.2.2, Method II*).

Alkalinity. To 10 ml of solution S add 0.2 ml of *phenolphthalein solution R*. Not more than 1.0 ml of *0.1 M hydrochloric acid* is required to change the colour of the indicator, (n_2).

Glycerol and alcohol-soluble substances: maximum 1.0 per cent.

Shake 1.000 g with 25 ml of *alcohol R* for 10 min. Filter. Evaporate the filtrate on a water-bath and dry the residue at 70 °C for 1 h. The residue weighs not more than 10 mg.

Chlorides (*2.4.4*): maximum 200 ppm.

Dilute 2.5 ml of solution S to 15 ml with *water R*.

Phosphates (*2.4.11*): maximum 0.1 per cent.

Dilute 1 ml of solution S to 10 ml with *water R*. Dilute 1 ml of this solution to 100 ml with *water R*.

Sulphates (*2.4.13*): maximum 500 ppm.

Dilute 3 ml of solution S to 15 ml with *water R*.

Iron (*2.4.9*): maximum 20 ppm.

Dilute 5 ml of solution S to 10 ml with *water R*.

Heavy metals (*2.4.8*): maximum 20 ppm.

Dilute 10 ml of solution S to 20 ml with *water R*. 12 ml of the solution complies with limit test A. Prepare the standard using 10 ml of *lead standard solution (1 ppm Pb) R*.

Water (*2.5.12*): 25.0 per cent to 35.0 per cent, determined on 0.100 g.

ASSAY

Dissolve 0.250 g in 30 ml of *water R*. Titrate with *0.05 M sulphuric acid*, determining the end-point potentiometrically (*2.2.20*), (n_1).

Calculate the percentage content of sodium glycerophosphate (anhydrous substance) from the expression:

$$\frac{216.0\left(n_1 - \frac{n_2}{4}\right)}{m\,(100 - a)}$$

a = percentage content of water,

n_1 = volume of *0.05 M sulphuric acid* used in the assay, in millilitres,

n_2 = volume of *0.1 M hydrochloric acid* used in the test for alkalinity, in millilitres,

m = mass of the substance to be examined, in grams.

07/2004:2048

SORBITOL, LIQUID, PARTIALLY DEHYDRATED

Sorbitolum liquidum partim deshydricum

DEFINITION

Liquid sorbitol, partially dehydrated is obtained by acid-catalysed partial internal dehydration of liquid sorbitol. It contains not less than 68.0 per cent *m/m* and not more than 85.0 per cent *m/m* of anhydrous substances, composed of a mixture of mainly D-sorbitol and 1,4-sorbitan with mannitol, hydrogenated oligo- and disaccharides, and sorbitans.

Content (nominal value):

- 1,4-sorbitan ($C_6H_{12}O_5$): minimum 15.0 per cent (anhydrous substance),
- D-sorbitol ($C_6H_{14}O_6$): minimum 25.0 per cent (anhydrous substance).

The contents of 1,4-sorbitan and D-sorbitol are within 95.0 per cent to 105.0 per cent of the nominal values.

CHARACTERS

Appearance: clear, colourless, syrupy liquid.

Solubility: miscible with water, practically insoluble in mineral oils and vegetable oils.

IDENTIFICATION

Examine the chromatograms obtained in the assay.

Results: the 2 principal peaks in the chromatogram obtained with the test solution are similar in retention time and size to the peaks in the chromatogram obtained with reference solution (a).

TESTS

Solution S. Dilute the substance to be examined with *carbon dioxide-free water R* prepared from *distilled water R* to obtain a solution containing 50.0 per cent *m/m* of anhydrous substance.

Monographs Q - Z

Appearance of solution. Solution S is clear (*2.2.1*) and colourless (*2.2.2, Method II*).

Conductivity (*2.2.38*): maximum 20 μS·cm^{-1}.

Measure the conductivity of solution S, while gently stirring with a magnetic stirrer.

Reducing sugars: maximum 0.3 per cent, calculated as glucose (anhydrous substance).

To an amount of the substance to be examined equivalent to 3.3 g of anhydrous substance, add 3 ml of *water R*, 20.0 ml of *cupri-citric solution R* and a few glass beads. Heat so that boiling begins after 4 min. Maintain boiling for 3 min. Cool rapidly and add 100 ml of a 2.4 per cent *V/V* solution of *glacial acetic acid R* and 20.0 ml of *0.025 M iodine*. With continuous shaking, add 25 ml of a mixture of 6 ml of *hydrochloric acid R* and 94 ml of *water R*. When the precipitate has dissolved, titrate the excess of iodine with *0.05 M sodium thiosulphate* using 2 ml of *starch solution R*, added towards the end of the titration, as indicator. Not less than 12.8 ml of *0.05 M sodium thiosulphate* is required.

Nickel (*2.4.15*): maximum 1 ppm (anhydrous substance).

Water (*2.5.12*): 15.0 per cent to 32.0 per cent, determined on 0.10 g.

Microbial contamination. Total viable aerobic count (*2.6.12*) not more than 10^3 micro-organisms per gram and not more than 10^2 fungi per gram, determined by plate count. It complies with the tests for *Escherichia coli* and *Salmonella* (*2.6.13*).

ASSAY

Liquid chromatography (*2.2.29*).

Test solution. Dissolve 0.400 g of the substance to be examined in *water R* and dilute to 20.0 ml with the same solvent.

Reference solution (a). Dissolve 50.0 mg of *sorbitol CRS* and 20.0 mg of *1,4-sorbitan CRS* in *water R* and dilute to 5.0 ml with the same solvent.

Reference solution (b). Dissolve 0.100 g of *mannitol R* and 0.100 g of *sorbitol R* in *water R* and dilute to 10.0 ml with the same solvent.

Column:

- *size*: *l* = 0.3 m, Ø = 7.8 mm,
- *stationary phase*: *strong cation exchange resin (calcium form) R* (9 μm),
- *temperature*: 80 ± 5 °C.

Mobile phase: degassed *water R*.

Flow rate: 0.5 ml/min.

Detection: refractometer maintained at a constant temperature of about 30-35 °C.

Injection: 40 μl.

Relative retention with reference to D-sorbitol (retention time = about 25 min): 1,4-sorbitan = about 0.5; mannitol = about 0.8.

System suitability: reference solution (b):

- *resolution*: minimum 2.0 between the peaks due to mannitol and D-sorbitol.

Calculate the percentage contents of 1,4-sorbitan and D-sorbitol using the chromatogram obtained with reference solution (a) and the declared contents of *1,4-sorbitan CRS* and of *sorbitol CRS*.

LABELLING

The label states the content of D-sorbitol and the content of 1,4-sorbitan (= nominal values).

07/2004:2108

STAR ANISE OIL

Anisi stellati aetheroleum

DEFINITION

Essential oil obtained by steam distillation from the dry ripe fruits of *Illicium verum* Hook. fil.

CHARACTERS

Appearance: clear, colourless or pale yellow liquid.

IDENTIFICATION

First identification: *B*.

Second identification: *A*.

A. Thin-layer chromatography (*2.2.27*).

Test solution. Dissolve 1 g of the substance to be examined in *toluene R* and dilute to 10 ml with the same solvent.

Reference solution. Dissolve 10 μl of *linalol R*, 30 μl of *anisaldehyde R* and 200 μl of *anethole R* and in *toluene R* and dilute to 15 ml with the same solvent. Dilute 1 ml of this solution to 5 ml with *toluene R*.

Plate: *TLC silica gel F_{254} plate R*.

Mobile phase: *ethyl acetate R, toluene R* (7:93 *V/V*).

Application: 5 μl as bands of 10 mm (for normal TLC plates) or 2 μl as bands of 10 mm (for fine particle TLC plates).

Development: over a path of 15 cm (for normal TLC plates) or over a path of 6 cm (for fine particle size plates).

Drying: in air.

Detection A: examine in ultraviolet light at 254 nm.

Results A: see below the sequence of zones present in the chromatograms obtained with the reference solution and the test solution. Furthermore, other zones may be present in the chromatogram obtained with the test solution.

Top of the plate	
	A quenching zone, partly separated
Anethole: a quenching zone	A very strong quenching zone (anethole)
_______	_______
Anisaldehyde: a quenching zone	A quenching zone (anisaldehyde)
_______	_______
Reference solution	**Test solution**

Detection B: spray with *methyl 4-acetylbenzoate reagent R* and heat at 100-105 °C for 10 min; examine the still hot plate in daylight within 10 min.

Results B: see below the sequence of zones present in the chromatograms obtained with the reference solution and the test solution. Furthermore, other zones may be present in the chromatogram obtained with the test solution.

Monographs Q - Z

Top of the plate	
	A violet-brown zone, not fully separated
Anethole: a brown zone	A very strong brown zone (anethole)
_______	_______
Anisaldehyde: a yellow zone	A yellow zone (anisaldehyde)
_______	_______
Linalol: a grey zone	A grey zone (linalol)
Reference solution	**Test solution**

B. Examine the chromatograms obtained in the test for chromatographic profile.

Results: the characteristic peaks in the chromatogram obtained with the test solution are similar in retention time to those in the chromatogram obtained with the reference solution.

TESTS

Relative density (*2.2.5*): 0.979 to 0.985.

Refractive index (*2.2.6*): 1.553 to 1.556.

Freezing point (*2.2.18*): 15 °C to 19 °C.

Fenchone. Gas chromatography (*2.2.28*) as described in the test for chromatographic profile with the following modifications.

Test solution. Dissolve 400 µl of the substance to be examined in 2.0 ml of *hexane R*.

Reference solution (a). Dilute 10 µl of *fenchone R* to 1.2 g with *hexane R*.

Reference solution (b). Dilute 100 µl of reference solution (a) to 100 ml with *hexane R*.

System suitability: reference solution (b):

– *signal-to-noise ratio*: minimum 10 for the principal peak.

Limit:

– *fenchone*: maximum 0.01 per cent.

Pseudoisoeugenyl 2-methylbutyrate. Gas chromatography (*2.2.28*) as described in the test for chromatographic profile with the following modifications.

Test solution. The substance to be examined.

Reference solution (a). Dilute 10 mg of the test solution to 1.000 g with *hexane R*. Dilute 0.5 ml of this solution to 100 ml with *hexane R*.

Reference solution (b). Anise oil CRS.

System suitability:

– the chromatogram obtained with reference solution (b) is similar to the chromatogram provided with *anise oil CRS*.

– *signal-to-noise ratio*: minimum 10 for the principal peak in the chromatogram obtained with reference solution (a).

Limit: locate the peak due to pseudoisoeugenyl 2-methylbutyrate by comparison with the chromatogram provided with *anise oil CRS*.

– *pseudoisoeugenyl 2-methylbutyrate*: maximum 0.01 per cent.

Fatty oils and resinified essential oils (*2.8.7*). It complies with the test for fatty oils and resinified essential oils.

Chromatographic profile. Gas chromatography (*2.2.28*): use the normalisation procedure.

Test solution. Dissolve 200 µl of the substance to be examined in 1.0 ml of *hexane R*.

Reference solution. To 1.0 ml of *hexane R*, add 20 µl of *linalol R*, 20 µl of *estragole R*, 20 µl of *α-terpineol R*, 60 µl of *anethole R* and 30 µl of *anisaldehyde R*.

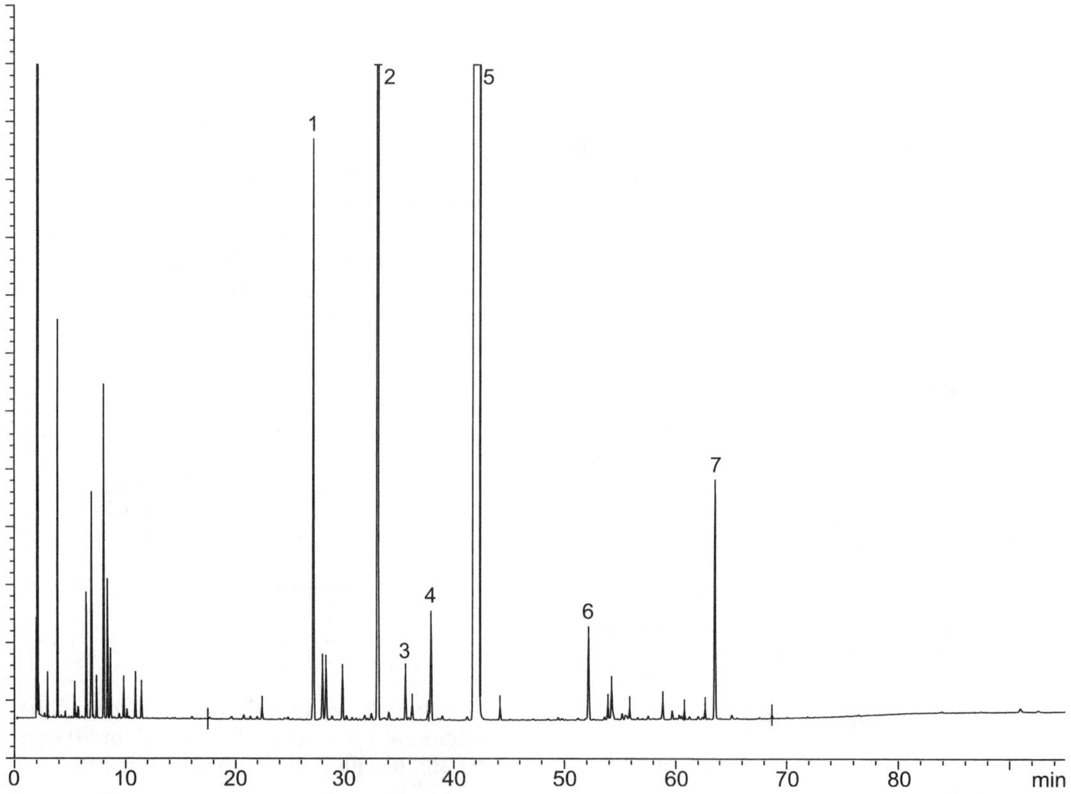

1. linalol
2. estragole
3. α-terpineol
4. *cis*-anethole
5. *trans*-anethole
6. anisaldehyde
7. foeniculin

Figure 2108.-1. – *Chromatogram for the test for chromatographic profile of star anise oil*

Column:

- *material*: fused silica,
- *size*: l = 30 m, Ø = 0.25 mm,
- *stationary phase*: *macrogol 20 000 R* (film thickness 0.25 µm).

Carrier gas: *helium for chromatography R*.

Flow rate: 1.0 ml/min.

Split ratio: 1:100.

Temperature:

	Time (min)	Temperature (°C)
Column	0 - 5	60
	5 - 80	60 → 210
	80 - 95	210
Injection port		200
Detector		220

Detection: flame ionisation.

Injection: 0.2 µl.

Elution order: order indicated in the composition of the reference solution; record the retention times of these substances.

System suitability: reference solution:

- *resolution*: minimum 1.5 between the peaks due to estragole and α-terpineol.

Using the retention times determined from the chromatogram obtained with the reference solution, locate the components of the reference solution in the chromatogram obtained with the test solution and locate *cis*-anethole and foeniculin using the chromatogram shown in Figure 2108.-1 (disregard any peak due to hexane).

Determine the percentage content of these components. The percentages are within the following ranges:

- *linalol*: 0.2 per cent to 2.5 per cent,
- *estragole*: 0.5 per cent to 6.0 per cent,
- *α-terpineol*: less than 0.3 per cent,
- *cis-anethole*: 0.1 per cent to 0.5 per cent,
- *trans-anethole*: 86 per cent to 93 per cent,
- *anisaldehyde*: 0.1 per cent to 0.5 per cent,
- *foeniculin*: 0.1 per cent to 3.0 per cent.

STORAGE

In a well-filled, airtight container, protected from light and at a temperature not exceeding 25 °C.

07/2004:0204

SUCROSE

Saccharum

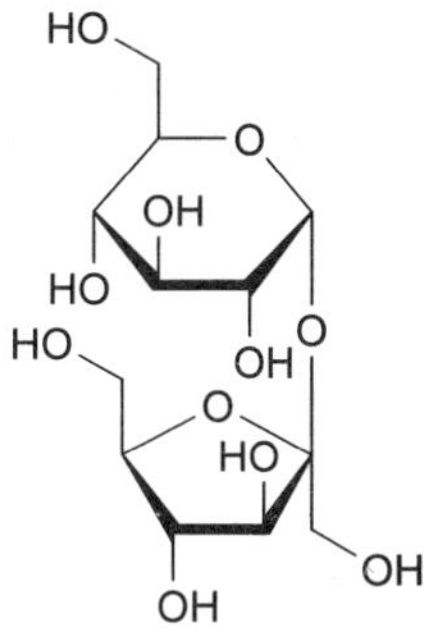

$C_{12}H_{22}O_{11}$ M_r 342.3

DEFINITION

β-D-Fructofuranosyl α-D-glucopyranoside.

It contains no additives.

CHARACTERS

Appearance: white, crystalline powder or shiny, colourless or white crystals.

Solubility: very soluble in water, slightly soluble in alcohol, practically insoluble in ethanol.

IDENTIFICATION

First identification: A.

Second identification: B, C.

A. Infrared absorption spectrophotometry (*2.2.24*).

Comparison: *sucrose CRS.*

B. Thin-layer chromatography (*2.2.27*).

Test solution. Dissolve 10 mg of the substance to be examined in a mixture of 2 volumes of *water R* and 3 volumes of *methanol R* and dilute to 20 ml with the same mixture of solvents.

Reference solution (a). Dissolve 10 mg of *sucrose CRS* in a mixture of 2 volumes of *water R* and 3 volumes of *methanol R* and dilute to 20 ml with the same mixture of solvents.

Reference solution (b). Dissolve 10 mg each of *fructose CRS, glucose CRS, lactose CRS* and *sucrose CRS* in a mixture of 2 volumes of *water R* and 3 volumes of *methanol R* and dilute to 20 ml with the same mixture of solvents.

Plate: *TLC silica gel G plate R.*

Mobile phase: *cold saturated boric acid solution R*, 60 per cent *V/V* solution of *glacial acetic acid R, ethanol R, acetone R, ethyl acetate R* (10:15:20:60:60 *V/V/V/V/V*).

Application: 2 µl.

Development: in an unsaturated tank over a path of 15 cm.

Drying: in a current of warm air.

Detection: spray with a solution of 0.5 g of *thymol R* in a mixture of 5 ml of *sulphuric acid R* and 95 ml of *alcohol R*. Heat the plate at 130 °C for 10 min.

System suitability: the chromatogram obtained with reference solution (b) shows 4 clearly separated spots.

Monographs Q - Z

Results: the principal spot in the chromatogram obtained with the test solution is similar in position, colour and size to the principal spot in the chromatogram obtained with reference solution (a).

C. Dilute 1 ml of solution S (see Tests) to 100 ml with *water R*. To 5 ml of the solution add 0.15 ml of freshly prepared *copper sulphate solution R* and 2 ml of freshly prepared *dilute sodium hydroxide solution R*. The solution is blue and clear and remains so after boiling. To the hot solution add 4 ml of *dilute hydrochloric acid R* and boil for 1 min. Add 4 ml of *dilute sodium hydroxide solution R*. An orange precipitate is formed immediately.

TESTS

Solution S. Dissolve 50.0 g in *carbon dioxide-free water R* prepared from *distilled water R* and dilute to 100 ml with the same solvent.

Appearance of solution. Solution S is clear (*2.2.1*).

Conductivity (*2.2.38*): maximum 35 µS·cm^{-1}.

Dissolve 31.3 g in *carbon dioxide-free water R* prepared from *distilled water R* and dilute to 100 ml with the same solvent. Measure the conductivity of the solution (C_1), while gently stirring with a magnetic stirrer, and that of the water used for preparing the solution (C_2). The readings must be stable within 1 per cent over a period of 30 s. Calculate the conductivity of the solution of the substance to be examined from the following expression:

$$C_1 - 0.35\,C_2$$

Specific optical rotation (*2.2.7*): + 66.3 to + 67.0.

Dissolve 26.0 g in *water R* and dilute to 100.0 ml with the same solvent.

Colour value: maximum 45.

Dissolve 50.0 g in 50.0 ml of *water R*. Mix, filter (diameter of pores 0.45 µm) and degas. Measure the absorbance (*2.2.25*) at 420 nm, using a cell of at least 4 cm (a cell length of 10 cm or more is preferred).

Calculate the colour value using the following expression:

$$\frac{A \times 1000}{b \times c}$$

A = absorbance measured at 420 nm,

b = path length in centimetres,

c = concentration of the solution, in grams per millilitre, calculated from the refractive index (*2.2.6*) of the solution; use Table 0204.-1 and interpolate the values if necessary.

Table 0204.-1

n_D^{20}	c (g/ml)
1.4138	0.570
1.4159	0.585
1.4179	0.600
1.4200	0.615
1.4221	0.630
1.4243	0.645
1.4264	0.661

System suitability:

– *repeatability*: the absolute difference between 2 results is maximum 3.

Dextrins. If intended for use in the preparation of large-volume infusions, it complies with the test for dextrins. To 2 ml of solution S add 8 ml of *water R*, 0.05 ml of *dilute hydrochloric acid R* and 0.05 ml of *0.05 M iodine*. The solution remains yellow.

Reducing sugars. To 5 ml of solution S in a test-tube about 150 mm long and 16 mm in diameter add 5 ml of *water R*, 1.0 ml of *1 M sodium hydroxide* and 1.0 ml of a 1 g/l solution of *methylene blue R*. Mix and place in a water-bath. After exactly 2 min, take the tube out of the bath and examine the solution immediately. The blue colour does not disappear completely. Ignore any blue colour at the air/solution interface.

Sulphites: maximum 10 ppm, calculated as SO_2.

Determine the sulphites content by a suitable enzymatic method based on the following reactions. Sulphite is oxidised by sulphite oxidase to sulphate and hydrogen peroxide which in turn is reduced by nicotinamide-adenine dinucleotide-peroxidase in the presence of reduced nicotinamide-adenine dinucleotide (NADH). The amount of NADH oxidised is proportional to the amount of sulphite.

Test solution. Dissolve 4.0 g of the substance to be examined in freshly prepared *distilled water R* and dilute to 10.0 ml with the same solvent.

Reference solution. Dissolve 4.0 g of the substance to be examined in freshly prepared *distilled water R*, add 0.5 ml of *sulphite standard solution (80 ppm SO_2) R* and dilute to 10.0 ml with freshly prepared *distilled water R*.

Blank solution. Freshly prepared *distilled water R*.

Separately introduce 2.0 ml each of the test solution, the reference solution and the blank in 10 mm cuvettes and add the reagents as described in the instructions in the kit for sulphite determination. Measure the absorbance (*2.2.25*) at the absorption maximum at about 340 nm before and at the end of the reaction time and subtract the value obtained with the blank.

The absorbance difference of the test solution is not greater than half the absorbance difference of the reference solution.

Lead: maximum 0.5 ppm.

Atomic absorption spectrometry (*2.2.23, Method II*).

Test solution. Dissolve 1.5 g of the substance to be examined in 1.5 ml of *deionised distilled water R* in a digestion tube(1). Add 0.75 ml of *lead-free nitric acid R1* and slowly warm to 90-95 °C, avoiding spattering. Heat for about 60 min, add again 0.75 ml of *lead-free nitric acid R1*. Heat until all brown vapours have dissipated and any reddish tint is gone (about 60 min). Cool. Add 0.5 ml of *strong hydrogen peroxide solution R* dropwise and heat at 90-95 °C for

(1) An acid-cleaned high density polyethylene tube, a polypropylene tube, a teflon tube or a quartz tube is suitable.

15 min. Cool. Add again 0.5 ml of *strong hydrogen peroxide solution R* dropwise, heat at 90-95 °C for 60 min and cool. Repeat these operations until a clear, light yellow solution is obtained. Dilute to 10.0 ml with *deionised distilled water R*. Store in capped plastic vials.

Reference solutions. Prepare 3 reference solutions in the same manner as the test solution but adding 0.5 ml, 1.0 ml and 1.5 ml respectively of *lead standard solution (0.5 ppm Pb) R1* in addition to the 1.5 g of the substance to be examined.

Blank solution. Prepare a blank in the same manner as for the test solution but without the substance to be examined.

Zero-setting solution. *Deionised distilled water R*.

Apparatus. Suitable graphite furnace atomic absorption spectrometer equipped with a background compensation system, an autosampler and pyrolytically-coated tubes or with pyrolytic graphite platforms.

Source: hollow-cathode lamp or electrodeless discharge lamp.

Gas:

– *argon R* as the purge gas,
– air as alternate gas during the charring step.

Flow rate: to be adapted according to the apparatus; usually between 200 ml/min and 300 ml/min.

Wavelength: 283.3 nm.

Method. Separately inject 20 µl each of the zero-setting solution, the blank solution, the test solution, the reference solutions, and add immediately 5 µl of *magnesium nitrate solution R1*, which is used as matrix modifier, to each of the solutions. Inject each solution in triplicate.

The ashing and atomisation temperatures and times vary according to the apparatus, the background compensation system, and the graphite tube etc. The following parameters are given for guidance and have to be adjusted.

Heat the furnace progressively to 200 °C and maintain the drying temperature at 200 °C for 30 s, the ashing temperature at 750 °C for 40 s after a 40 s temperature rise, and the atomisation temperature at 1800 °C for 10 s (0 s temperature rise). Clean out at 2600 °C for 7 s after a 1 s temperature rise. Use the zero-setting solution to set the instrument zero. Calculate the mean readings of the test solution and of the reference solutions subtracting the mean blank. If necessary, dilute with the zero-setting solution to obtain a reading within the linear range.

System suitability:

– the relative standard deviation of the 3 readings obtained for the triplicate injections of the test solution and the reference solutions to which the mean blank has been subtracted is not greater than 15 per cent.

Loss on drying (*2.2.32*): maximum 0.1 per cent, determined on 2.000 g by drying in an oven at 100-105 °C for 3 h.

Bacterial endotoxins (*2.6.14*): less than 0.25 IU/mg, if intended for use in the preparation of large-volume infusions.

LABELLING

The label states, where applicable, that the substance is suitable for use in the manufacture of large-volume parenteral dosage forms.

T

07/2004:0954

TEMAZEPAM

Temazepamum

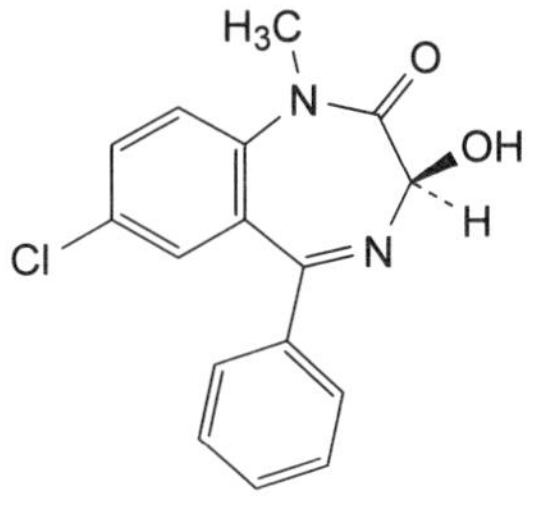

and enantiomer

$C_{16}H_{13}ClN_2O_2$ M_r 300.7

DEFINITION

(3*RS*)-7-Chloro-3-hydroxy-1-methyl-5-phenyl-1,3-dihydro-2*H*-1,4-benzodiazepin-2-one.

Content: 99.0 per cent to 101.0 per cent (dried substance).

CHARACTERS

Appearance: white or almost white, crystalline powder.

Solubility: practically insoluble in water, freely soluble in methylene chloride, sparingly soluble in alcohol.

IDENTIFICATION

Infrared absorption spectrophotometry (*2.2.24*).

Comparison: *Ph. Eur. reference spectrum of temazepam.*

TESTS

Impurity A: maximum 0.05 per cent.

Dissolve 0.400 g in *methylene chloride R* and dilute to 20.0 ml with the same solvent. The absorbance (*2.2.25*) is maximum 0.30 at 409 nm.

Related substances. Liquid chromatography (*2.2.29*).

Test solution. Dissolve 10.0 mg of the substance to be examined in a mixture of 1 volume of *water R* and 9 volumes of *methanol R* and dilute to 50.0 ml with the same mixture of solvents.

Reference solution (a). Dilute 1.0 ml of the test solution to 100.0 ml with a mixture of 1 volume of *water R* and 9 volumes of *methanol R*. Dilute 2.0 ml of the solution to 10.0 ml with a mixture of 1 volume of *water R* and 9 volumes of *methanol R*.

Reference solution (b). Dissolve 1 mg of *oxazepam R*, 1 mg of *temazepam impurity F CRS* and 1 mg of *temazepam impurity G CRS* in a mixture of 1 volume of *water R* and 9 volumes of *methanol R* and dilute to 25 ml with the same mixture of solvents.

Reference solution (c). Dissolve 1 mg of *temazepam impurity C CRS* and 1 mg of *temazepam impurity D CRS* with a mixture of 1 volume of *water R* and 9 volumes of *methanol R* and dilute to 25 ml with the same mixture of solvents.

Column:

- *size*: *l* = 0.15 m, Ø = 4.6 mm,
- *stationary phase*: *end-capped octadecylsilyl silica gel for chromatography R* (3.5 µm).

Mobile phase:

- *mobile phase A*: solution containing 4.9 g/l of *sodium dihydrogen phosphate R* and 0.63 g/l of *disodium hydrogen phosphate R* (pH 5.6),
- *mobile phase B*: *methanol R,*
- *mobile phase C*: *acetonitrile R,*

Time (min)	Mobile phase A (per cent *V/V*)	Mobile phase B (per cent *V/V*)	Mobile phase C (per cent *V/V*)
0 - 18	54	39	7
18 - 25	54 → 22	39 → 63	7 → 15
25 - 31	22	63	15
31 - 37	22 → 54	63 → 39	15 → 7

Flow rate: 1.5 ml/min.

Detection: spectrophotometer at 230 nm.

Injection: 20 µl.

Relative retention with reference to temazepam (retention time = about 16 min): impurity E = about 0.55; impurity F = about 0.67; impurity G = about 0.73; impurity B = about 0.8; impurity D = about 1.2; impurity C = about 1.3; impurity A = about 1.5.

System suitability: reference solution (b):

- *resolution*: minimum 1.5 between the peaks due to impurity F and impurity G,
- *peak-to-valley ratio*: minimum 1.7, where H_p = height above the baseline of the peak due to impurity G and H_v = height above the baseline of the lowest point of the curve separating this peak from the peak due to impurity B.

Limits:

- *correction factors*: for the calculation of contents, multiply the peak areas of the following impurities by the corresponding correction factor: impurity F = 3.2; impurity G = 3.1;
- *impurities B, C, D, E, F, G*: for each impurity, not more than the area of the principal peak in the chromatogram obtained with reference solution (a) (0.2 per cent);
- *any other impurity*: for each impurity, not more than 0.5 times the area of the principal peak in the chromatogram obtained with reference solution (a) (0.1 per cent);
- *total*: not more than 2.5 times the area of the principal peak in the chromatogram obtained with reference solution (a) (0.5 per cent);
- *disregard limit*: 0.25 times the area of the principal peak in the chromatogram obtained with reference solution (a) (0.05 per cent).

Loss on drying (*2.2.32*): maximum 0.5 per cent, determined on 1.000 g by drying in an oven at 100-105 °C for 4 h.

Sulphated ash (*2.4.14*): maximum 0.1 per cent, determined on 1.0 g.

ASSAY

Dissolve 0.250 g in 50 ml of *nitroethane R*. Titrate with *0.1 M perchloric acid*, determining the end-point potentiometrically (*2.2.20*).

1 ml of *0.1 M perchloric acid* is equivalent to 30.07 mg of $C_{16}H_{13}ClN_2O_2$.

STORAGE

Protected from light.

IMPURITIES

Specified impurities (see note for information p. xli): A, B, C, D, E, F, G.

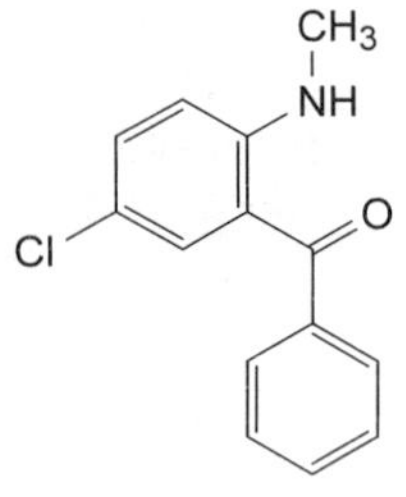

A. [5-chloro-2-(methylamino)phenyl]phenylmethanone,

B. oxazepam,

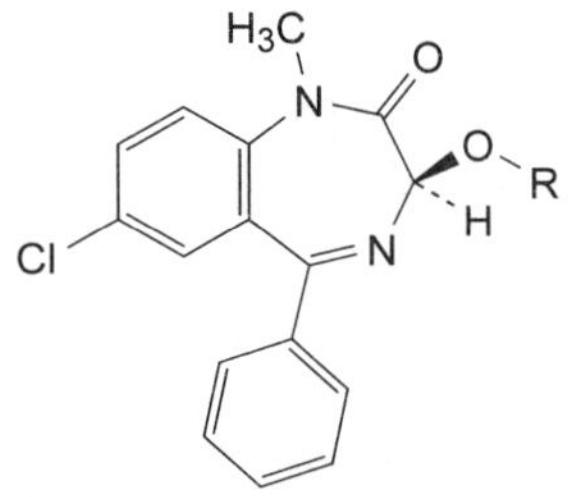

C. R = CO-CH_3: (3*RS*)-7-chloro-1-methyl-2-oxo-5-phenyl-2,3-dihydro-1*H*-1,4-benzodiazepin-3-yl acetate,

D. R = CH_3: (3*RS*)-7-chloro-3-methoxy-1-methyl-5-phenyl-1,3-dihydro-2*H*-1,4-benzodiazepin-2-one,

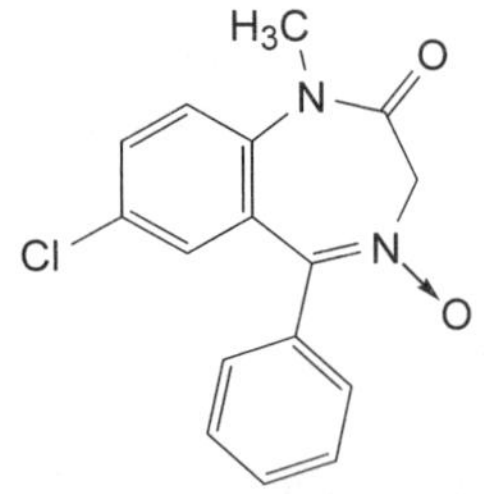

E. 7-chloro-1-methyl-5-phenyl-1,3-dihydro-2*H*-1,4-benzodiazepin-2-one 4-oxide,

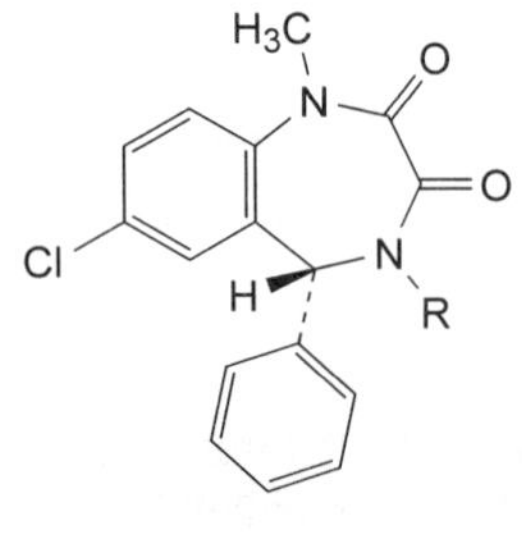

F. R = H: (5*RS*)-7-chloro-1-methyl-5-phenyl-4,5-dihydro-1*H*-1,4-benzodiazepine-2,3-dione,

G. R = CH_3: (5*RS*)-7-chloro-1,4-dimethyl-5-phenyl-4,5-dihydro-1*H*-1,4-benzodiazepine-2,3-dione.

07/2004:1373

TESTOSTERONE

Testosteronum

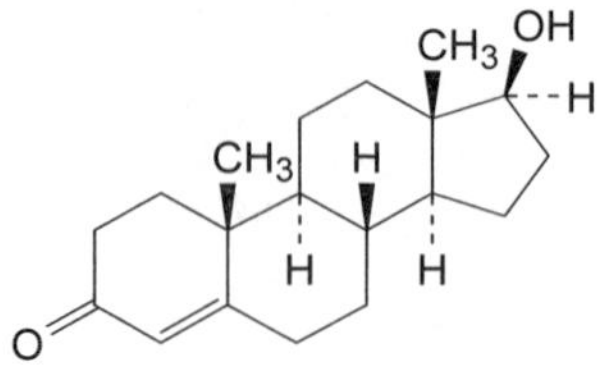

$C_{19}H_{28}O_2$ M_r 288.4

DEFINITION

17β-Hydroxyandrost-4-en-3-one.

Content: 97.0 per cent to 103.0 per cent (dried substance).

CHARACTERS

Appearance: white crystalline powder, or colourless or yellowish-white crystals.

Solubility: practically insoluble in water, freely soluble in alcohol and in methylene chloride, practically insoluble in fatty oils.

mp: about 155 °C.

IDENTIFICATION

Infrared absorption spectrophotometry (*2.2.24*).

Comparison: *testosterone CRS*.

TESTS

Specific optical rotation (*2.2.7*): + 106 to + 114 (dried substance).

Dissolve 0.250 g in *ethanol R* and dilute to 25.0 ml with the same solvent.

Impurities D and F. Thin-layer chromatography (*2.2.27*).

Test solution. Dissolve 0.100 g of the substance to be examined in *methanol R* and dilute to 10 ml with the same solvent.

Reference solution (a). Dissolve 1 mg of *stanolone R* in *methanol R* and dilute to 10 ml with the same solvent. In 1 ml of this solution, dissolve 10 mg of *testosterone for impurity D identification CRS* (testosterone spiked with about 1 per cent of impurity D).

Reference solution (b). Dilute 1.0 ml of the test solution to 100.0 ml with *methanol R*.

Reference solution (c). Dilute 2.0 ml of reference solution (b) to 10.0 ml with *methanol R*.

Reference solution (d). Dilute 1.0 ml of reference solution (b) to 10.0 ml with *methanol R*.

Plate: *TLC silica gel F_{254} plate R* (6-8 µm).

Preconditioning (in the dark): add about 5 g of powdered *silver nitrate R* to 100 ml of *methanol R*. Stir the suspension for 30 min. Filter or decant the suspension and immerse the plate in the silver nitrate solution for at least 30 min. Dry at 75 °C for 30 min.

A pre-conditioned plate can be stored in the dark for 5-7 days.

Mobile phase: *acetic acid R, ethanol R, dioxan R, methylene chloride R* (1:2:10:90 *V/V/V/V*).

Application: 2 µl.

Development: in a saturated tank over 3/4 of the plate.

Drying: allow to stand at room temperature and protected from light for 30 min.

Detection: spray with a 200 g/l solution of *toluenesulphonic acid R* in *ethanol R* and heat at 105 °C for 10 min. Examine in ultraviolet light at 365 nm.

System suitability: the chromatogram obtained with reference solution (a) shows 3 clearly separated spots; impurity D Rf = about 0.5; testosterone Rf = about 0.65; impurity F Rf = about 0.7.

Limits:

- *impurity D*: any spot due to impurity D is not more intense than the spot in the chromatogram obtained with reference solution (c) (0.2 per cent),
- *impurity F*: any spot due to impurity F is not more intense than the spot in the chromatogram obtained with reference solution (d) (0.1 per cent).

Related substances. Liquid chromatography (*2.2.29*).

Test solution. Dissolve 0.100 g of the substance to be examined in *methanol R* and dilute to 10.0 ml with the same solvent.

Reference solution (a). Dissolve 10 mg of *testosterone for system suitability CRS* (containing impurities C and I) in 1 ml of *methanol R*.

Reference solution (b). Dilute 1.0 ml of the test solution to 20.0 ml with *methanol R*. Dilute 1.0 ml of this solution to 10.0 ml with *methanol R*.

Reference solution (c). Dilute 2.0 ml of reference solution (b) to 10.0 ml with *methanol R*.

Column:

- *size*: l = 0.25 m, Ø = 4.6 mm,
- *stationary phase*: spherical *end-capped octadecylsilyl silica gel for chromatography R* (5 µm) with a pore size of 15 nm,
- *temperature*: 40 °C.

Mobile phase:

- *mobile phase A*: *water for chromatography R*, *methanol R* (45:55 *V/V*),
- *mobile phase B*: *methanol R*,

Time (min)	Mobile phase A (per cent *V/V*)	Mobile phase B (per cent *V/V*)
0 - 4	100	0
4 - 24	100 → 60	0 → 40
24 - 53	60 → 0	40 → 100
53 - 55	0	100
55 - 56	0 → 100	100 → 0
56 - 75	100	0

Flow rate: 1.0 ml/min.

Detection: spectrophotometer at 254 nm.

Injection: 20 µl.

Relative retention with reference to testosterone (retention time = about 18 min): impurity G = about 0.6; impurity H = about 0.8; impurity A = about 0.9; impurity I = about 0.95; impurity C = about 1.2; impurity E = about 1.7; impurity J = about 2.1; impurity B = about 2.5.

System suitability: reference solution (a):

- *resolution*: minimum baseline separation between the peaks due to impurity I and testosterone.

Limits: use the chromatogram obtained with reference solution (a) to identify the peaks due to impurities C and I:

- *correction factor*: for the calculation of content, multiply the peak area of impurity I by 2.9,
- *impurity C*: not more than the area of the principal peak in the chromatogram obtained with reference solution (b) (0.5 per cent),
- *impurity I*: not more than twice the area of the principal peak in the chromatogram obtained with reference solution (c) (0.2 per cent),
- *impurities A, B, E, G, H, J*: for each impurity, not more than the area of the principal peak in the chromatogram obtained with reference solution (c) (0.1 per cent),
- *any other impurity*: for each impurity, not more than the area of the principal peak in the chromatogram obtained with reference solution (c) (0.1 per cent),
- *total*: not more than 1.2 times the area of the principal peak in the chromatogram obtained with reference solution (b) (0.6 per cent),
- *disregard limit*: 0.5 times the area of the principal peak in the chromatogram obtained with reference solution (c) (0.05 per cent).

Loss on drying (*2.2.32*): maximum 1.0 per cent, determined on 0.500 g by drying in an oven at 100-105 °C for 2 h.

ASSAY

Dissolve 50.0 mg in *alcohol R* and dilute to 100.0 ml with the same solvent. Dilute 2.0 ml to 100.0 ml with *alcohol R*. Measure the absorbance (*2.2.25*) at the absorption maximum at 241 nm.

Calculate the content of $C_{19}H_{28}O_2$ taking the specific absorbance to be 569.

STORAGE

Protected from light.

IMPURITIES

Specified impurities (see note for information p. xli): A, B, C, D, E, F, G, H, I, J.

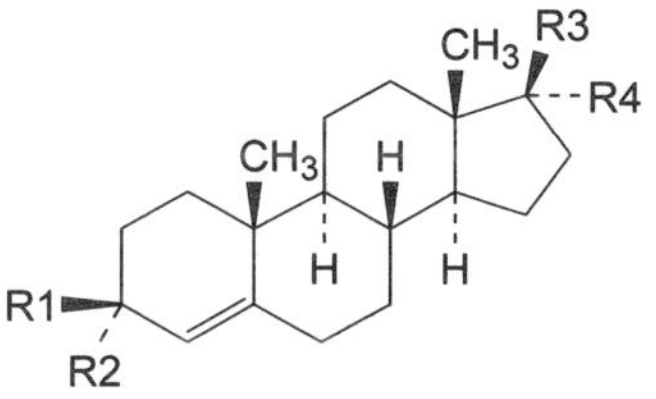

A. R1 + R2 = R3 + R4 = O: androst-4-ene-3,17-dione (androstenedione),

C. R1 + R2 = O, R3 = H, R4 = OH: 17α-hydroxyandrost-4-en-3-one (epitestosterone),

D. R1 = R3 = OH, R2 = R4 = H: androst-4-ene-3β,17β-diol (Δ4-androstenediol),

E. R1 + R2 = O, R3 = O-CO-CH_3, R4 = H: 3-oxoandrost-4-en-17β-yl acetate (testosterone acetate),

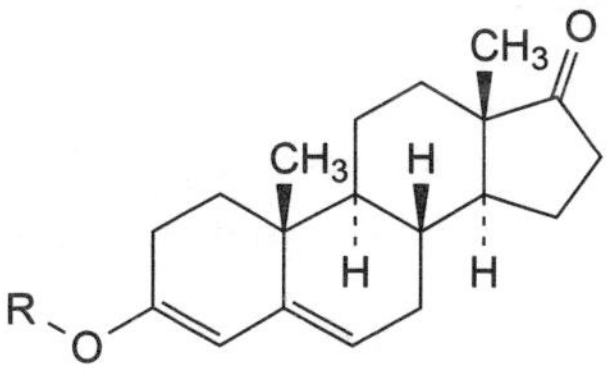

B. R = C_2H_5: 3-ethoxyandrosta-3,5-dien-17-one (androstenedione ethylenolether),

J. R = CH_3: 3-methoxyandrosta-3,5-dien-17-one (androstenedione methylenolether),

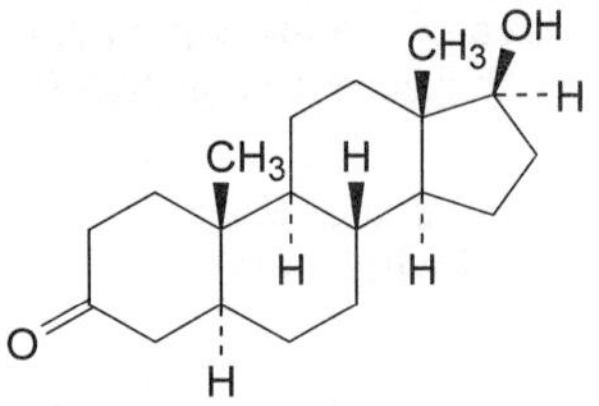

F. 17β-hydroxy-5α-androstan-3-one (androstanolone, stanolone),

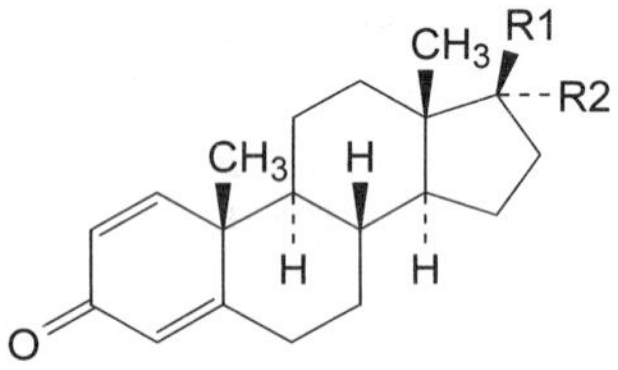

G. R1 + R2 = O: androsta-1,4-diene-3,17-dione (androstadienedione).

H. R1 = OH, R2 = H: 17β-hydroxyandrosta-1,4-dien-3-one (boldenone),

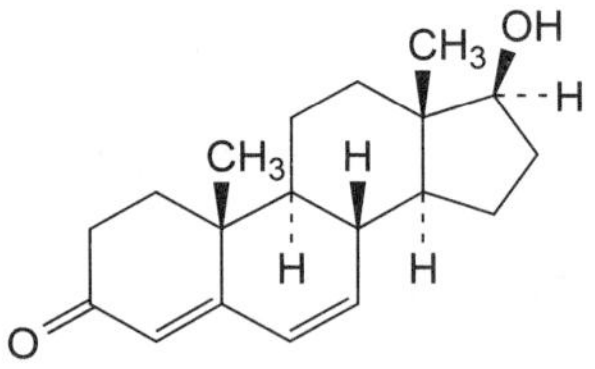

I. 17β-hydroxyandrosta-4,6-dien-3-one (Δ6-testosterone).

07/2004:1767

TILIDINE HYDROCHLORIDE HEMIHYDRATE

Tilidini hydrochloridum hemihydricum

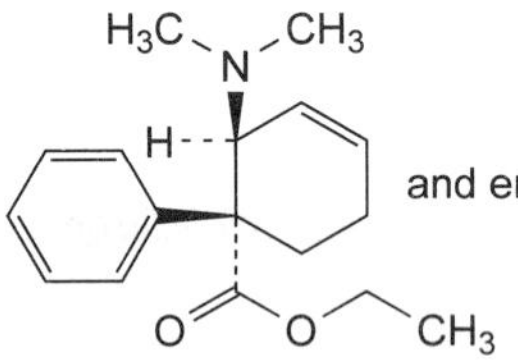

$C_{17}H_{24}ClNO_2,{}^1/_2H_2O$ M_r 318.9

DEFINITION

Ethyl (1*RS*,2*SR*)-2-(dimethylamino)-1-phenylcyclohex-3-enecarboxylate hydrochloride hemihydrate.

Content: 99.0 per cent to 101.0 per cent (anhydrous substance).

A suitable antioxidant may be added.

CHARACTERS

Appearance: white or almost white, crystalline powder.

Solubility: freely soluble in water, very soluble in methylene chloride, freely soluble in alcohol.

IDENTIFICATION

A. Infrared absorption spectrophotometry (*2.2.24*).

Comparison: *Ph. Eur. reference spectrum of tilidine hydrochloride hemihydrate.*

B. It gives reaction (a) of chlorides (*2.3.1*).

TESTS

Solution S. Dissolve 1.0 g in *carbon dioxide-free water R* and dilute to 20 ml with the same solvent.

Appearance of solution. Solution S is clear (*2.2.1*) and not more intensely coloured than reference solution Y_7 (*2.2.2, Method II*).

Acidity or alkalinity. To 20 ml of solution S add 0.2 ml of *0.01 M sodium hydroxide*. The pH is not less than 4.1. Add 0.4 ml of *0.01 M hydrochloric acid*. The pH is not more than 4.3.

Related substances. Liquid chromatography (*2.2.29*).

The following chromatogram is published for information.

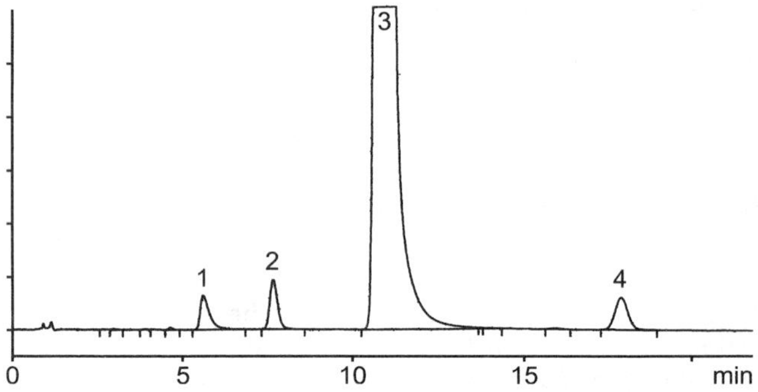

1. impurity C 2. impurity B 3. tilidine 4. impurity A

Figure 1767.-1. – *Chromatogram for the test for related substances of tilidine hydrochloride hemihydrate*

Test solution. Dissolve 50.0 mg of the substance to be examined in *water R* and dilute to 50.0 ml with the same solvent.

Reference solution (a). Dilute 0.5 ml of the test solution to 100.0 ml with *water R*.

Reference solution (b). Dilute 2.0 ml of reference solution (a) to 10.0 ml with *water R*.

Precolumn:

– *size*: *l* = 4 mm, Ø = 4.0 mm,
– *stationary phase*: spherical *octadecylsilyl silica gel for chromatography R* (5 µm).

Column:

– *size*: *l* = 0.125 m, Ø = 4.0 mm,
– *stationary phase*: spherical *octadecylsilyl silica gel for chromatography R* (5 µm).

Mobile phase: mix equal volumes of *acetonitrile R* and a 0.98 g/l solution of *ammonium carbonate R*.

Flow rate: 0.8 ml/min.

Detection: spectrophotometer at 220 nm.

Injection: 10 µl.

Run time: twice the retention time of tilidine.

Relative retention with reference to tilidine (retention time = about 11 min): impurity D = about 0.4; impurity C = about 0.5; impurity B = about 0.7; impurity A = about 1.5.

Limits:

– *impurities A, B, C*: for each impurity, not more than the area of the principal peak in the chromatogram obtained with reference solution (a) (0.5 per cent),
– *any other impurity*: for each impurity, not more than the area of the principal peak in the chromatogram obtained with reference solution (b) (0.1 per cent),
– *total*: not more than the area of the principal peak in the chromatogram obtained with reference solution (a) (0.5 per cent),

- *disregard limit*: 0.5 times the area of the principal peak in the chromatogram obtained with reference solution (b) (0.05 per cent).

Heavy metals (*2.4.8*): maximum 20 ppm.

Dissolve 2.0 g in 20 ml of *water R*. 12 ml of the solution complies with limit test A. Prepare the standard using *lead standard solution (2 ppm Pb) R*.

Water (*2.5.12*): 2.5 per cent to 3.1 per cent, determined on 0.300 g.

Bacterial endotoxins (*2.6.14*): less than 0.25 IU/mg, if intented for use in the manufacture of parenteral dosage forms without a further appropriate procedure for the removal of bacterial endotoxins.

ASSAY

Dissolve 0.250 g in a mixture of 10 ml of *anhydrous acetic acid R* and 50 ml of *acetic anhydride R*. Titrate with *0.1 M perchloric acid*, determining the end-point potentiometrically (*2.2.20*).

1 ml of *0.1 M perchloric acid* is equivalent to 30.99 mg of $C_{17}H_{24}ClNO_2$.

STORAGE

Protected from light.

LABELLING

The label states:

- where applicable, that the substance is free from bacterial endotoxins,
- where applicable, the name and concentration of any added antioxidant.

IMPURITIES

Specified impurities (see note for information p. xli): A, B, C.

Other detectable impurities: D.

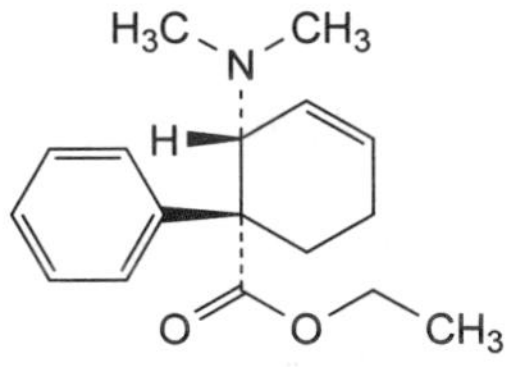

A. ethyl (1*RS*,2*RS*)-2-(dimethylamino)-1-phenylcyclohex-3-enecarboxylate,

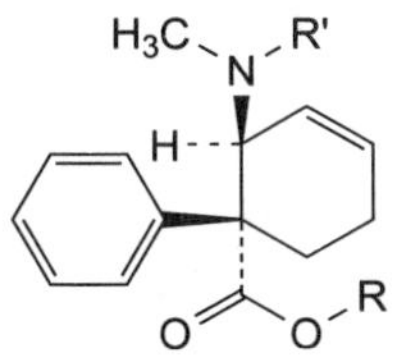

B. R = R′ = CH_3: methyl (1*RS*,2*SR*)-2-(dimethylamino)-1-phenylcyclohex-3-enecarboxylate,

C. R = C_2H_5, R′ = H: ethyl (1*RS*,2*SR*)-2-(methylamino)-1-phenylcyclohex-3-enecarboxylate,

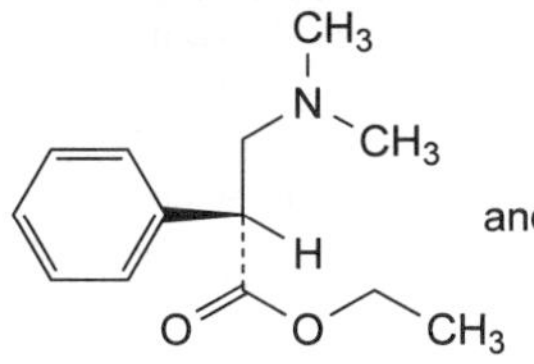

D. ethyl (2*RS*)-3-dimethylamino-2-phenylpropanoate.

04/2004:1770
corrected

TRIBUTYL ACETYLCITRATE

Tributylis acetylcitras

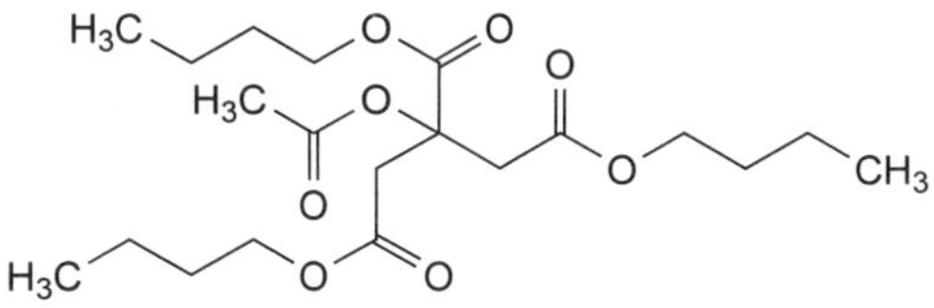

$C_{20}H_{34}O_8$ M_r 402.5

DEFINITION

Tributyl 2-(acetyloxy)propane-1,2,3-tricarboxylate.

Content: 99.0 per cent to 101.0 per cent (anhydrous substance).

CHARACTERS

Appearance: clear, oily liquid.

Solubility: not miscible with water, miscible with alcohol and with methylene chloride.

IDENTIFICATION

Infrared absorption spectrophotometry (*2.2.24*).

Comparison: *Ph. Eur. reference spectrum of tributyl acetylcitrate.*

TESTS

Appearance. The substance to be examined is clear (*2.2.1*) and not more intensely coloured than reference solution BY_6 (*2.2.2, Method II*).

Acidity. Dilute 10 g with 10 ml of previously neutralised *alcohol R*, add 0.5 ml of *bromothymol blue solution R2*. Not more than 0.3 ml of *0.1 M sodium hydroxide* is required to change the colour of the indicator to blue.

Refractive index (*2.2.6*): 1.442 to 1.445.

Related substances. Gas chromatography (*2.2.28*).

Test solution. Dissolve 1.0 g of the substance to be examined in *methylene chloride R* and dilute to 20.0 ml with the same solvent.

Reference solution (a). Dissolve 50 mg of the substance to be examined and 50 mg of *tributyl citrate R* in *methylene chloride R* and dilute to 20.0 ml with the same solvent.

Reference solution (b). Dilute 1.0 ml of the test solution to 20.0 ml with *methylene chloride R*. Dilute 1.0 ml of this solution to 25.0 ml with *methylene chloride R*.

Column:

- *material*: fused silica,
- *size*: *l* = 30 m, Ø = 0.53 mm,
- *stationary phase*: *poly[(cyanopropyl)(methyl)][(phenyl)(methyl)]siloxane R* (film thickness 1.0 µm).

Carrier gas: *helium for chromatography R*.

Linear velocity: 36 cm/s.

Split ratio: 1:20.

Temperature:

- *column*: 200 °C,
- *injection port and detector*: 250 °C.

Detection: flame ionisation.

Injection: 1 µl.

Run time: twice the retention time of tributyl acetylcitrate.

Monographs Q - Z

Relative retention with reference to tributyl acetylcitrate (retention time = abou 26 min): impurity B = about 0.83; impurity A = about 0.87.

System suitability: reference solution (a):

- *resolution*: minimum 2.0 between the peaks due to impurity A and tributyl acetylcitrate.

Limits:

- *impurities A, B*: for each impurity, not more than the area of the principal peak in the chromatogram obtained with reference solution (b) (0.2 per cent),
- *any other impurity*: for each impurity, not more than 0.5 times the area of the principal peak in the chromatogram obtained with reference solution (b) (0.1 per cent),
- *total*: not more than 2.5 times the area of the principal peak in the chromatogram obtained with reference solution (b) (0.5 per cent),
- *disregard limit*: 0.25 times the area of the principal peak in the chromatogram obtained with reference solution (b) (0.05 per cent).

Heavy metals (*2.4.8*): maximum 10 ppm.

2.0 g complies with limit test F. Prepare the standard using 2 ml of *lead standard solution (10 ppm Pb) R*.

Water (*2.5.12*): maximum 0.25 per cent, determined on 2.00 g.

Sulphated ash (*2.4.14*): maximum 0.1 per cent, determined on 1.0 g.

ASSAY

Introduce 1.500 g into a 250 ml borosilicate glass flask. Add 25 ml of *2-propanol R*, 50 ml of *water R*, 25.0 ml of *1 M sodium hydroxide* and a few glass beads. Heat under a reflux condenser for 1 h. Allow to cool. Add 1 ml of *phenolphthalein solution R1* and titrate with *1 M hydrochloric acid.* Carry out a blank titration.

1 ml of *1 M sodium hydroxide* is equivalent to 100.6 mg of $C_{20}H_{34}O_8$.

IMPURITIES

Specified impurities (see note for information p. xli): A, B.

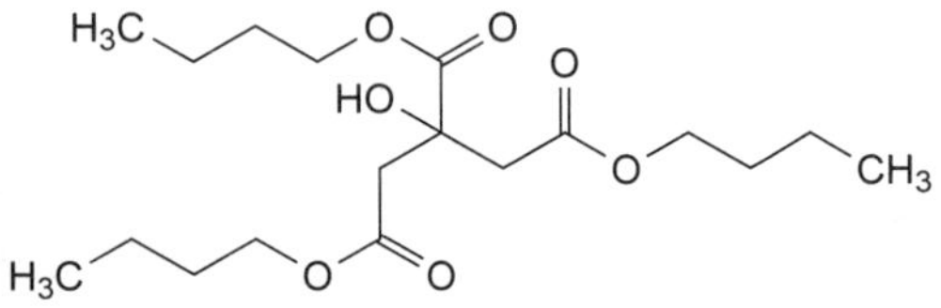

A. tributyl 2-hydroxypropane-1,2,3-tricarboxylate (tributyl citrate),

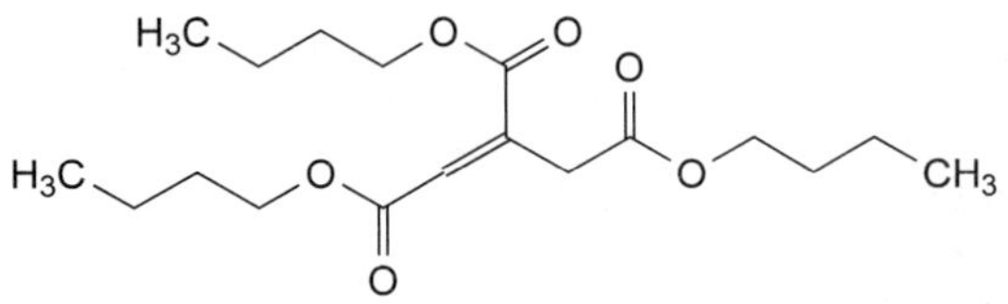

B. tributyl propene-1,2,3-tricarboxylate (tributyl aconitate).

Monographs Q - Z

07/2004:1377

TRIFLUSAL

Triflusalum

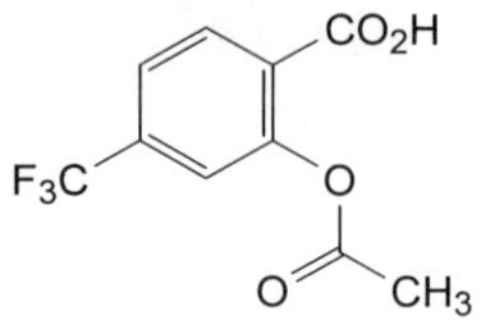

$C_{10}H_7F_3O_4$ M_r 248.2

DEFINITION

2-(Acetyloxy)-4-(trifluoromethyl)benzoic acid.

Content: 98.5 per cent to 101.5 per cent (dried substance).

CHARACTERS

Appearance: white or almost white, crystalline powder.

Solubility: practically insoluble in water, very soluble in ethanol, freely soluble in methylene chloride.

mp: about 118 °C, with decomposition.

IDENTIFICATION

Infrared absorption spectrophotometry (*2.2.24*).

Preparation: discs.

Comparison: *triflusal CRS.*

TESTS

Related substances. Liquid chromatography (*2.2.29*).

Test solution. Dissolve 0.20 g of the substance to be examined in *acetonitrile R* and dilute to 20.0 ml with the same solvent. *Prepare the solution immediately before use.*

Reference solution (a). Dissolve 5.0 mg of *triflusal impurity B CRS* in *acetonitrile R* and dilute to 10.0 ml with the same solvent.

Reference solution (b). Dilute 1.0 ml of reference solution (a) to 25.0 ml with *acetonitrile R.*

Reference solution (c). Dissolve 2.5 mg of the substance to be examined in *acetonitrile R,* add 5 ml of reference solution (a) and dilute to 10 ml with *acetonitrile R. Prepare the solution immediately before use.*

Column:

- *size*: l = 0.15 m, Ø = 4.0 mm,
- *stationary phase*: *octadecylsilyl silica gel for chromatography R* (4-5 µm).

Mobile phase:

- *mobile phase A*: *acetonitrile R,*
- *mobile phase B*: 0.5 per cent *V/V* solution of *phosphoric acid R,*

Time (min)	Mobile phase A (per cent *V/V*)	Mobile phase B (per cent *V/V*)
0 - 20	20 → 70	80 → 30
20 - 25	70	30
25 - 26	70 → 20	30 → 80
26 - 30	20	80

Flow rate: 1.2 ml/min.

Detection: spectrophotometer at 237 nm.

Injection: 10 µl of the test solution and reference solutions (b) and (c).

Relative retention with reference to triflusal (retention time = about 13 min): impurity A = about 0.3; impurity B = about 1.2; impurity C = about 1.3; impurity D = about 1.6.

System suitability: reference solution (c):

– *resolution*: minimum 3.0 between the peaks due to triflusal and impurity B.

Limits:

– *impurity B*: not more than 1.5 times the area of the corresponding peak in the chromatogram obtained with reference solution (b) (0.3 per cent),

– *total of impurities other than B*: not more than 0.5 times the area of the peak due to impurity B in the chromatogram obtained with reference solution (b) (0.1 per cent),

– *disregard limit*: 0.1 times the area of the peak due to impurity B in the chromatogram obtained with reference solution (b) (0.02 per cent).

Heavy metals (*2.4.8*): maximum 10 ppm.

Dissolve 2.0 g in 12 ml of *alcohol R* and dilute to 20 ml with *water R*. 12 ml complies with limit test B. Prepare the standard using lead standard solution (1 ppm Pb) obtained by diluting *lead standard solution (100 ppm Pb) R* with a mixture of 2 volumes of *water R* and 3 volumes of *alcohol R*.

Loss on drying (*2.2.32*): maximum 0.5 per cent, determined on 1.000 g by drying in a desiccator *in vacuo* over *diphosphorus pentoxide R*.

Sulphated ash (*2.4.14*): maximum 0.1 per cent, determined on 1.0 g in a platinum crucible.

ASSAY

Dissolve 0.200 g in 50 ml of *ethanol R*. Titrate with *0.1 M sodium hydroxide*, determining the end-point potentiometrically (*2.2.20*).

1 ml of *0.1 M sodium hydroxide* is equivalent to 24.82 mg of $C_{10}H_7F_3O_4$.

STORAGE

In an airtight container, at a temperature not exceeding 25 °C.

IMPURITIES

Specified impurities (see note for information p. xli): B.

Other detectable impurities: A, C, D.

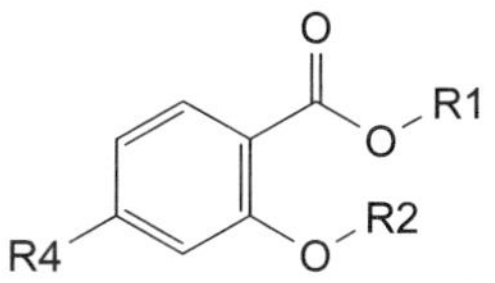

A. R1 = H, R2 = CO-CH_3, R4 = CO_2H: 2-(acetyloxy)benzene-1,4-dicarboxylic acid (2-acetoxyterephthalic acid),

B. R1 = R2 = H, R4 = CF_3: 2-hydroxy-4-(trifluoromethyl)benzoic acid (4-(trifluoromethyl)salicylic acid),

C. R1 = R2 = CO-CH_3, R4 = CF_3: acetic 2-(acetyloxy)-4-(trifluoromethyl)benzoic anhydride,

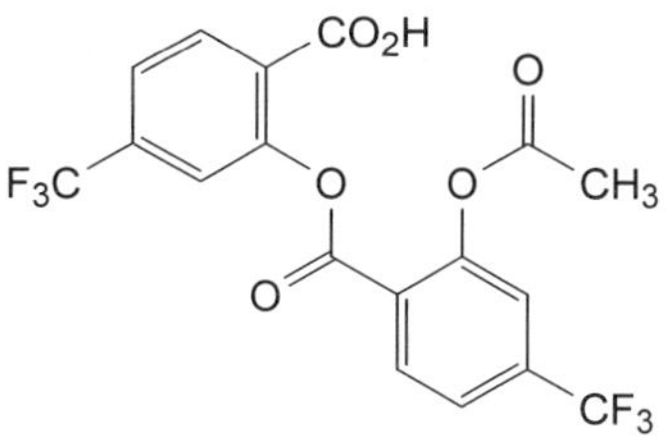

D. 2-[[2-(acetyloxy)-4-(trifluoromethyl)benzoyl]oxy]-4-(trifluoromethyl)benzoic acid.

07/2004:1662

TYROTHRICIN

Tyrothricinum

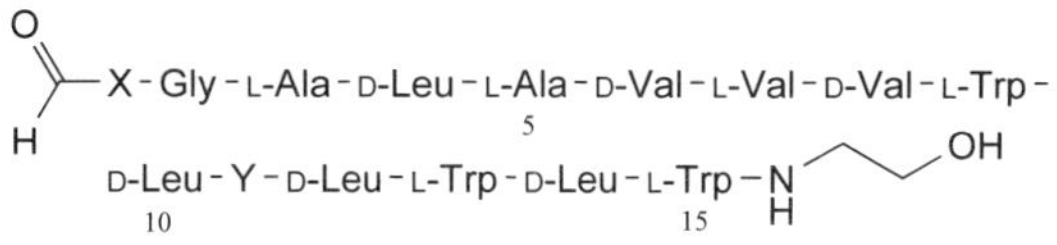

Gramicidin	Mol. formula	M_r	X	Y
A1	$C_{99}H_{140}N_{20}O_{17}$	1882	L-Val	L-Trp
A2	$C_{100}H_{142}N_{20}O_{17}$	1896	L-Ile	L-Trp
C1	$C_{97}H_{139}N_{19}O_{18}$	1859	L-Val	L-Tyr
C2	$C_{98}H_{141}N_{19}O_{18}$	1873	L-Ile	L-Tyr

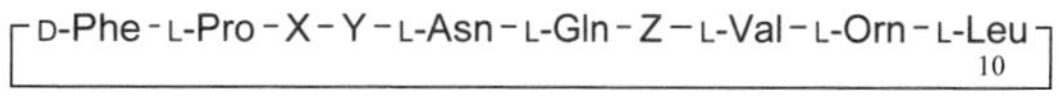

Tyrocidin	Mol. formula	M_r	X	Y	Z
A	$C_{66}H_{88}N_{13}O_{13}$	1271	L-Phe	D-Phe	L-Tyr
B	$C_{68}H_{89}N_{14}O_{13}$	1311	L-Trp	D-Phe	L-Tyr
C	$C_{70}H_{90}N_{15}O_{13}$	1350	L-Trp	D-Trp	L-Tyr
D	$C_{72}H_{91}N_{16}O_{12}$	1373	L-Trp	D-Trp	L-Trp
E	$C_{66}H_{88}N_{13}O_{12}$	1255	L-Phe	D-Phe	L-Phe

DEFINITION

Mixture of antimicrobial linear and cyclic polypeptides, isolated from the fermentation broth of *Bacillus brevis* Dubos. It consists mainly of gramicidins and tyrocidins as described above; other related compounds may be present in smaller amounts.

Potency: 180 IU/mg to 280 IU/mg (dried substance).

CHARACTERS

Appearance: white or almost white powder.

Solubility: practically insoluble in water, soluble in alcohol and in methanol.

IDENTIFICATION

First identification: B.

Second identification: A.

A. Thin-layer chromatography (*2.2.27*).

Test solution. Dissolve 5 mg of the substance to be examined in 4.0 ml of *alcohol R*.

Reference solution. Dissolve 5 mg of *tyrothricin CRS* in 4.0 ml of *alcohol R*.

Plate: *TLC silica gel F_{254} plate R.*

Mobile phase: *methanol R, butanol R, water R, acetic acid R, butyl acetate R* (2.5:7.5:12:20:40 *V/V/V/V/V*).

Application: 1 µl.

Development: over 2/3 of the plate.

Drying: in a current of warm air.

Detection A: examine in ultraviolet light at 254 nm.

Results A: the principal spots or groups of principal spots in the chromatogram obtained with the test solution are similar in position and size to the principal spots or groups of principal spots in the chromatogram obtained with the reference solution. The upper group corresponds to gramicidins, the lower group to tyrocidins.

Detection B: spray with *dimethylaminobenzaldehyde solution R2.* Heat the plate in a current of warm air until the spots appear.

System suitability: reference solution:

– the chromatogram shows 2 clearly separated spots or groups of spots.

Results B: the principal spots or groups of principal spots in the chromatogram obtained with the test solution are similar in position, colour and size to the principal spots or groups of principal spots in the chromatogram obtained with the reference solution. The upper group corresponds to gramicidins, the lower group to tyrocidins.

B. It complies with the test for composition (see Tests).

TESTS

Composition. Liquid chromatography (*2.2.29*): use the normalisation procedure. *Prepare the solutions immediately before use.*

Test solution. Dissolve 25 mg of the substance to be examined in 10 ml of *methanol R* and dilute to 25.0 ml with the mobile phase.

Reference solution (a). Dissolve 25 mg of *tyrothricin CRS* in 10 ml of *methanol R* and dilute to 25.0 ml with the mobile phase.

Reference solution (b). Dilute 1.0 ml of reference solution (a) to 50.0 ml with the mobile phase.

Column:

– *size*: *l* = 0.25 m, Ø = 4.6 mm,
– *stationary phase*: *octadecylsilyl silica gel for chromatography R* (5 µm),
– *temperature*: 60 °C.

Mobile phase: 0.79 g/l solution of *ammonium sulphate R, methanol R* (25:75 *V/V*).

Flow rate: 1.2 ml/min.

Detection: spectrophotometer at 280 nm.

Injection: 25 µl.

Run time: 6 times the retention time of gramicidin A1.

Use the chromatogram obtained with reference solution (a) and the chromatogram supplied with *tyrothricin CRS* to identify the peaks due to gramicidin A1, gramicidin A2 and the tyrocidins.

Relative retention with reference to gramicidin A1 (retention time = about 10 min): gramicidin C1 = about 0.8; gramicidin C2 = about 0.9; gramicidin A2 = about 1.1; tyrocidins = about 1.5 to 6.

System suitability: reference solution (a):

– *resolution*: minimum 1.5 between the peaks due to gramicidin A1 and gramicidin A2.

Composition:

– *sum of gramicidins*: 25 per cent to 50 per cent,
– *sum of tyrocidins*: 50 per cent to 70 per cent,
– *total*: minimum 85 per cent,
– *disregard limit*: the sum of the areas of the peaks due to gramicidins in the chromatogram obtained with reference solution (b).

Loss on drying (*2.2.32*): maximum 4.0 per cent, determined on 1.000 g by drying under high vacuum at 60 °C for 3 h.

Sulphated ash (*2.4.14*): maximum 1.5 per cent, determined on 1.0 g.

ASSAY

Carry out the microbiological assay of antibiotics (*2.7.2*) using the turbidimetric method. Use *gramicidin CRS* as the reference substance.

Test solution. Prepare a solution of tyrothricin containing about the same amount of gramicidin as the corresponding solution of *gramicidin CRS* i.e. 5 times more concentrated.

STORAGE

In an airtight container, protected from light.

V

01/2002:0573
corrected

VERAPAMIL HYDROCHLORIDE

Verapamili hydrochloridum

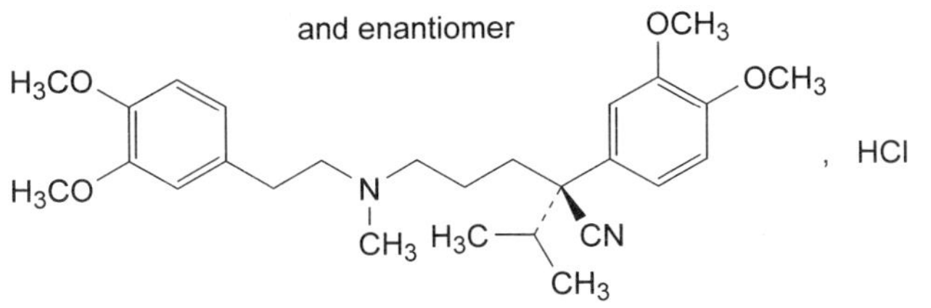

$C_{27}H_{39}ClN_2O_4$ M_r 491.1

DEFINITION

Verapamil hydrochloride contains not less than 99.0 per cent and not more than the equivalent of 101.0 per cent of (2*RS*)-2-(3,4-dimethoxyphenyl)-5-[[2-(3,4-dimethoxyphenyl)ethyl](methyl)amino]-2-(1-methylethyl)pentanenitrile hydrochloride, calculated with reference to the dried substance.

CHARACTERS

A white, crystalline powder, soluble in water, freely soluble in methanol, sparingly soluble in alcohol.

It melts at about 144 °C.

IDENTIFICATION

First identification: B, D.

Second identification: A, C, D.

A. Dissolve 20.0 mg in *0.01 M hydrochloric acid* and dilute to 100.0 ml with the same acid. Dilute 5.0 ml of this solution to 50.0 ml with *0.01 M hydrochloric acid*. Examined between 210 nm and 340 nm (*2.2.25*), the solution shows 2 absorption maxima, at 229 nm and 278 nm, and a shoulder at 282 nm. The ratio of the absorbance at the maximum at 278 nm to that at the maximum at 229 nm is 0.35 to 0.39.

B. Examine by infrared absorption spectrophotometry (*2.2.24*), comparing with the spectrum obtained with *verapamil hydrochloride CRS*. Examine the substances prepared as discs.

C. Examine by thin-layer chromatography (*2.2.27*), using as the coating substance a suitable silica gel with a fluorescent indicator having an optimal intensity at 254 nm.

Test solution. Dissolve 10 mg of the substance to be examined in *methylene chloride R* and dilute to 5 ml with the same solvent.

Reference solution (a). Dissolve 20 mg of *verapamil hydrochloride CRS* in *methylene chloride R* and dilute to 10 ml with the same solvent.

Reference solution (b). Dissolve 5 mg of *papaverine hydrochloride CRS* in reference solution (a) and dilute to 5 ml with the same solution.

Apply separately to the plate 5 µl of each solution. Develop over a path of 15 cm using a mixture of 15 volumes of *diethylamine R* and 85 volumes of *cyclohexane R*. Allow the plate to dry in air and examine in ultraviolet light at 254 nm. The principal spot in the chromatogram obtained with the test solution is similar in position and size to the principal spot in the chromatogram obtained with reference solution (a). The test is not valid unless the chromatogram obtained with reference solution (b) shows 2 clearly separated principal spots.

D. It gives reaction (b) of chlorides (*2.3.1*).

TESTS

Solution S. Dissolve 1.0 g in *carbon dioxide-free water R* while gently heating and dilute to 20.0 ml with the same solvent.

Appearance of solution. Solution S is clear (*2.2.1*) and colourless (*2.2.2, Method II*).

pH (*2.2.3*). The pH of solution S is 4.5 to 6.0.

Optical rotation (*2.2.7*). The angle of optical rotation, determined on solution S, is − 0.10° to + 0.10°.

Related substances. Examine by liquid chromatography (*2.2.29*).

Test solution. Dissolve 25.0 mg of the substance to be examined in the initial mobile phase composition and dilute to 10.0 ml with the same mobile phase.

Reference solution (a). Dissolve 5 mg of *verapamil hydrochloride CRS*, 5 mg of *verapamil impurity I CRS* and 5 mg of *verapamil impurity M CRS* in the initial mobile phase composition and dilute to 20 ml with the same mobile phase. Dilute 1 ml of this solution to 10 ml with the initial mobile phase composition.

Reference solution (b). Dilute 1.0 ml of the test solution to 100.0 ml with the initial mobile phase composition. Dilute 1.0 ml of this solution to 10.0 ml with the same mobile phase.

The chromatographic procedure may be carried out using:

– a stainless steel column 0.25 m long and 4.6 mm in internal diameter packed with *end-capped palmitamidopropylsilyl silica gel for chromatography R* (5 µm),

– as mobile phase at a flow rate of 1.5 ml/min a double isocratic programme using the following conditions:

Mobile phase A. A 6.97 g/l solution of *dipotassium hydrogen phosphate R* adjusted to pH 7.20 with *phosphoric acid R*,

Mobile phase B. *Acetonitrile R*,

Time (min)	Mobile phase A (per cent *V/V*)	Mobile phase B (per cent *V/V*)	Comment
0 - 22	63	37	first isocratic step
22 - 27	63 → 35	37 → 65	switch to second isocratic step
27 - 35	35	65	second isocratic step
35 - 36	35 → 63	65 → 37	switch to initial mobile phase
36 - 50	63	37	equilibration

– as detector a spectrophotometer set at 278 nm.

Equilibrate the column with the initial mobile phase composition for about 60 min.

Inject 10 µl of reference solution (a). When the chromatogram is recorded in the prescribed conditions the retention times are: verapamil, about 16 min, verapamil impurity I, about 21 min and verapamil impurity M about 32 min, eluting as a doublet. The test is not valid unless the resolution between the peaks corresponding to verapamil and verapamil impurity I is at least 5.0 and verapamil impurity M elutes from the column.

Adjust the sensitivity of the system so that the height of principal peak in the chromatogram obtained with 10 µl of the reference solution (b) is at least 15 per cent of the full scale of the recorder.

Inject separately 10 µl of the test solution and 10 µl of reference solution (b). In the chromatogram obtained with the test solution: the area of any peak, apart from the principal peak, is not greater than the area of the principal peak in the chromatogram obtained with reference solution (b) (0.1 per cent); the sum of the areas of the peaks, apart from the principal peak, is not greater than 3 times the area of the principal peak in the chromatogram obtained with reference solution (b) (0.3 per cent). Disregard any peak with an area less than 0.1 times the area of the principal peak in the chromatogram obtained with reference solution (b).

Heavy metals (*2.4.8*). 1.0 g complies with limit test C for heavy metals (10 ppm). Prepare the standard using 1 ml of *lead standard solution (10 ppm Pb) R.*

Loss on drying (*2.2.32*). Not more than 0.5 per cent, determined on 1.000 g by drying in an oven at 100 °C to 105 °C.

Sulphated ash (*2.4.14*). Not more than 0.1 per cent, determined on 1.0 g.

ASSAY

Dissolve 0.400 g in 50 ml of *ethanol R* and add 5.0 ml of *0.01 M hydrochloric acid.* Titrate with *0.1 M sodium hydroxide,* determining the end-point potentiometrically (*2.2.20*). Measure the volume of titrant required between the 2 points of inflexion.

1 ml of *0.1 M sodium hydroxide* is equivalent to 49.11 mg of $C_{27}H_{39}ClN_2O_4$.

STORAGE

Store protected from light.

IMPURITIES

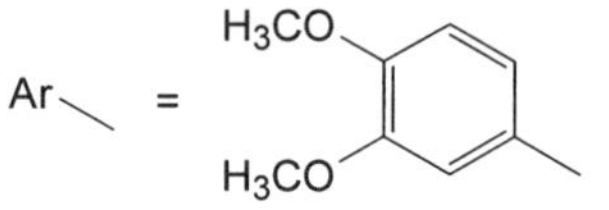

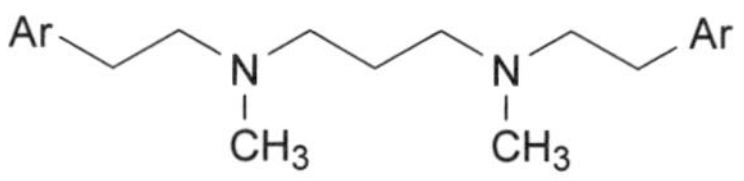

A. *N,N'*-bis[2-(3,4-dimethoxyphenyl)ethyl]-*N,N'*-dimethylpropane-1,3-diamine,

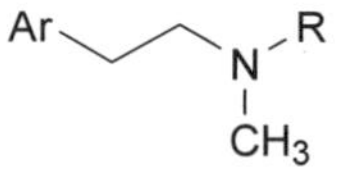

B. R = H: 2-(3,4-dimethoxyphenyl)-*N*-methylethanamine,

C. R = CH_3: 2-(3,4-dimethoxyphenyl)-*N,N*-dimethylethanamine,

D. R = CH_2-CH_2-CH_2-Cl: 3-chloro-*N*-[2-(3,4-dimethoxyphenyl)ethyl]-*N*-methylpropan-1-amine,

E. Ar-CH_2OH: (3,4-dimethoxyphenyl)methanol,

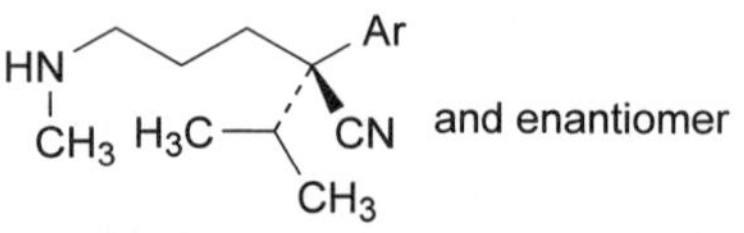

F. (2*RS*)-2-(3,4-dimethoxyphenyl)-5-(methylamino)-2-(1-methylethyl)pentanenitrile,

G. Ar-CHO: 3,4-dimethoxybenzaldehyde,

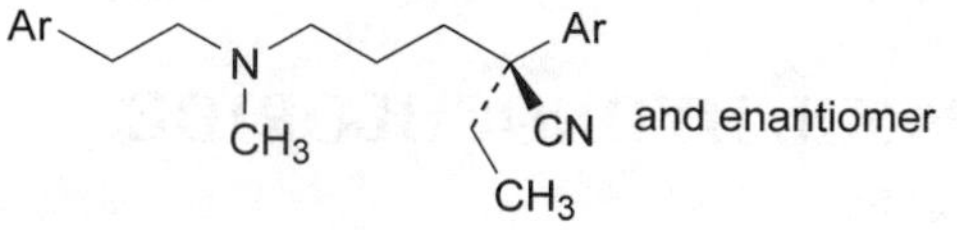

H. (2*RS*)-2-(3,4-dimethoxyphenyl)-5-[[2-(3,4-dimethoxyphenyl)ethyl](methyl)amino]-2-ethylpentanenitrile,

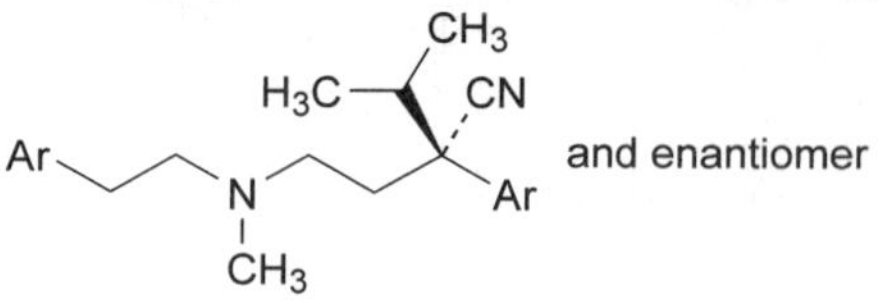

I. (2*RS*)-2-(3,4-dimethoxyphenyl)-2-[2-[[2-(3,4-dimethoxyphenyl)ethyl](methyl)amino]ethyl]-3-methylbutanenitrile,

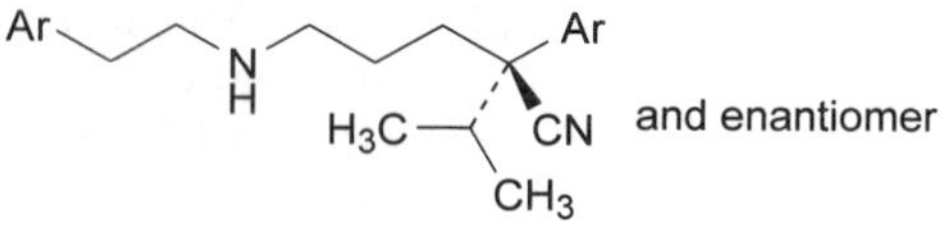

J. (2*RS*)-2-(3,4-dimethoxyphenyl)-5-[[2-(3,4-dimethoxyphenyl)ethyl]amino]-2-(1-methylethyl)pentanenitrile (*N*-norverapamil),

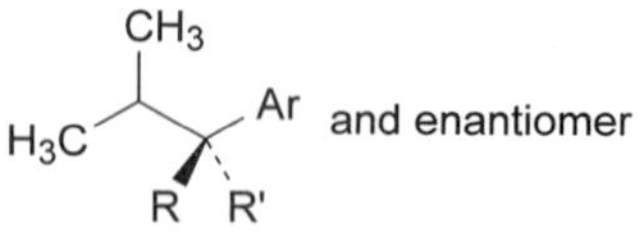

K. R = H, R′ = CN: (2*RS*)-2-(3,4-dimethoxyphenyl)-3-methylbutanenitrile,

L. R+ R′ = O: 1-(3,4-dimethoxyphenyl)-2-methylpropan-1-one,

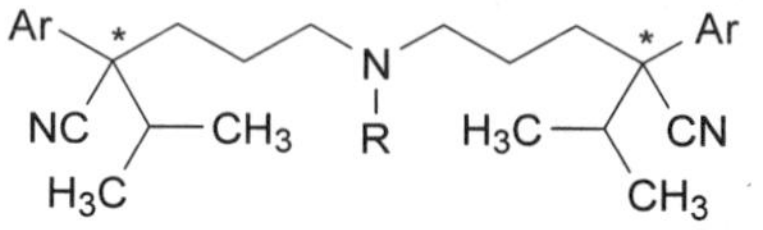

M. R = CH_2-CH_2-Ar: 5,5′-[[2-(3,4-dimethoxyphenyl)ethyl]imino]bis[2-(3,4-dimethoxyphenyl)-2-(1-methylethyl)pentanenitrile],

N. R = CH_3: 5,5′-(methylimino)bis[2-(3,4-dimethoxyphenyl)-2-(1-methylethyl)pentanenitrile],

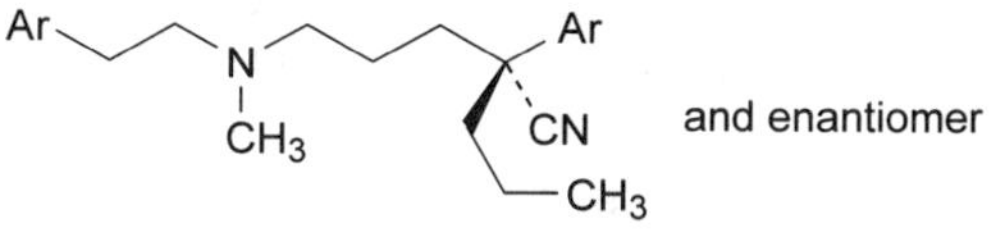

O. (2*RS*)-2-(3,4-dimethoxyphenyl)-5-[2-[2-(3,4-dimethoxyphenyl)ethyl](methyl)amino]- 2-propylpentanenitrile,

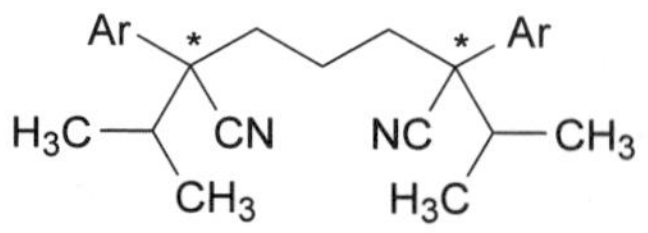

P. 2,6-bis(3,4-dimethoxyphenyl)-2,6-bis(1-methylethyl)-heptane-1,7-dinitrile.

W

07/2004:0169

WATER FOR INJECTIONS

Aqua ad iniectabilia

H_2O M_r 18.02

DEFINITION

Water for the preparation of medicines for parenteral administration when water is used as vehicle (water for injections in bulk) and for dissolving or diluting substances or preparations for parenteral administration (sterilised water for injections).

Water for injections in bulk

PRODUCTION

Water for injections in bulk is obtained from water that complies with the regulations on water intended for human consumption laid down by the competent authority or from purified water by distillation in an apparatus of which the parts in contact with the water are of neutral glass, quartz or suitable metal and which is fitted with an effective device to prevent the entrainment of droplets. The correct maintenance of the apparatus is essential. The first portion of the distillate obtained when the apparatus begins to function is discarded and the distillate is collected.

During production and subsequent storage, appropriate measures are taken to ensure that the total viable aerobic count is adequately controlled and monitored. Appropriate alert and action limits are set so as to detect adverse trends. Under normal conditions, an appropriate action limit is a total viable aerobic count (*2.6.12*) of 10 micro-organisms per 100 ml when determined by membrane filtration, using agar medium S, using at least 200 ml of water for injections in bulk and incubating at 30-35 °C for 5 days. For aseptic processing, stricter alert limits may need to be applied.

Total organic carbon (*2.2.44*): maximum 0.5 mg/l.

Conductivity. Determine the conductivity off-line or in-line under the following conditions.

EQUIPMENT

Conductivity cell:

- electrodes of a suitable material such as stainless steel;
- cell constant: within 2 per cent of the given value determined using a certified reference solution with a conductivity less than 1500 $\mu S \cdot cm^{-1}$.

Conductometer: resolution 0.1 $\mu S \cdot cm^{-1}$ on the lowest range.

System calibration (conductivity cell and conductometer):

- against one or more suitable certified standard solutions;
- tolerance: 3 per cent of the measured conductivity plus 0.1 $\mu S \cdot cm^{-1}$.

Conductometer calibration: by means of precision resistors or equivalent devices, after disconnecting the conductivity cell, for all ranges used for conductivity measurement and cell calibration (with an accuracy of at least ± 0.1 per cent of the stated value, traceable to the official standard).

If in-line conductivity cells cannot be dismantled, system calibration may be performed against a calibrated conductivity cell placed close to the cell to be calibrated in the water flow.

PROCEDURE

Stage 1

1. Measure the conductivity without temperature compensation, recording simultaneously the temperature. Temperature-compensated measurement may be performed after suitable validation.

2. Using Table 0169.-1, find the closest temperature value that is not greater than the measured temperature. The corresponding conductivity value is the limit at that temperature.

3. If the measured conductivity is not greater than the value in Table 0169.-1, the water to be examined meets the requirements of the test for conductivity. If the conductivity is higher than the value in Table 0169.-1, proceed with stage 2.

Table 0169.-1. – *Stage 1 - Temperature and conductivity requirements (for non-temperature-compensated conductivity measurements)*

Temperature (°C)	Conductivity ($\mu S \cdot cm^{-1}$)
0	0.6
5	0.8
10	0.9
15	1.0
20	1.1
25	1.3
30	1.4
35	1.5
40	1.7
45	1.8
50	1.9
55	2.1
60	2.2
65	2.4
70	2.5
75	2.7
80	2.7
85	2.7
90	2.7
95	2.9
100	3.1

Stage 2

4. Transfer a sufficient amount of the water to be examined (100 ml or more) to a suitable container, and stir the test sample. Adjust the temperature, if necessary, and while maintaining it at 25 ± 1 °C, begin vigorously agitating the test sample while periodically observing the conductivity. When the change in conductivity (due to uptake of atmospheric carbon dioxide) is less than 0.1 $\mu S.cm^{-1}$ per 5 min, note the conductivity.

5. If the conductivity is not greater than 2.1 $\mu S.cm^{-1}$, the water to be examined meets the requirements of the test for conductivity. If the conductivity is greater than 2.1 $\mu S.cm^{-1}$, proceed with stage 3.

Monographs Q - Z

Stage 3

6. Perform this test within approximately 5 min of the conductivity determination in step 5 under stage 2, while maintaining the sample temperature at 25 ± 1 °C. Add a recently prepared saturated solution of *potassium chloride R* to the test sample (0.3 ml per 100 ml of the test sample), and determine the pH (*2.2.3*) to the nearest 0.1 pH unit.
7. Using Table 0169.-2, determine the conductivity limit at the measured pH value in step 6. If the measured conductivity in step 4 under stage 2 is not greater than the conductivity requirements for the pH determined, the water to be examined meets the requirements of the test for conductivity. If either the measured conductivity is greater than this value or the pH is outside the range of 5.0-7.0, the water to be examined does not meet the requirements of the test for conductivity.

Table 0169.-2. — *Stage 3 - pH and conductivity requirements (for atmosphere and temperature equilibrated samples)*

pH	Conductivity ($\mu S \cdot cm^{-1}$)
5.0	4.7
5.1	4.1
5.2	3.6
5.3	3.3
5.4	3.0
5.5	2.8
5.6	2.6
5.7	2.5
5.8	2.4
5.9	2.4
6.0	2.4
6.1	2.4
6.2	2.5
6.3	2.4
6.4	2.3
6.5	2.2
6.6	2.1
6.7	2.6
6.8	3.1
6.9	3.8
7.0	4.6

In order to ensure the appropriate quality of the water, validated procedures and in-process-monitoring of the electrical conductivity and regular microbial monitoring are applied.

Water for injections in bulk is stored and distributed in conditions designed to prevent growth of micro-organisms and to avoid any other contamination.

CHARACTERS

Appearance: clear and colourless liquid.

TESTS

Nitrates: maximum 0.2 ppm.

Place 5 ml in a test-tube immersed in iced water, add 0.4 ml of a 100 g/l solution of *potassium chloride R*, 0.1 ml of *diphenylamine solution R* and, dropwise with shaking, 5 ml of *nitrogen-free sulphuric acid R*. Transfer the tube to a water-bath at 50 °C. After 15 min, any blue colour in the solution is not more intense than that in a reference solution prepared at the same time in the same manner using a mixture of 4.5 ml of *nitrate-free water R* and 0.5 ml of *nitrate standard solution (2 ppm* NO_3*) R*.

Aluminium (*2.4.17*): maximum 10 ppb, if intended for use in the manufacture of dialysis solutions.

Prescribed solution. To 400 ml of the water to be examined add 10 ml of *acetate buffer solution pH 6.0 R* and 100 ml of *distilled water R*.

Reference solution. Mix 2 ml of *aluminium standard solution (2 ppm Al) R*, 10 ml of *acetate buffer solution pH 6.0 R* and 98 ml of *distilled water R*.

Blank solution. Mix 10 ml of *acetate buffer solution pH 6.0 R* and 100 ml of *distilled water R*.

Heavy metals (*2.4.8*): maximum 0.1 ppm.

Heat 200 ml in a glass evaporating dish on a water-bath until the volume is reduced to 20 ml. 12 ml of the concentrated solution complies with limit test A. Prepare the standard using 10 ml of *lead standard solution (1 ppm Pb) R*.

Bacterial endotoxins (*2.6.14*): less than 0.25 IU/ml.

Sterilised water for injections

DEFINITION

Water for injections in bulk that has been distributed into suitable containers, closed and sterilised by heat in conditions which ensure that the product still complies with the test for bacterial endotoxins. Sterilised water for injections is free from any added substances.

Examined in suitable conditions of visibility, it is clear and colourless.

Each container contains a sufficient quantity of water for injections to permit the nominal volume to be withdrawn.

TESTS

Acidity or alkalinity. To 20 ml add 0.05 ml of *phenol red solution R*. If the solution is yellow, it becomes red on the addition of 0.1 ml of *0.01 M sodium hydroxide*; if red, it becomes yellow on the addition of 0.15 ml of *0.01 M hydrochloric acid*.

Conductivity: maximum 25 $\mu S \cdot cm^{-1}$ for containers with a nominal volume of 10 ml or less; maximum 5 $\mu S \cdot cm^{-1}$ for containers with a nominal volume greater than 10 ml.

Use equipment and the calibration procedure as defined under Water for injections in bulk.

Oxidisable substances. Boil 100 ml with 10 ml of *dilute sulphuric acid R*. Add 0.2 ml of *0.02 M potassium permanganate* and boil for 5 min. The solution remains faintly pink.

Chlorides (*2.4.4*): maximum 0.5 ppm for containers with a nominal volume of 100 ml or less.

15 ml complies with the limit test for chlorides. Prepare the standard using a mixture of 1.5 ml of *chloride standard solution (5 ppm Cl) R* and 13.5 ml of *water R*. Examine the solutions down the vertical axes of the tubes.

Nitrates: maximum 0.2 ppm.

Place 5 ml in a test-tube immersed in iced water, add 0.4 ml of a 100 g/l solution of *potassium chloride R,* 0.1 ml of *diphenylamine solution R* and, dropwise with shaking, 5 ml of *nitrogen-free sulphuric acid R*. Transfer the tube to a water-bath at 50 °C. After 15 min, any blue colour in the solution is not more intense than that in a reference solution prepared at the same time in the same manner using a mixture of 4.5 ml of *nitrate-free water R* and 0.5 ml of *nitrate standard solution (2 ppm* NO_3*) R*.

Sulphates. To 10 ml add 0.1 ml of *dilute hydrochloric acid R* and 0.1 ml of *barium chloride solution R1*. The solution shows no change in appearance for at least 1 h.

Aluminium (*2.4.17*): maximum 10 ppb, if intended for use in the manufacture of dialysis solutions.

Prescribed solution. To 400 ml of the water to be examined add 10 ml of *acetate buffer solution pH 6.0 R* and 100 ml of *distilled water R*.

Reference solution. Mix 2 ml of *aluminium standard solution (2 ppm Al) R,* 10 ml of *acetate buffer solution pH 6.0 R* and 98 ml of *distilled water R*.

Blank solution. Mix 10 ml of *acetate buffer solution pH 6.0 R* and 100 ml of *distilled water R*.

Ammonium: maximum 0.2 ppm.

To 20 ml add 1 ml of *alkaline potassium tetraiodomercurate solution R*. After 5 min, examine the solution down the vertical axis of the tube. The solution is not more intensely coloured than a standard prepared at the same time by adding 1 ml of *alkaline potassium tetraiodomercurate solution R* to a mixture of 4 ml of *ammonium standard solution (1 ppm* NH_4*) R* and 16 ml of *ammonium-free water R*.

Calcium and magnesium. To 100 ml add 2 ml of *ammonium chloride buffer solution pH 10.0 R,* 50 mg of *mordant black 11 triturate R* and 0.5 ml of *0.01 M sodium edetate*. A pure blue colour is produced.

Heavy metals (*2.4.8*): maximum 0.1 ppm.

Heat 200 ml in a glass evaporating dish on a water-bath until the volume is reduced to 20 ml. 12 ml of the concentrated solution complies with limit test A. Prepare the standard using 10 ml of *lead standard solution (1 ppm Pb) R*.

Residue on evaporation: maximum 4 mg (0.004 per cent) for containers with a nominal volume of 10 ml or less; maximum 3 mg (0.003 per cent) for containers with a nominal volume greater than 10 ml.

Evaporate 100 ml to dryness on a water-bath and dry in an oven at 100-105 °C.

Particulate contamination: sub-visible particles (*2.9.19*). It complies with test A or test B, as appropriate.

Sterility (*2.6.1*). It complies with the test for sterility.

Bacterial endotoxins (*2.6.14*): less than 0.25 IU/ml.

07/2004:1927

WATER, HIGHLY PURIFIED

Aqua valde purificata

H_2O M_r 18.02

DEFINITION

Water intended for use in the preparation of medicinal products where water of high biological quality is needed, except where *Water for injections (0169)* is required.

PRODUCTION

Highly purified water is obtained from water that complies with the regulations on water intended for human consumption laid down by the competent authority.

Current production methods include for example double-pass reverse osmosis coupled with other suitable techniques such as ultrafiltration and deionisation. Correct operation and maintenance of the system is essential.

During production and subsequent storage, appropriate measures are taken to ensure that the total viable aerobic count is adequately controlled and monitored. Appropriate alert and action limits are set so as to detect adverse trends. Under normal conditions, an appropriate action limit is a total viable aerobic count (*2.6.12*) of 10 micro-organisms per 100 ml when determined by membrane filtration, using agar medium S, at least 200 ml of highly purified water and incubating at 30-35 °C for 5 days.

Total organic carbon (*2.2.44*): maximum 0.5 mg/l.

Conductivity. Determine the conductivity off-line or in-line under the following conditions.

EQUIPMENT

Conductivity cell:

– electrodes of a suitable material such as stainless steel;

– cell constant: within 2 per cent of the given value determined using a certified reference solution with a conductivity less than 1500 $\mu S{\cdot}cm^{-1}$.

Conductometer: resolution 0.1 $\mu S{\cdot}cm^{-1}$ on the lowest range.

System calibration (conductivity cell and conductometer):

– against one or more suitable certified standard solutions;

– tolerance: 3 per cent of the measured conductivity plus 0.1 $\mu S{\cdot}cm^{-1}$.

Conductometer calibration: by means of precision resistors or equivalent devices after disconnecting the conductivity cell, for all ranges used for conductivity measurement and cell calibration (with an accuracy of at least ± 0.1 per cent of the stated value, traceable to the official standard).

If in-line conductivity cells cannot be dismantled, system calibration may be performed against a calibrated conductivity cell placed close to the cell to be calibrated in the water flow.

PROCEDURE

Stage 1

1. Measure the conductivity without temperature compensation, recording simultaneously the temperature. Temperature-compensated measurement may be performed after suitable validation.

2. Using Table 1927.-1, find the closest temperature value that is not greater than the measured temperature. The corresponding conductivity value is the limit at that temperature.

3. If the measured conductivity is not greater than the value in Table 1927.-1, the water to be examined meets the requirements of the test for conductivity. If the conductivity is higher than the value in Table 1927.-1, proceed with stage 2.

Table 1927.-1. – *Stage 1 - Temperature and conductivity requirements (for non-temperature-compensated conductivity measurements)*

Temperature (°C)	Conductivity (µS·cm^{-1})
0	0.6
5	0.8
10	0.9
15	1.0
20	1.1
25	1.3
30	1.4
35	1.5
40	1.7
45	1.8
50	1.9
55	2.1
60	2.2
65	2.4
70	2.5
75	2.7
80	2.7
85	2.7
90	2.7
95	2.9
100	3.1

Stage 2

4. Transfer a sufficient amount of the water to be examined (100 ml or more) to a suitable container, and stir the test sample. Adjust the temperature, if necessary, and while maintaining it at 25 ± 1 °C, begin vigorously agitating the test sample while periodically observing the conductivity. When the change in conductivity (due to uptake of atmospheric carbon dioxide) is less than 0.1 µS·cm^{-1} per 5 min, note the conductivity.

5. If the conductivity is not greater than 2.1 µS·cm^{-1}, the water to be examined meets the requirements of the test for conductivity. If the conductivity is greater than 2.1 µS·cm^{-1}, proceed with stage 3.

Stage 3

6. Perform this test within approximately 5 min of the conductivity determination in step 5 under stage 2, while maintaining the sample temperature at 25 ± 1 °C. Add a recently prepared saturated solution of *potassium chloride R* to the test sample (0.3 ml per 100 ml of the test sample), and determine the pH (*2.2.3*) to the nearest 0.1 pH unit.

7. Using Table 1927.-2, determine the conductivity limit at the measured pH value in step 6. If the measured conductivity in step 4 under stage 2 is not greater than the conductivity requirements for the pH determined, the water to be examined meets the requirements of the test for conductivity. If either the measured conductivity is greater than this value or the pH is outside the range of 5.0-7.0, the water to be examined does not meet the requirements of the test for conductivity.

Table 1927.-2. – *Stage 3 - pH and conductivity requirements (for atmosphere and temperature equilibrated samples)*

pH	Conductivity (µS·cm^{-1})
5.0	4.7
5.1	4.1
5.2	3.6
5.3	3.3
5.4	3.0
5.5	2.8
5.6	2.6
5.7	2.5
5.8	2.4
5.9	2.4
6.0	2.4
6.1	2.4
6.2	2.5
6.3	2.4
6.4	2.3
6.5	2.2
6.6	2.1
6.7	2.6
6.8	3.1
6.9	3.8
7.0	4.6

In order to ensure the appropriate quality of the water, validated procedures and in-process monitoring of the electrical conductivity and regular microbial monitoring are applied.

Highly purified water is stored in bulk and distributed in conditions designed to prevent growth of micro-organisms and to avoid any other contamination.

CHARACTERS

Appearance: clear and colourless liquid.

TESTS

Nitrates: maximum 0.2 ppm.

Place 5 ml in a test-tube immersed in iced water, add 0.4 ml of a 100 g/l solution of *potassium chloride R*, 0.1 ml of *diphenylamine solution R* and, dropwise with shaking, 5 ml of *nitrogen-free sulphuric acid R*. Transfer the tube to a water-bath at 50 °C. After 15 min, any blue colour in the solution is not more intense than that in a reference solution prepared at the same time in the same manner using a mixture of 4.5 ml of *nitrate-free water R* and 0.5 ml of *nitrate standard solution (2 ppm* NO_3*) R*.

Aluminium (*2.4.17*): maximum 10 ppb, if intended for use in the manufacture of dialysis solutions.

Prescribed solution. To 400 ml of the water to be examined add 10 ml of *acetate buffer solution pH 6.0 R* and 100 ml of *distilled water R*.

Reference solution. Mix 2 ml of *aluminium standard solution (2 ppm Al) R*, 10 ml of *acetate buffer solution pH 6.0 R* and 98 ml of *distilled water R*.

Blank solution. Mix 10 ml of *acetate buffer solution pH 6.0 R* and 100 ml of *distilled water R*.

Heavy metals (*2.4.8*): maximum 0.1 ppm.

Heat 200 ml in a glass evaporating dish on a water-bath until the volume is reduced to 20 ml. 12 ml of the concentrated solution complies with limit test A. Prepare the standard using 10 ml of *lead standard solution (1 ppm Pb) R.*

Bacterial endotoxins (*2.6.14*): less than 0.25 IU/ml.

LABELLING

The label states, where applicable, that the substance is suitable for use in the manufacture of dialysis solutions.

07/2004:0008

WATER, PURIFIED

Aqua purificata

H_2O M_r 18.02

DEFINITION

Water for the preparation of medicines other than those that are required to be both sterile and apyrogenic, unless otherwise justified and authorised.

Purified water in bulk

PRODUCTION

Purified water in bulk is prepared by distillation, by ion exchange, by reverse osmosis or by any other suitable method from water that complies with the regulations on water intended for human consumption laid down by the competent authority.

During production and subsequent storage, appropriate measures are taken to ensure that the total viable aerobic count is adequately controlled and monitored. Appropriate alert and action limits are set so as to detect adverse trends. Under normal conditions, an appropriate action limit is a total viable aerobic count (*2.6.12*) of 100 micro-organisms per millilitre, determined by membrane filtration, using agar medium S and incubating at 30-35 °C for 5 days. The size of the sample is to be chosen in relation to the expected result.

In addition, the test for total organic carbon (*2.2.44*) with a limit of 0.5 mg/l or alternatively the following test for oxidisable substances is carried out: to 100 ml add 10 ml of *dilute sulphuric acid R* and 0.1 ml of *0.02 M potassium permanganate* and boil for 5 min; the solution remains faintly pink.

Conductivity. Determine the conductivity off-line or in-line under the following conditions.

EQUIPMENT

Conductivity cell:

- electrodes of a suitable material such as stainless steel;
- cell constant: within 2 per cent of the given value determined using a certified reference solution with a conductivity less than 1500 $\mu S{\cdot}cm^{-1}$.

Conductometer: resolution 0.1 $\mu S{\cdot}cm^{-1}$ on the lowest range.

System calibration (conductivity cell and conductometer):

- against one or more suitable certified standard solutions;
- tolerance: 3 per cent of the measured conductivity plus 0.1 $\mu S{\cdot}cm^{-1}$.

Conductometer calibration: by means of precision resistors or equivalent devices, after disconnecting the conductivity cell, for all ranges used for conductivity measurement and cell calibration (with an accuracy of at least ± 0.1 per cent of the stated value, traceable to the official standard).

If in-line conductivity cells cannot be dismantled, system calibration may be performed against a calibrated conductivity cell placed close to the cell to be calibrated in the water flow.

PROCEDURE

Measure the conductivity without temperature compensation, recording simultaneously the temperature. Temperature-compensated measurement may be performed after suitable validation.

The water to be examined meets the requirements if the measured conductivity at the recorded temperature is not greater than the value in Table 0008.-1.

Table 0008.-1. – *Temperature and conductivity requirements*

Temperature (°C)	Conductivity ($\mu S{\cdot}cm^{-1}$)
0	2.4
10	3.6
20	4.3
25	5.1
30	5.4
40	6.5
50	7.1
60	8.1
70	9.1
75	9.7
80	9.7
90	9.7
100	10.2

For temperatures not listed in Table 0008.-1, calculate the maximal permitted conductivity by interpolation between the next lower and next higher data points in the table.

Purified water in bulk is stored and distributed in conditions designed to prevent growth of micro-organisms and to avoid any other contamination.

CHARACTERS

Appearance: clear and colourless liquid.

TESTS

Nitrates: maximum 0.2 ppm.

Place 5 ml in a test-tube immersed in iced water, add 0.4 ml of a 100 g/l solution of *potassium chloride R*, 0.1 ml of *diphenylamine solution R* and, dropwise with shaking, 5 ml of *nitrogen-free sulphuric acid R*. Transfer the tube to a water-bath at 50 °C. After 15 min, any blue colour in the solution is not more intense than that in a reference solution prepared at the same time in the same manner using a mixture of 4.5 ml of *nitrate-free water R* and 0.5 ml of *nitrate standard solution (2 ppm NO_3) R.*

Aluminium (*2.4.17*): maximum 10 ppb, if intended for use in the manufacture of dialysis solutions.

Prescribed solution. To 400 ml of the water to be examined add 10 ml of *acetate buffer solution pH 6.0 R* and 100 ml of *distilled water R.*

Reference solution. Mix 2 ml of *aluminium standard solution (2 ppm Al) R*, 10 ml of *acetate buffer solution pH 6.0 R* and 98 ml of *distilled water R.*

Blank solution. Mix 10 ml of *acetate buffer solution pH 6.0 R* and 100 ml of *distilled water R.*

Heavy metals (*2.4.8*): maximum 0.1 ppm.

Heat 200 ml in a glass evaporating dish on a water-bath until the volume is reduced to 20 ml. 12 ml of the concentrated solution complies with limit test A. Prepare the standard using 10 ml of *lead standard solution (1 ppm Pb) R*.

Bacterial endotoxins (*2.6.14*): less than 0.25 IU/ml, if intended for use in the manufacture of dialysis solutions without a further appropriate procedure for removal of bacterial endotoxins.

LABELLING

The label states, where applicable, that the substance is suitable for use in the manufacture of dialysis solutions.

Purified water in containers

DEFINITION

Purified water in bulk that has been filled and stored in conditions designed to assure the required microbiological quality. It is free from any added substances.

CHARACTERS

Appearance: clear and colourless liquid.

TESTS

It complies with the tests prescribed in the section on Purified water in bulk and with the following additional tests.

Acidity or alkalinity. To 10 ml, freshly boiled and cooled in a borosilicate glass flask, add 0.05 ml of *methyl red solution R*. The solution is not coloured red.

To 10 ml add 0.1 ml of *bromothymol blue solution R1*. The solution is not coloured blue.

Oxidisable substances. To 100 ml add 10 ml of *dilute sulphuric acid R* and 0.1 ml of *0.02 M potassium permanganate* and boil for 5 min. The solution remains faintly pink.

Chlorides. To 10 ml add 1 ml of *dilute nitric acid R* and 0.2 ml of *silver nitrate solution R2*. The solution shows no change in appearance for at least 15 min.

Sulphates. To 10 ml add 0.1 ml of *dilute hydrochloric acid R* and 0.1 ml of *barium chloride solution R1*. The solution shows no change in appearance for at least 1 h.

Ammonium: maximum 0.2 ppm.

To 20 ml add 1 ml of *alkaline potassium tetraiodomercurate solution R*. After 5 min, examine the solution down the vertical axis of the tube. The solution is not more intensely coloured than a standard prepared at the same time by adding 1 ml of *alkaline potassium tetraiodomercurate solution R* to a mixture of 4 ml of *ammonium standard solution (1 ppm NH_4) R* and 16 ml of *ammonium-free water R*.

Calcium and magnesium. To 100 ml add 2 ml of *ammonium chloride buffer solution pH 10.0 R*, 50 mg of *mordant black 11 triturate R* and 0.5 ml of *0.01 M sodium edetate*. A pure blue colour is produced.

Residue on evaporation: maximum 0.001 per cent.

Evaporate 100 ml on a water-bath and dry in an oven at 100-105 °C. The residue weighs a maximum of 1 mg.

Microbial contamination. Total viable aerobic count (*2.6.12*) not more than 10^2 micro-organisms per millilitre, determined by membrane filtration, using agar medium B.

LABELLING

The label states, where applicable, that the substance is suitable for use in the manufacture of dialysis solutions.

RADIOPHARMACEUTICAL PREPARATIONS

07/2004:0563

SODIUM IODIDE (^{123}I) INJECTION

Natrii iodidi (^{123}I) solutio iniectabilis

DEFINITION

Sterile solution containing iodine-123 in the form of sodium iodide; it may contain sodium thiosulphate or some other suitable reducing agent and a suitable buffer.

Content: 90 per cent to 110 per cent of the declared iodine-123 radioactivity at the date and hour stated on the label.

PRODUCTION

Iodine-123 is obtained by proton irradiation of xenon enriched in xenon-124 (minimum 98 per cent) followed by the decay of xenon-123 which is formed directly and by the decay of caesium-123. No carrier iodide is added.

CHARACTERS

Appearance: clear, colourless solution.

Half-life and nature of radiation of iodine-123: see *Table of physical characteristics of radionuclides (5.7)*.

IDENTIFICATION

A. Gamma-ray spectrometry.

Results: the spectrum obtained with the preparation to be examined does not differ significantly from that of a standardised iodine-123 solution. The most prominent gamma photon has an energy of 0.159 MeV and is accompanied by the principal X-ray of 0.027 MeV.

B. Examine the chromatograms obtained in the test for radiochemical purity.

Results: the principal peak in the radiochromatogram obtained with the test solution is similar in retention time to the principal peak in the chromatogram obtained with reference solution (a).

TESTS

pH (*2.2.3*): 7.0 to 10.0.

Sterility. It complies with the test for sterility prescribed in the monograph on *Radiopharmaceutical preparations (0125)*. The preparation may be released for use before completion of the test.

RADIONUCLIDIC PURITY

Iodine-123: minimum 99.65 per cent of the total radioactivity.

Gamma-ray spectrometry.

Determine the relative amounts of iodine-123, iodine-125, tellurium-121 and other radionuclidic impurities present. For the detection of tellurium-121 and iodine-125, retain the preparation to be examined for a sufficient time to allow iodine-123 to decay to a level which permits the detection of radionuclidic impurities. No radionuclides with a half-life longer than that of iodine-125 are detected.

The preparation may be released for use before completion of the test.

RADIOCHEMICAL PURITY

[^{123}I]iodide. Liquid chromatography (*2.2.29*).

Test solution. Dilute the preparation to be examined with a 2 g/l solution of *sodium hydroxide R* to a radioactive concentration suitable for the detector. Add an equal volume of a solution containing 1 g/l of *potassium iodide R*, 2 g/l of *potassium iodate R* and 10 g/l of *sodium hydrogen carbonate R* and mix.

Reference solution (a). Dilute 1 ml of a 26.2 mg/l solution of *potassium iodide R* to 10 ml with *water R*.

Reference solution (b). Dilute 1 ml of a 24.5 mg/l solution of *potassium iodate R* to 10 ml with *water R*. Mix equal volumes of this solution and reference solution (a).

Column:
- *size*: l = 0.25 m, Ø = 4.0 mm,
- *stationary phase*: *octadecylsilyl silica gel for chromatography R* (5 µm),
- *temperature*: constant between 20 °C and 30 °C.

Mobile phase: dissolve 5.85 g of *sodium chloride R* in 1000 ml of *water R*, add 0.65 ml of *octylamine R* and adjust to pH 7.0 with *dilute phosphoric acid R*; add 50 ml of *acetonitrile R* and mix.

Flow rate: 1.5 ml/min.

Detection: spectrophotometer at 220 nm and a radioactivity detector connected in series.

Injection: 20 µl.

Run time: 12 min.

Relative retention with reference to iodide (retention time = about 5 min): iodate = 0.2 to 0.3.

System suitability: reference solution (b):
- *resolution*: minimum 2 between the peaks due to iodide and iodate in the chromatogram recorded with the spectrophotometer.

Limit: examine the chromatogram obtained with the test solution using the radioactivity detector and locate the peak due to iodide by comparison with the chromatogram obtained with reference solution (a) using the spectrophotometer:
- *[^{123}I]iodide*: minimum 95 per cent of the total radioactivity.

RADIOACTIVITY

Determine the radioactivity using a calibrated instrument.

LABELLING

The label states any substance added.

IMPURITIES

A. [^{123}I]iodate ion.

07/2004:0938

SODIUM IODIDE (^{131}I) CAPSULES FOR DIAGNOSTIC USE

Natrii iodidi (^{131}I) capsulae ad usum diagnosticum

DEFINITION

Capsules for diagnostic use containing iodine-131 in the form of sodium iodide on a solid support; they may contain sodium thiosulphate or some other suitable reducing agents and a suitable buffering substance. A package contains 1 or more capsules.

Content:
- iodine-131: maximum 37 MBq per capsule; the average radioactivity determined in the test for uniformity of content is 90 per cent to 110 per cent of the declared iodine-131 radioactivity at the date and hour stated on the label;
- iodide: maximum 20 µg per capsule.

PRODUCTION

Iodine-131 is obtained by neutron irradiation of tellurium or by extraction from uranium fission products. No carrier iodide is added.

CHARACTERS

Half-life and nature of radiation of iodine-131: see *Table of physical characteristics of radionuclides (5.7)*.

IDENTIFICATION

A. Gamma-ray spectrometry.

Results: the spectrum obtained with the preparation to be examined does not differ significantly from that of a standardised iodine-131 solution. The most prominent gamma photon has an energy of 0.365 MeV.

B. Examine the chromatograms obtained in the test for radiochemical purity.

Results: the principal peak in the radiochromatogram obtained with test solution (b) is similar in retention time to the principal peak in the chromatogram obtained with reference solution (a).

TESTS

Disintegration: the contents of the capsule dissolve completely within 15 min.

In a water-bath at 37 °C, warm in a small beaker about 20 ml of a 2.0 g/l solution of *potassium iodide R*. Add a capsule to be examined. Stir magnetically at 20 r/min.

Uniformity of content. Determine the radioactivity of each of not fewer than 10 capsules. Calculate the average radioactivity per capsule. The radioactivity of no capsule differs by more than 10 per cent from the average, the relative standard deviation is not greater than 3.5 per cent.

Iodide. Liquid chromatography (*2.2.29*).

Test solution (a). Dissolve a capsule to be examined in 10 ml of *water R*. Filter through a 0.2 µm filter.

Test solution (b). Dissolve a capsule to be examined in *water R*. Filter through a 0.2 µm filter and dilute the filtrate with a 2 g/l solution of *sodium hydroxide R* to a radioactive concentration suitable for the detector. Add an equal volume of a solution containing 1 g/l of *potassium iodide R*, 2 g/l of *potassium iodate R* and 10 g/l of *sodium hydrogen carbonate R* and mix.

Reference solution (a). Dilute 1 ml of a 26.2 mg/l solution of *potassium iodide R* to 10 ml with *water R*.

Reference solution (b). Dilute 1 ml of a 24.5 mg/l solution of *potassium iodate R* to 10 ml with *water R*. Mix equal volumes of this solution and reference solution (a).

Blank solution. Prepare a solution containing 2 mg/ml of each constituent stated on the label, apart from iodide.

Column:

- *size*: l = 0.25 m, Ø = 4.0 mm,
- *stationary phase*: *octadecylsilyl silica gel for chromatography R* (5 µm),
- *temperature*: constant between 20 °C and 30 °C.

Mobile phase: dissolve 5.85 g of *sodium chloride R* in 1000 ml of *water R*, add 0.65 ml of *octylamine R* and adjust to pH 7.0 with *dilute phosphoric acid R*; add 50 ml of *acetonitrile R* and mix.

Flow rate: 1.5 ml/min.

Detection: spectrophotometer at 220 nm and radioactivity detector connected in series.

Injection: 20 µl of test solution (a), reference solutions (a) and (b) and the blank solution.

Run time: 12 min.

Relative retention with reference to iodide (retention time = about 5 min): iodate = 0.2 to 0.3.

System suitability:

- in the chromatogram obtained with the blank solution, none of the peaks has a retention time similar to that of the peak due to iodide,
- *resolution*: minimum 2 between the peaks due to iodide and iodate in the chromatogram obtained with reference solution (b) recorded with the spectrophotometer.

Limit: examine the chromatograms obtained with the spectrophotometer:

- *iodide*: not more than the area of the corresponding peak in the chromatogram obtained with reference solution (a) (20 µg/capsule).

RADIONUCLIDIC PURITY

Iodine-131: minimum 99.9 per cent of the total radioactivity.

Gamma-ray spectrometry.

Determine the relative amounts of iodine-131, iodine-133, iodine-135 and other radionuclidic impurities present.

RADIOCHEMICAL PURITY

[^{131}I]iodide. Liquid chromatography (*2.2.29*) as described in the test for iodide with the following modifications.

Injection: 20 µl of test solution (b) and reference solution (a).

Limit: examine the chromatogram obtained with the test solution using the radioactivity detector and locate the peak due to iodide by comparison with the chromatogram obtained with reference solution (a) using the spectrophotometer:

- *[^{131}I]iodide*: minimum 95 per cent of the total radioactivity.

RADIOACTIVITY

Determine the radioactivity of the package using a calibrated instrument.

LABELLING

The label states any substance added and the number of capsules in the package.

IMPURITIES

A. [^{131}I]iodate ion.

HOMOEOPATHIC PREPARATIONS

01/2002:1599
corrected

ARSENIOUS TRIOXIDE FOR HOMOEOPATHIC PREPARATIONS

Arsenii trioxidum ad praeparationes homoeopathicae

As_2O_3 A_r 197.8

DEFINITION

Content: 99.5 per cent to 100.5 per cent of As_2O_3.

CHARACTERS

Appearance: white or almost white powder.

Solubility: practically insoluble to sparingly soluble in water. It dissolves in solutions of alkali hydroxides and carbonates.

IDENTIFICATION

A. Dissolve 20 mg in 1 ml of *dilute hydrochloric acid R*, add 4 ml of *water R* and 0.1 ml of *sodium sulphide solution R*. The resulting yellow precipitate is soluble in *dilute ammonia R1*.

B. Dissolve 20 mg in 1 ml of *hydrochloric acid R1*, add 5 ml of *hypophosphorous reagent R* and heat for 15 min on a water-bath. A black precipitate develops.

TESTS

Appearance of solution. A 100 g/l solution in *dilute ammonia R1* is clear (*2.2.1*) and colourless (*2.2.2, Method II*).

Sulphides. Dissolve 1.0 g in 10.0 ml of *dilute sodium hydroxide solution R*. Add 0.05 ml of *lead acetate solution R*. Any colour in the test solution is not more intense than that in a standard prepared at the same time and in the same manner using a mixture of 10.0 ml of a 0.015 g/l solution of *sodium sulphide R* in *dilute sodium hydroxide solution R* and 0.05 ml of *lead acetate solution R* (20 ppm).

ASSAY

Dissolve 40.0 mg in a mixture of 10 ml of *water R* and 10 ml of *dilute sodium hydroxide solution R*. Add 10 ml of *dilute hydrochloric acid R* and 3 g of *sodium hydrogen carbonate R* and mix. Add 1 ml of *starch solution R* and titrate with *0.05 M iodine*.

1 ml of *0.05 M iodine* is equivalent to 4.946 mg of As_2O_3.

INDEX

To aid users the index includes a reference to the supplement where the latest version of a text can be found.

For example: Alfacalcidol..**4.2**-2656

means the monograph Alfacalcidol can be found on page 2656 of Supplement 4.2.

Note that where no reference for a supplement is made, the text can be found in the principal volume.

Monographs deleted from the Fourth Edition are not included in the index; a cumulative list of deleted texts is found in the Contents of this supplement, page xliv.

Numerics/Symbols

A

B

Index

D

F

Index

H

I

Index

M

Index

Index

N

O

Q

R

S

T

Index

W

X

Y

Z

KEY TO MONOGRAPHS

Monograph (new or revised) is applicable from 1 January 2002

Monograph reference number

Correction to be taken into account from the publication date of the supplement

01/2002:0884
corrected

CARBIMAZOLE

Carbimazolum

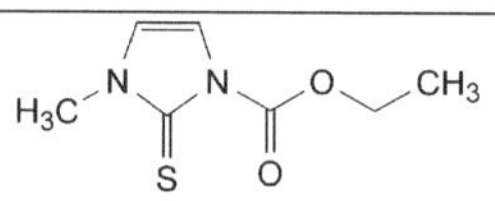

$C_7H_{10}N_2O_2S$ M_r 186.2

Chemical name in accordance with IUPAC nomenclature rules

DEFINITION

Ethyl 3-methyl-2-thioxo-2,3-dihydro-1*H*-imidazole-1-carboxylate.

Content: 98.0 per cent to 102.0 per cent (dried substance).

CHARACTERS

Appearance: white or yellowish-white, crystalline powder.

Solubility: slightly soluble in water, soluble in acetone and in alcohol.

Application of the first and second identification is defined in the General Notices (chapter 1)

IDENTIFICATION

First identification: B.

Second identification: A, C, D.

A. Melting point (*2.2.14*): 122 °C to 125 °C.

B. Infrared absorption spectrophotometry (*2.2.24*).

Preparation: discs.

Comparison: *carbimazole CRS.*

Chemical reference substance available from the Secretariat (see inside front cover)

C. Thin-layer chromatography (*2.2.27*).

Test solution. Dissolve 10 mg of the substance to be examined in *methylene chloride R* and dilute to 10 ml with the same solvent.

Reference solution. Dissolve 10 mg of *carbimazole CRS* in *methylene chloride R* and dilute to 10 ml with the same solvent.

Plate: *TLC silica gel GF_{254} plate R.*

Mobile phase: *acetone R, methylene chloride R* (20:80 *V/V*).

Reagents described in chapter 4

Application: 10 µl.

Development: over a path of 15 cm.

Drying: in air for 30 min.

Detection: examine in ultraviolet light at 254 nm.

Results: the principal spot in the chromatogram obtained with the test solution is similar in position and size to the principal spot in the chromatogram obtained with the reference solution.

D. Dissolve about 10 mg in a mixture of 50 ml of *water R* and 0.05 ml of *dilute hydrochloric acid R*. Add 1 ml of *potassium iodobismuthate solution R*. A red precipitate is formed.

TESTS

Impurity A and other related substances. Liquid chromatography (*2.2.29*).

Reference to a general chapter

Test solution. Dissolve 5.0 mg of the substance to be examined in 10.0 ml of a mixture of 20 volumes of *acetonitrile R* and 80 volumes of *water R*. Use this solution within 5 min of preparation.

Reference solution (a). Dissolve 5 mg of *thiamazole R* and 0.10 g of *carbimazole CRS* in a mixture of 20 volumes of *acetonitrile R* and 80 volumes of *water R* and dilute to 100.0 ml with the same mixture of solvents. Dilute 1.0 ml of this solution to 10.0 ml with a mixture of 20 volumes of *acetonitrile R* and 80 volumes of *water R*.

Reference solution (b). Dissolve 5.0 mg of *thiamazole R* in a mixture of 20 volumes of *acetonitrile R* and 80 volumes of *water R* and dilute to 10.0 ml with the same mixture of solvents. Dilute 1.0 ml of this solution to 100.0 ml with a mixture of 20 volumes of *acetonitrile R* and 80 volumes of *water R*.

Column:

- *size*: *l* = 0.15 m, Ø = 3.9 mm,
- *stationary phase*: *octadecylsilyl silica gel for chromatography R* (5 µm).

Mobile phase: *acetonitrile R, water R* (10:90 *V/V*).

Flow rate: 1 ml/min.

Detection: spectrophotometer at 254 nm.

Injection: 10 µl.

Run time: 1.5 times the retention time of carbimazole.

Retention time: carbimazole = about 6 min.

System suitability: reference solution (a):

- *resolution*: minimum 5.0 between the peaks due to impurity A and carbimazole.

Limits:

- *impurity A*: not more than half the area of the principal peak in the chromatogram obtained with reference solution (b) (0.5 per cent),
- *any other impurity*: not more than 0.1 times the area of the principal peak in the chromatogram obtained with reference solution (b) (0.1 per cent).

Loss on drying (*2.2.32*): maximum 0.5 per cent, determined on 1.000 g by drying in a desiccator over *diphosphorus pentoxide R* at a pressure not exceeding 0.7 kPa for 24 h.

Sulphated ash (*2.4.14*): maximum 0.1 per cent, determined on 1.0 g.

ASSAY

Dissolve 50.0 mg in *water R* and dilute to 500.0 ml with the same solvent. To 10.0 ml add 10 ml of *dilute hydrochloric acid R* and dilute to 100.0 ml with *water R*. Measure the absorbance (*2.2.25*) at the maximum at 291 nm. Calculate the content of $C_7H_{10}N_2O_2S$ taking the specific absorbance to be 557.

IMPURITIES

Specified impurities: A.

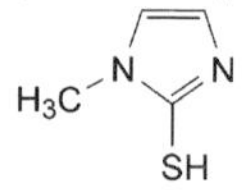

A. 1-methyl-1*H*-imidazole-2-thiol (thiamazole).

List of impurities controlled by the tests (see chapter 1 General Notices, the monograph Substances for pharmaceutical use (2034) and the note for information page xli)